# CONTEMPORARY ISSUES IN PERINATAL EDUCATION

Providing essential knowledge and understanding that midwives, health visitors, nursery nurses and lay birth and early parenting educators need to deliver effective and evidence-based education to all new parents and families, this book explores key issues in perinatal education.

Bringing together research and thinking around preconception and birth, infant sleep, nutrition, attachment and development, it also includes chapters on topics of growing importance, such as preconception education, LGBTQ+ parent education, the role of parenting advice, parent education across different cultures and teaching antenatal classes online. Each chapter includes a key knowledge update and pointers for practice.

This wide-ranging and practical text is an important read for all those supporting new parents from pregnancy through the first 1000 days, especially those delivering antenatal care and birth and early parenting education.

**Mary Nolan** is well known for her work in perinatal education. She has published numerous articles and several books in the field, the most recent being *Parent Education for the Critical 1000 Days*. She has been Professor of Perinatal Education at the University of Worcester for 15 years and Honorary Professor at Nottingham University for 10 years. Prior to her University appointment, she worked as a birth and early parenting educator and trainer across the UK and in France, Belgium, Germany, Australia and New Zealand. In 2013, she was one of the founders of the *International Journal of Birth and Parent Education* and its first Editor-in-Chief.

**Shona Gore** has facilitated antenatal and perinatal courses in the UK for those in the transition to parenthood during a 30-year career in childbirth education, relationship and birth education in schools (including for children with special learning needs) and workshops in adult education for NHS and Early Years' Practitioners. In association with the Universities of Bedfordshire and Worcester, she has devised and taught courses to train NCT practitioners from entrance to degree level. In 2013, with Mary Nolan (Editor-in-Chief), she founded the *International Journal of Birth and Parent Education*.

# CONTEMPORARY ISSUES IN PERINATAL EDUCATION

## Knowledge into Practice

*Edited by*
*Mary Nolan and Shona Gore*

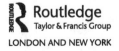

Routledge
Taylor & Francis Group

LONDON AND NEW YORK

Cover image: © Getty Images

First published 2023
by Routledge
4 Park Square, Milton Park, Abingdon, Oxon OX14 4RN

and by Routledge
605 Third Avenue, New York, NY 10158

*Routledge is an imprint of the Taylor & Francis Group, an informa business*

*British Library Cataloguing-in-Publication Data*
A catalogue record for this book is available from the British Library

*Library of Congress Cataloging-in-Publication Data*
A catalog record has been requested for this book

ISBN: 978-1-032-12252-6 (hbk)
ISBN: 978-1-032-12251-9 (pbk)
ISBN: 978-1-003-22377-1 (ebk)

DOI: 10.4324/9781003223771

Typeset in Bembo
by codeMantra

# CONTENTS

# FIGURES

# TABLES

# CONTRIBUTORS

**Alanna E.F. Rudzik** is Associate Professor at the Department of Anthropology, State University of New York College at Oneonta, USA.

**Amanda Benham** is a Dietitian in private practice, specialising in plant-based nutrition and paediatrics, Australia.

**Amy Bryson** is a Community Peer Support Co-ordinator for The Breastfeeding Network, UK.

**Angela D. Staples** is Assistant Professor in the Psychology Department at Eastern Michigan University, USA.

**Anna Malmquist** is Associate Professor in Social Psychology at Linköping University, Sweden.

**Cathy Green** is a Midwife working with the Homebirth Team at Birmingham Women's Hospital, UK.

**Chris May** is an Antenatal Facilitator at the Family Action Centre in the College of Health, Medicine and Wellbeing, The University of Newcastle, Australia.

**Elizabeth Smith** is Breastfeeding Advocacy Lead for Scotland, UK, and a Queen's Nurse.

**Erin K. McClain** is Assistant Director and Research Associate in the Collaborative for Maternal and Infant Health, School of Medicine, University of North Carolina at Chapel Hill, USA.

**Frances Brett** is Course Leader and Teacher in Education at Shrewsbury Colleges Group, UK.

**Gillian Harris** is Consultant Clinical Psychologist, and Honorary Senior Research Fellow at the University of Birmingham, UK.

**Graham F. Welch** is Chair of Music Education at the International Music Education Research Centre, Institute of Education, University College London, UK.

**Graham Music** is Consultant Child and Adult Psychotherapist at The Tavistock and Portman NHS Foundation Trust, UK.

**Hanan Hussein** is Honorary Tutor at the University of Birmingham, and Principal Clinical Psychologist at Birmingham and Solihull Mental Health Trust, UK.

**Hanna Rouhe** is Senior Consultant in Obstetrics at the Department of Obstetrics and Gynaecology, Helsinki University and Helsinki University Hospital, Finland.

**Helen Ball** is Director of the Durham Infancy and Sleep Centre, UK.

**Helen Knight** is an Antenatal Teacher, UK.

**Hen Otley** is a Child and Adolescent Psychotherapist, UK.

**Isabelle Karimov** is an Antenatal Teacher in Belgium.

**Janet Balaskas** is Founder of the Active Birth Movement, UK.

**Jennifer St George** is Senior Lecturer in Health Sciences at the College of Health, Medicine and Wellbeing, The University of Newcastle, Australia.

**Jenny S. Radesky** is Assistant Professor in the Division of Developmental Behavioral Pediatrics, Department of Pediatrics at the University of Michigan Medical School, Ann Arbor MI, USA.

**Joan A. Friedman** is Senior Psychoanalyst at the Institute of Contemporary Psychoanalysis, Los Angeles, USA.

**Jonathan Sher** is Senior Fellow at the Queen's Nursing Institute Scotland, UK, and Programme Lead for 'Healthier Pregnancies, Better Lives'.

**Katherine Rosenblum** is Clinical and Developmental Psychologist at the University of Michigan Medical School, Ann Arbor MI, USA.

**Kathleen Hodkinson** is Assistant Professor of Psychology at Webster Vienna Private University, Austria.

**Kathleen Roche-Nagi** is Managing Director of Approachable Parenting, UK.

**Kathryn Stagg** is an International Board Certified Lactation Consultant, and Founder and Trustee of Breastfeeding Twins and Triplets charity, UK.

**Kathryn Thomson** is a Trainee Clinical Psychologist, Cardiff and Vale University Health Board, UK.

**Katrin Kristjansdottir** is Director of the Counseling Center, Webster Vienna Private University, Austria.

**Kay Cram** is a Consultant Perinatal Educator, UK.

**Leah LaLonde** is a Doctoral Fellow at Eastern Michigan University, USA.

**Lorna Davies** is Principal Lecturer in Midwifery at Otago Polytechnic, New Zealand.

**Megan M. McClelland** is Professor and Director of the Hallie E. Ford Center for Healthy Children & Families at Oregon State University, USA.

**Michele Stranger Hunter** is Founder of the One Key Question® initiative and formerly Executive Director of the Oregon Foundation for Reproductive Health, USA.

**Rachel H. Farr** is Associate Professor in Psychology at the University of Kentucky, USA.

**Raija-Leena Punamäki** is Professor of Psychology at Tampere University, Finland.

**Richard Fletcher** is Associate Professor at the Family Action Centre, College of Health, Medicine and Wellbeing, The University of Newcastle, Australia.

**Riikka Airo** is Special Psychologist and Psychotherapist Coach at Psychotherapy Tunnetila, Finland.

**Robin Balbernie** is a Child Psychotherapist and Infant Mental Health Specialist, UK.

**Samantha L. Tornello** is Assistant Professor of Human Development and Family Studies at Pennsylvania State University, USA.

**Sarah Edwards** is Scottish Programme Manager for The Breastfeeding Network, UK.

**Sarah Verbiest** is Adjunct Assistant Professor in the Department of Maternal and Child Health at the University of North Carolina at Chapel Hill, USA.

**Shauna L. Tominey** is Associate Professor of Practice and Parenting Education Specialist at Oregon State University, USA.

**Shona Gore** is a Consultant Perinatal Educator, UK.

**Sofia Klittmark** is an Analyst at the Department of Behavioural Sciences and Learning, Linköping University, Sweden.

**Svea G. Olsen** is a Postdoctoral Scholar at Oregon State University, USA.

**Tara Acevedo** is a Researcher at Webster Vienna Private University, Austria.

**Terhi Saisto** is Senior Consultant in Perinataology at the Department of Obstetrics and Gynaecology, Helsinki University and Helsinki University Hospital, Finland.

**Yasmin Shikara** is a Research Assistant at Approachable Parenting, UK.

# PREFACE

This book celebrates some of the best writing from the *International Journal of Birth and Parent Education* from its inception in 2013 to 2022. All the chapters were originally editorials or articles in the Journal, and all have been carefully updated by the authors. It is the role and the privilege of health and social care professionals working in the critical 1000 days from conception to two years, and the many committed and skilled lay people who also provide birth and early parenting education, to share information with parents at a transformative time of their lives. Their work requires knowledge and understanding of the best evidence available on the many topics that parents want to know about, and skills to be able to get the best out of antenatal and postnatal groups and engage one-to-one with parents facing huge challenges in their transition to parenthood. This book provides readers with the up-to-date evidence they need, provided by authors skilled at communicating complex topics in accessible language. It also looks at how practitioners can translate knowledge into practice – focusing on what parents need to know, want to know and how they want to learn. It is, we hope, highly responsive to the early intervention agenda – recognising that anything we can do to educate and support parents in their job of bringing up babies and toddlers is highly likely to impact positively on the life trajectories of those children. It is our aim in presenting the following chapters to support you to support parents.

Mary Nolan and Shona Gore
April 2022

# PART I

# Preconception Education

## Introduction to Part I

In the second decade of the twenty-first century, as in every other, a newborn baby's future health and wellbeing have already been determined, at least in part, by the genetic cards she has been dealt and by the environment of the womb in which she has spent her first nine months of life. As she enters the world, her physical and mental wellbeing is further shaped by the way in which she is parented and the opportunities her parents can give her.

In her early babyhood, does she become firmly attached to the key people in her life – her parents, grandparents or other special carers? Is she breast-fed? Are her basic needs for cleanliness, warmth and safety met? Do her parents chat to her? Is she weaned onto a nutritious diet? As she grows, does she have opportunities for learning about the world beyond home and school? Is she introduced to the natural world? Is she encouraged by her parents in her school work? Does she learn about healthy relationships and see them enacted by the people around her?

The answers to all of these questions will determine whether she is well prepared for her first pregnancy (and equally so if the baby we're thinking about is a boy). If she has been brought up to make her own (supported) choices and to accept the responsibility for her decisions, she will probably *choose* when to have a baby rather than let it 'just happen'. If her body is healthy as a result of a child-hood of positive nutrition and frequent exercise, she will be predisposed to have a healthy pregnancy. If she is fortunate enough to enjoy positive mental health because, as a child, she has always been confident that help from key people would be there for her if she needed it, she will be strong to meet the challenges of new motherhood.

DOI: 10.4324/9781003223771-1

So, the parenting that this baby will provide for her babies depends critically on her own time in the womb and on her experience of childhood, that is, what has happened to her or not happened to her during the period we now call the 'critical 1000 days'. Her state of health and wellbeing in the months leading up to her first pregnancy will also be critical. The chapters included in this opening section of the book stress the importance and the urgency of providing education and care to girls, women, boys and men *well before* they become parents in order that, when their time comes, they stand the best chance of enjoying a healthy pregnancy and offering their baby the best possible start in life.

As birth and early parenting educators and carers, we need to seize the opportunities presented by 'ordinary' encounters with women of reproductive age to ask, 'Would you like to become pregnant in the next year?' The answer to this question can be a springboard for care that is tailored to the needs of this particular woman at this moment in her childbearing years – whether she wants to delay pregnancy, become pregnant or avoid it entirely.

A life-course approach to preconception health, education and care is essential because it is only by taking the long view of parenting that can we level the playing field for babies and ensure an equitable start for every single new life. The final chapter in this section looks at educating about breastfeeding in Early Years settings. Challenging the cultural norm of bottle feeding at a very early age may be a powerful means of encouraging our youngest children to become the breastfeeding mothers of the next generation.

# 1

# PRECONCEPTION HEALTH, EDUCATION AND CARE

## The Earliest Intervention

*Jonathan Sher*

\*\*\*

Everyone who aspires to have a child desires a safe pregnancy, a thriving baby and a rewarding parenthood. Those universal positive goals are good news because no one needs to 'sell' people on their value and importance. The bad news is that, too often, those desirable outcomes are not achieved. Many unwelcome pregnancy and birth results are preventable, but not prevented.

The challenge is to help an ever-growing proportion of prospective mothers and fathers actually get what they already want in relation to their reproductive lives. The key is *preparing* early, wisely and consistently for pregnancy and parenthood through preconception health, education and care across the life course.

\*\*\*

Those earliest weeks, months and years – although beyond conscious recollection – continue to inform and affect all of us throughout our lives. These are the foundational experiences that profoundly shape (and occasionally mis-shape) our development from childhood through adulthood. This is not to assert that later experiences don't 'count' or have little impact. That would be nonsense. But what happens (or fails to happen) early in life does truly and enduringly matter.

'Being parented' is the cornerstone upon which our lived experiences accumulate and are constructed. The deepest roots of how we think, feel and act as parents during our adulthood can be found in how we ourselves were parented. Thus, 'parent education' actually begins not with our first child, but rather at the start of our own lives.

DOI: 10.4324/9781003223771-2

What we experienced at the dawn of our days creates the mental and emotional template – the default setting – for our later attitudes and behaviours. People who enjoyed happy, nurturing, healthy and loving parenting tend to replicate that positive pattern with their own children. Conversely, those who hated, or perceive themselves as harmed by, the parenting they received tend to diligently strive to parent in ways as different as possible from that negative legacy. Whether we reject, modify or emulate, the point is that our first parenting 'classes' occurred while still a fetus, an infant, a toddler and a young child.

Awareness and understanding of this 'fact of life' has three crucial implications for professionals, policymakers and opinion leaders.

First, potential, expectant and new mothers and fathers are no more 'empty vessels' to be filled with our expert knowledge and good advice about parenthood than children are empty vessels to be filled by classroom teaching and the formal curricula.

The time is overdue to take each individual's experiences, knowledge and concerns seriously as the basis for building and maintaining two-way relationships of trust and respect. That involves far more listening than lecturing, more humility than hubris and more person-centred approaches than 'one size fits all' practices.

Of course, accurate information, reliable, robust evidence and ground-breaking research are, and will continue to be, vitally important. The challenge is to move beyond our collective history of regarding and treating (even if inadvertently) the ostensible beneficiaries of our expertise as people who should passively 'hear and heed' our well-intentioned professional advice. Compassionate, culturally competent, respectful relationships are the irreplaceable key to personal growth, professional success and social progress.

Second, powerful 'teachable moments' for influencing parents and parenting already exist across the life course, not just during the antenatal or postnatal periods. To cite one of numerous examples, supporting positive attachment/attunement between infants and their mothers, fathers and carers not only benefits all concerned in the here and now, but also lays an excellent foundation for how those very young children will eventually parent their own babies. Similarly, the attitudes and intentions about breastfeeding – first developed in childhood and solidified during adolescence – are powerful predictors of eventual breastfeeding behaviour.

The public health response to the COVID-19 pandemic included a recurring message to wash hands thoroughly and often. For children, this helped to 'join the dots' between their actions and their health. Along with playing outdoors, eating nutritious food and other measures to promote health and prevent illness, these efforts are modern manifestations of the old proverb that 'As the twig is bent, so is the tree inclined'. They also instil a sense of *agency* by underscoring that what a girl or boy does (or fails to do) is directly connected to staying healthy or falling ill which, in turn, makes the world seem less random and discourages a *que sera sera* attitude towards their health and wellbeing. Without the foundation of feeling empowered and understanding one's own right/ability to make important decisions about personal wellbeing, the psychological and practical framework for 'choosing' (or avoiding) parenthood as adults can be very weak. Building habits of mind, habits of behaviour and 'habits of the heart' are integral elements of a life-course approach to preconception health, education and care – as well as to preparing for pregnancy and parenthood.

Third, as professionals and societies, we need to radically redefine the meaning of 'early' in order to both reduce existing inequities and prevent gaps from opening in the first place. 'Early' interventions generally refer to actions taken after a baby is born. Too often, that is too late to fundamentally alter an infant's life chances. For example, a baby born with lifelong, life-limiting neurodevelopmental conditions – such as fetal alcohol spectrum disorder (FASD) – will experience diminished health and wellbeing, no matter how lovingly and intelligently parented or how many first-rate early interventions are received.

Across the globe, there are valuable and successful efforts underway to close existing gaps during early childhood in terms of health/wellbeing indicators and socioeconomic status. And it is imperative to continue efforts to reduce poverty, overcome inequalities and advance social justice. However, it is at least equally wise and less costly (in both human and financial terms) to take meaningful action much earlier than is commonly the case, i.e. before birth and, especially, before pregnancy. The overall health and wellbeing of mothers at the time of conception remains the most reliable predictor of pregnancy and birth outcomes. It is no secret that women who are happy, healthy, enjoying good lives and well prepared for pregnancy are much more likely to have better birth outcomes than their less fortunate, stressed counterparts who are leading chaotic lives and ill-prepared for pregnancy.

And so, the preconception period is when 'early intervention' should really begin and when primary prevention can be most potent.

Many risk factors are best mitigated and many health promotion activities are best accomplished – from stopping smoking to achieving a healthy weight, from improving mental health to weaning off teratogenic medications – well in advance of pregnancy.

Some crucial issues can *only* be resolved during the preconception or inter-conception periods. Preventing neural tube defects (NTDs) is a classic and powerful example. The neural tube – which will become the brain, spine and central nervous system – is fundamentally formed (or malformed) around the end of the first month after conception; that is, before women may even know they are pregnant. NTDs not only cause such lifelong conditions as spina bifida, but also result in a higher number of miscarriages, stillbirths and post-screening terminations.

For decades, it has been known that an adequate level of blood folate (Vitamin B9) can prevent the majority of neural tube defects. However, that level is rarely achievable by diet alone. Even with folic acid (Vitamin B9) supplements, it takes months to obtain this preventative benefit. That protection can only happen prior to conception. The case for mandatory fortification of flour or other staple foods with folic acid – as 88 countries have already done – rests upon the reality that many pregnancies are neither planned nor prepared for. Moreover, voluntary folic acid supplementation programmes have, for a variety of reasons, not had the widespread impact sought.

## Practitioner Guidance

The 'traffic light' poster, 'Practitioner Guidance on Preconception/Interconception Health Care', summarises key lessons from the preconception/interconception literature and international practice. It is intended to spark conversations about, and by, professionals, providers and organisations relating to the final stage of preparing for pregnancy and parenthood. Thus, it does not reflect the emphasis that should be accorded to a life-course approach, i.e. what could, and should, be considered, talked about and acted upon much earlier in women's and men's lives.

Telling people what to do is usually unsuccessful and neither as respectful nor as ethical as engaging people in discussions about topics of mutual interest or concern. For example, just telling a woman not to get pregnant while she is in an abusive or coercive relationship is, at best, a waste of breath. By contrast, asking her in sensitive and appropriate ways about her relationship with her partner (the prospective father) may lead to better understanding of the root causes of her dilemmas/difficulties and direct assistance or referrals to sources of help she would find welcome and helpful.

## Thinking about Preconception Health, Education and Care

One fundamental reason there has been relatively little coherent, consistent work in the area of preconception health, education and care across the Organisation for Economic Co-operation and Development (OECD) countries is that it largely has been and remains a 'blind spot'. If the great majority of policymakers, practitioners and other relevant individuals and organisations don't even 'see' it, then, inevitably, myriad opportunities for constructive, empowering, impactful action will be missed.

There are understandable reasons for this blind spot, which range from over-full professional workloads (and thus, no incentive to think about new activities, even if sensible and promising) to empty coffers (as it is assumed that significant action must be costly). In addition, rolling back public and political ideas about what constitutes 'early' from pre-school to pre-birth is seen as difficult enough without trying to encourage thinking and acting *pre-pregnancy* which is viewed by some as simply 'too hard'.

Perhaps the biggest impediment to taking preconception health, education and care seriously is, however, cultural, rather than pragmatic. It is a cultural norm in most OECD countries to see only two realities, i.e. avoiding pregnancy or being pregnant. With the exception of people having fertility issues, the middle ground between 'avoiding and being' remains largely invisible. Such middle ground consists of actively thinking about, and preparing for, pregnancy and parenthood.

That cultural norm, in turn, reflects a widespread 'que sera sera' attitude about becoming pregnant (and about parenthood). Why bother thinking about preconception health, education and care when it is passively accepted that roughly half of all pregnancies will continue to be unintended, unplanned or mistimed? Why do we collectively think that this very high proportion of 'accidental' pregnancies will simply continue unabated? We do not think that even such longstanding and complex realities as poverty or inequality are beyond our collective wit and will to reduce. So, why don't we think and feel the same about unforeseen conception and ill-prepared pregnancies?

The urgent need to improve preconception and interconception health, education and care is largely unrecognised. Yet, our societies can no longer afford, in human, public policy or financial terms, the costs of *laissez faire* attitudes and cultural blind spots that result in negative pregnancy and birth outcomes that were preventable, but not actually prevented.

## If It Takes a Village to Raise a Child, What Does It Take to Prepare and Support That Child's Mother and Father?

The short answer is that it takes a social movement uniting relevant individuals, communities, civic groups, agencies, institutions, professions and voluntary organisations. The fundamental understanding within such an informal alliance is that 'while nobody can do everything, everybody can do something' to transform preconception health, education and care across the life course from a good idea into a meaningful reality. The cumulative impact of an ever-growing number of positive, effective actions in this arena – large and small; national, regional and local; governmental and non-governmental – has the potential to be enormous.

Too many women, men and babies are 'dealt a bad hand' in the preconception 'game' that ends up causing them pain, creating long-term difficulties and sometimes even costing them their lives. Individually and collectively, we can all make a difference for the better by keeping some of those 'bad hands' from ever being dealt.

## Practice Pointers

Some suggestions for how to help people who will ever have a child get what they already deeply desire: a safe pregnancy, a thriving baby and a rewarding parenthood.

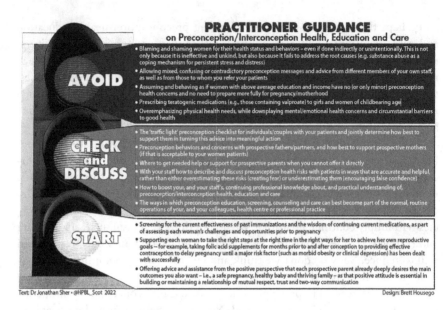

**PRACTITIONER GUIDANCE**
on Preconception/Interconception Health, Education and Care

**AVOID**
- Blaming and shaming women for their health status and behaviors – even if done indirectly or unintentionally. This is not only because it is ineffective and unkind, but also because it fails to address the root causes (e.g. substance abuse as a coping mechanism for persistent stress and distress)
- Allowing mixed, confusing or contradictory preconception messages and advice from different members of your own staff, as well as from those to whom you refer your patients
- Assuming and behaving as if women with above average education and income have no (or only minor) preconception health concerns and no need to prepare more fully for pregnancy/motherhood
- Prescribing teratogenic medications (e.g., those containing valproate) to girls and women of childbearing age
- Overemphasizing physical health needs, while downplaying mental/emotional health concerns and circumstantial barriers to good health

**CHECK and DISCUSS**
- The 'traffic light' preconception checklist for individuals/couples with your patients and jointly determine how best to support them in turning this advice into meaningful action
- Preconception behaviors and concerns with prospective fathers/partners, and how best to support prospective mothers (if that is acceptable to your women patients)
- Where to get needed help or support for prospective parents when you cannot offer it directly
- With your staff how to describe and discuss preconception health risks with patients in ways that are accurate and helpful, rather than either overestimating these risks (creating fear) or underestimating them (encouraging false confidence)
- How to boost your, and your staff's, continuing professional knowledge about, and practical understanding of, preconception/interconception health, education and care
- The ways in which preconception education, screening, counseling and care can best become part of the normal, routine operations of your, and your colleagues, health centre or professional practice

**START**
- Screening for the current effectiveness of past immunizations and the wisdom of continuing current medications, as part of assessing each woman's challenges and opportunities prior to pregnancy
- Supporting each woman to take the right steps at the right time in the right ways for her to achieve her own reproductive goals – for example, taking folic acid supplements for months prior to and after conception to providing effective contraception to delay pregnancy until a major risk factor (such as morbid obesity or clinical depression) has been dealt with successfully
- Offering advice and assistance from the positive perspective that each prospective parent already deeply desires the main outcomes you also want – i.e., a safe pregnancy, healthy baby and thriving family – as that positive attitude is essential in building or maintaining a relationship of mutual respect, trust and two-way communication

Text: Dr Jonathan Sher • @HPBL_Scot 2022          Design: Brett Housego

**FIGURE 1.1** Practitioner Guidance.
*Source*: Author

- Add an antenatal, and then a preconception, version of an already successful service dealing with postnatal depression or other mental health concerns.
- Create a peer support group among expectant fathers alongside an existing one for mothers-to-be.
- Ensure new mothers with drug or alcohol dependency will be encouraged and supported to make informed choices about birth-spacing, contraception alternatives and treatment possibilities.
- Challenge and then end the cruel and ineffective tendency to name, shame and blame people – especially women – for adverse pregnancy and birth outcomes that were largely, if not entirely, beyond their control. It is extraordinarily rare for prospective parents to make poor choices or take negative actions because they are driven by the desire to harm their baby.
- Enhance services to individuals in prison, and their partners, to include preconception education and respectful, person-centred counselling about parenthood.
- Encourage primary care providers and key specialists to opportunistically explore the desires of potential parents to avoid, delay or prepare for pregnancy as a routine element of their practice – and then to either directly help or signpost them to trustworthy sources of advice and assistance.

# 2

# IMPROVING HEALTH AND WELL-BEING BEFORE, BETWEEN AND BEYOND PREGNANCY

*Sarah Verbiest and Erin K. McClain*

Preconception, reproductive, and preventive healthcare are foundational to well-being. Practitioners who provide services to people of reproductive age have many strategies to consider in offering equitable, quality, respectful whole-person care.

★

Narrowly defined, preconception health is the physical, social, and emotional health of a person before pregnancy. Broadening the definition with a reproductive justice lens expands this to supporting the health and well-being of people of reproductive age, regardless of their intention to become a parent. Well-being is an essential building block for a person, their community, and their current/future family if that is their goal. There are many broad recommendations for improving health and wellness for people of reproductive age. In 2014, a national meeting of experts in the United States suggested that preconception care should be integrated into clinical and preventive care – reiterating the 'every woman, every time' approach (Before, Between & Beyond Pregnancy, 2021). They also underscored the importance of providing quality, actionable health information and education to a diverse group of people. Equally, the recommendations included developing clinical care supports and tools, harnessing the potential of technology and health information systems, and encouraging researchers, public health professionals, and practitioners to develop measures to improve clinical care and community services (Johnson et al., 2014). This approach was reiterated in a 2016 article that focused on the importance of a health equity and health justice perspective as foundational to preconception health programs, resources, and care (Verbiest et al., 2016). More recently, 'Preconception Health and Care: A Life Course Approach', by Shawe et al. (2020), offered a series of

DOI: 10.4324/9781003223771-3

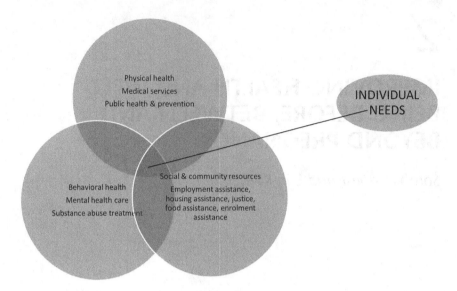

**FIGURE 2.1**   A Visual Depiction of Whole-Person Care.

recommendations. The first highlighted the importance of access to continuous, quality, culturally appropriate, comprehensive care across the life course. The authors emphasized the potential that preconception health programs have to advance reproductive justice and equitable health outcomes for people and their families. They called for practitioners to engage with the populations they serve to co-create new strategies for providing care and urged governments and philanthropic organizations to fund these ideas. Finally, they encouraged a collective investment in building healthy and economically sound communities and then collecting population and clinical data to measure change and reveal disparities (Shawe et al., 2020).

In September 2021, the National Preconception Health and Health Care Initiative led by the University of North Carolina at Chapel Hill's Schools of Social Work and Medicine convened a national, virtual summit entitled 'Future Forward: Equity Centered Wellness'. The event highlighted diverse voices and underscored the necessity of taking a holistic view of the healthcare and wellness supports and resources that people, families, and communities need. People want and need comprehensive care that considers their mental and social well-being as well as their physical health. There is a desire for services that are tailored to each person's unique needs and circumstances, and which are provided in a way that inspires hope and supports individuals' reproductive health goals. Healthcare providers, public health leaders, and community leaders need to pay attention to the conditions that support health and to assure that programs and strategies honor diversity and advance equitable outcomes for all people regardless of their identity.

Figure 2.1 offers a visual depiction of whole-person care. This considers the complete needs of individuals and helps connect them with the information, treatment, and services needed to support each individual's well-being. This requires improving cross-system connections, data sharing, service coordination, financial flexibility, and collaborative leadership (Maxwell et al., 2014).

The recommendations and approach described are intended to push the health and social care sectors toward innovative thinking and action. Practitioners who work with people of reproductive age, birthing people, and new families have a unique opportunity to provide intergenerational whole-person care. Four strategies are suggested below. The specific approach within each strategy will vary based on the practitioner's role, training, and opportunities for engagement with people of reproductive age.

## Strategy 1: Support Access to Quality, Preventive Care and Mental Health Services across the Life Course

Millions of women across the globe do not receive regular, preventive healthcare, including routine screening for health conditions, health education and promotion, and access to interventions (Johnson et al., 2014). While the United States' healthcare system has a robust standard of preventive care and interventions for children – and interest in extending that to adolescents – only recently has there been an effort to identify and fund routine preventive services for women (Women's Preventive Services Initiative, 2016). Access to regular care, including mental health and behavioral health, is an essential component of preconception wellness.

Women who have experienced difficulties conceiving, miscarriage, stillbirth, or early infant loss are often under-served and under-recognized by maternal and child health practitioners. Yet, this cohort of women are likely to be the people who have the greatest need for whole-person care. Many may be living with one or more chronic conditions and struggling to coordinate their care across specialists. Preconception health messages need to be carefully tailored to recognize their unique needs in their desire to become a parent.

Research has also shown that mothers who have newborns who require intensive nursery care are more likely than mothers of healthy babies to have experienced a traumatic birth and to have one or more chronic conditions. They are also at higher risk of experiencing depression and anxiety. This is another group of women who need increased services and coordinated care (Verbiest et al., 2020).

One way to meet these needs is to opportunistically use existing opportunities, such as connecting parents and caregivers to appropriate services during a pediatric visit for their child as well as encouraging home visitors and community health workers to help prepare people to make the most of upcoming healthcare encounters.

## Practice Pointers

- Providers and their teams should support seamless transitions of care from regular preventive care and family planning through prenatal care and postpartum care (if appropriate to that person's goals) and back to preventive care. All populations of people, regardless of pregnancy goals, benefit when healthcare systems and providers work in concert to support their care. Offering additional services such as care coordination for people with chronic conditions, including physical, mental, and behavior conditions, would be beneficial. Seamless care includes sharing of medical records and health information across providers and ensuring clear communication when multiple providers are involved in a person's care. One important care transition that is often overlooked is when adolescents move from pediatric to adult care providers.
- Qualitative work highlights the many instances of miscarriage, infertility, and infant loss experienced by women with chronic conditions. This suggests that professionals need to listen and respond to grief and loss, as well as to partner with the woman to identify and secure access to practitioners who can support her in this journey.
- Help people make the most of their healthcare encounters, including building their confidence to ask questions.
- Identify mental health hotline numbers and resources in your country to share with patients. For example, in the United States, the JED Foundation hosts many resources for young adults (https://jedfoundation.org/mental-health-resource-center/) and the Mental Health First Aid program offers resources and training (https://www.mentalhealthfirstaid.org). Many are free, anonymous and provide 24/7 access via text, chat, email, telehealth, and more.
- One important note: while whole-person care includes support in areas such as housing, jobs, and education, health practitioners should screen for the social determinants of health only if they can offer meaningful referrals or follow-up assistance.

## Strategy 2: Provide Messages and Education in a Way That Models 'You Matter'

The days of handing a person a one-page list of 'dos and don'ts' for preconception health as the only educational tool are over. While plain language guidance is important, telling a person to 'lose weight', or 'reduce stress', or 'change medications' is not helpful on its own. In fact, this can generate new sources of stress for people who may wish to make these changes but do not have the resources to do so. Further, images used in educational materials that focus on people who are thin, attractive, members of the country's dominant culture (e.g., in the USA, white people), and engaging in activities that require financial resources, do not connect with many of the people who need access to information and support. A detailed report on preconception health communications was published with recommendations in 2018 (The Lancet, 2018).

People want information and advice tailored to their unique needs and circumstances. They want action steps that are doable with reasonable goals, shared in a language that works for them. Being mindful of concepts of adult learning and literacy can make materials more accessible to more people. Improving accessibility may include providing messages in a variety of formats, including video, audio, and written text, as well as using pictures and icons to provide context clues for written messages to engage readers with lower levels of literacy. Messaging that combines information from experts, such as physicians and midwives, with perspectives from the intended beneficiaries, for instance on how to use the expert information, can be powerful and effective. Receiving and responding to feedback from the people being served as well as the practitioners who might use the tools is essential. Asking for that feedback early and often will ultimately save time and resources by creating messages and tools that resonate with each community.

The Show Your Love Campaign (www. showyourlovetoday.com) in the United States was created to reach young adults with a variety of health messages. Instead of focusing on preconception health, the resources are designed to focus on health and wellness overall, with specific information when there are special considerations for people who wish to become pregnant. The images and language were carefully selected to highlight social justice considerations.

## Practice Pointers

- Support ALL people to better understand fertility and reproduction by taking time to offer and discuss resources and education.
- Build health and social care providers' skills in shared decision-making conversations and motivational interviewing as ways to help people identify clear, actionable strategies that they can undertake.
- Use positive framing and messages of self-care and self-love. Be ready to encourage people on their journey, recognize their strengths, and help them troubleshoot when they run into barriers.
- Pay attention to social media and consider proactively posting and sharing quality resources, videos, apps, and materials. Make sure that images reflect the diversity of your community. Many seek health information on social media, so sharing creative and trustworthy social media sources can be helpful.
- Whole-person care means considering each individual's social circumstances as well as mental and physical health. It should take into account people's desire and ability to modify behaviors and assist each person to be clear about their priorities.
- Consider taking a family approach in identifying and supporting positive behavior change.

## Strategy 3: Create Opportunities to Talk about a Woman's/ Person's/Couple's Interest in Becoming Parents

Opening the door for people to talk about their thoughts and wishes for becoming parents can be a powerful relationship builder and a way to provide tailored care. However, conversations about reproduction are also inherently value laden. People have opinions about who should become parents based on relationship status, age, economic status, parity, health status, and racial and ethnic identities. Practitioners should reflect on their own biases and acknowledge the ways these can affect how they approach prospective parents. It is essential that practitioners believe – and behave in ways that reflect this belief – that they are there first to listen and then to provide support for the person in achieving their goal, not to try to change their goal.

This conversation works best when it feels natural – for example, at an annual health check, in a contraception clinic, or when closing out postpartum care. Ideally, it is approached in the context of a good patient–provider relationship. It can be a difficult conversation for people who may be struggling with infertility (primary or secondary) or who have experienced a miscarriage or major relationship challenges. As such, consider asking whether this is the right time for them to have the conversation. Remember, it is not unusual for plans and wishes to change. Further, it is important for people to understand it is okay to 'not know' or to not already have a reproductive life plan. The conversation itself, and providing relevant information, can help them think more clearly about their future.

It is generally advisable to use a standard approach to asking all patients about their reproductive goals, as a consistent, system-wide approach can help decrease inequities in screening and service provision. There are several different models for asking patients about their reproductive desires. One model that is being used extensively in the United States is the PATH Framework developed by Envision Sexual and Reproductive Health (Envision SRH, 2020):

## The Path Framework

**P**arenthood/Pregnancy
**A**ttitude
**T**iming
**H**ow important is pregnancy prevention?

1  Do you think you might like to have (more) children at some point?
2  When do you think that might be?
3  How important is it to you to prevent pregnancy (until then)?

The PATH questions have been used with women, men, transgender, and gender non-binary/gender fluid folks, as well as those who are in heterosexual and queer relationships, at all ages across the reproductive years. By using a standardized set of questions that are both person-centered and do not communicate provider bias, the PATH approach opens the door to a nuanced conversation that takes into account current desires for (more) children, future goals, and timing. This leads to more opportunities to support people in receiving quality care, including tailored education, decisional support and advice, and access to appropriate resources. Positive outcomes, such as better contraceptive method matching, reduced fetal exposure to teratogenic medications, and timely fertility-related counseling and treatment, can follow. If this framework is used in a nonclinical setting or a setting where contraceptive or infertility services are not available, it is important to make sure that appropriate referrals to required services are part of the follow-up.

## Practice Pointers

- Asking about people's reproductive goals and desires can be a powerful tool to learn more about the context of their lives and build a stronger relationship between practitioner and patient/client.
- Practitioners must interrogate their own biases, specifically about who should have children and how families are made.
- Using a standardized, person-centered framework when asking people about their goals can help reduce inequities.
- If asking questions about reproductive goals, have a plan for following up, including making referrals for necessary services.

## Strategy 4: Provide Respectful Care

Preconception, preventive, and reproductive healthcare creates the opportunity to benefit at least two generations. When conversations are approached thoughtfully, they can build trust and confidence, which in turn can lead to improved health outcomes. When such conversations are not respectful, sensitive, and person-centered, they can cause harm, pain and lead to health disparities.

Whole-person care requires practitioners to demonstrate a nuanced approach. For example, women who are overweight or obese experience frequent discrimination in care. Before making a quick recommendation to lose weight, consider other factors in her life that could influence weight – medications, lack of sleep, high stress, chronic conditions, or lack of access to a safe place to exercise. Further, 'normal' weight may not reflect what is considered to be healthy and beautiful in different cultures. Practitioners can approach this conversation by asking the person how they feel about their weight and go from there.

A trauma-informed approach to care is important given the level of violence that women across the globe experience, including intimate partner violence, military sexual trauma, rape and other forms of sexual assault, child abuse and neglect, terrorism, natural disasters, and street violence. Violence, whether physical or emotionally harmful or life-threatening, has lasting adverse effects on a person's ability to function. Trauma-Informed Care principles include the four Rs:

- Realize the prevalence of traumatic events and the widespread impact of trauma
- Recognize the signs and symptoms of trauma
- Respond by integrating knowledge about trauma into policies, procedures, and practices
- Resist re-traumatization. It is important for practitioners to understand their own trauma in order to provide this essential care.

## Practice Pointers

- Understand about how your service/clinic/program is perceived by people in communities who are experiencing health disparities. History does matter.
- Seek training opportunities for yourself and make them available for your team. Take time to learn more about the people you serve who experience health disparities. Consider how your identity and experience impact your ability to provide equitable care.
- Ask people about their pronouns. Never assume how someone looks is how they identify, including race/ethnicity. Be sure screening tools are welcoming to different sexualities in a non-judgmental way. Recognize that people in the LGBTQ+ community are more likely to have unplanned pregnancies and suffer from unmet health needs than other groups.
- Provide resources and have conversations in the language of the people you serve. Employ people with similar identities to the people you serve.
- Collect and review data from your service/program to see if you are providing care in a way that results in equitable outcomes. If you see differences, take time to explore why these might be happening, including talking with the people you are serving and reviewing patient satisfaction data. Be open to making changes.
- Consider using these phrases: 'I believe you'; 'I see you'; 'I trust you to be the expert about your own body'; 'I'm here to support you no matter what. I want to help you reach your goals'. Acknowledge that it is 'okay to not be okay'.

## Summary

There are many opportunities for supporting the complete health and well-being of people before, between, and beyond pregnancy. Practitioners have an important role to play given their unique relationships with the people and families who could benefit from preconception or inter-conception education and care. Whole-person care means that practitioners and their organizations need to build partnerships with other agencies and sectors to provide the best services possible. Partnerships that are multi-directional and involve agencies really understanding each other's processes and policies, as well as the services provided, can more easily withstand personnel changes and help smooth the way for people to receive comprehensive, whole-person care.

In many communities, necessary resources, funding, and/or policies may not be in place to fully support the care and structures needed to enable people's preconception health, education, and care. Practitioners can be powerful advocates in their local community for policies and funding decisions that support people in leading healthy lives. In some communities, this may mean supporting funding to improve the built environment, such as provision of sidewalks and parks for people to exercise and reduce stress. In others, practitioners may need to advocate and educate on the need for essential healthcare funding and infrastructure.

The most important strategy is the one where you can begin! Identify what will work best for your organization and your clients and then get started. Regularly checking in with the people you serve, paying attention to practitioner biases and seeking to mitigate their effect, and keeping whole-person-centered care at the heart of your work will allow you to better support the people you serve across their reproductive years.

## Acknowledgments

The authors would like to thank Suzanne Woodward and Katherine Bryant, Collaborative for Maternal and Infant Health, School of Medicine, University of North Carolina at Chapel Hill, for their assistance with this chapter.

## References

Before, Between & Beyond Pregnancy (2021) Module 2: Every woman, every time – integrating health promotion into primary care. Available at: https://beforeandbeyond. org/modules/module-2-everywoman-every-time/ <accessed July 12, 2020>

Envision SRH (2020) The PATH Framework. Available at: https://www.envisionsrh. com/path-framework <accessed November 12, 2021>

Johnson, K., Balluff, M., Abresch, C. Verbiest, S., Atrash, H. (2014) Summary of findings from the reconvened Select Panel on Preconception Health and Health Care. Available at: https://beforeandbeyond.org/wp-content/uploads/2014/03/002192_Preconception-Health-Report-Booklet_5th.pdf <accessed November 16, 2021>

Maxwell, J., Tobey, R., Barron, C., Bateman, C., Ward, M. (2014) National approaches to whole-person care in the safety net. Available at: https://publications.jsi. com/JSIInternet/Inc/Common/download_pub.cfm?id=14261&lid=3 <accessed November 16, 2021>

Shawe, J., Steegers, E.A.P., Verbiest, S. (2020) Preconception Health and Care: A life course approach. Basingstoke: Springer.

The Lancet (2018) Preconception health. (series) Available at: thelancet.com/series/preconception-health <accessed 29 November, 2021>

Verbiest, S., Ferrari, R., Tucker, C., McClain, E.K., Charles, N. et al. (2020) Health needs of mothers of infants in a neonatal intensive care unit: A mixed-methods study. Annals of Internal Medicine, 1(173): S37–S44.

Verbiest, S., McClain, E., Woodward, S. (2016) Advancing preconception health in the United States: Strategies for change. *Upsala Journal of Medical Sciences*, 121(4): 222–226.

Women's Preventive Services Initiative (2016) Available at: https://www.womenspreventivehealth.org/about/ <accessed 21 November, 2021>

# 3

# WOULD YOU LIKE TO BECOME PREGNANT IN THE NEXT YEAR? THE ONE KEY QUESTION® INITIATIVE IN THE UNITED STATES

*Michele Stranger Hunter*

This is the story about changing standard US medical practice from ignoring pre-pregnancy issues in primary care to initiating open conversations with women about preconception and contraception, listening carefully, and responding appropriately and respectfully to their concerns. While the context of healthcare in the United States is different in the United Kingdom and Europe, the need to initiate conversations about potential, rather than actual, pregnancies is vital for practitioners everywhere to improve outcomes for children and their families.

\*

Nearly a century ago, the equally revered and reviled 'father of psychoanalysis', Sigmund Freud, admitted:

> The great question that has never been answered, and which I have not yet been able to answer, despite my thirty years of research into the feminine soul, is 'What does a woman want?'

Given it is primarily women who have the capacity to become pregnant and give birth, what they want is often related to their current desires about pregnancy. While a small percentage of those who want to become pregnant have fertility issues, there is a much larger group who become pregnant at the wrong time or under the wrong circumstances.

'Approximately half of all pregnancies are unintended'. For over four decades, I repeated this statistic to motivate practitioners and catalyze change in policies across the United States.

Despite advances in contraceptive methods, the increase in reproductive health practitioners, the promotion of conception as an informed choice, and

DOI: 10.4324/9781003223771-4

a lowering of barriers to accessing relevant information and services, the fact remains that the United States has not significantly moved the dial on planned versus unplanned pregnancy (Verbiest et al., 2016). The same is true of OECD (Organization for Economic Co-operation and Development) countries (Goossens et al., 2018).

'Unintended' conceptions are associated with most termination decisions, delayed prenatal care, high-risk pregnancies, and poor maternal and birth outcomes (Aiken et al., 2016). Interview and survey data from those with lived experience, however, seriously challenge the use of pregnancy intention as the indicator. A positive intention to become pregnant does not indicate preparation before conception and does not improve outcomes. The negative outcomes associated with 'unintended' pregnancy can be equally associated with 'unprepared' for pregnancy (Potter et al., 2019). Treatment of pre-existing conditions, avoidance of toxic medications, addition of folic acid prior to conception, and elimination of high-risk behaviors are all necessary to improve birth outcomes. Many poor results are avoidable. Without preconception counseling and care prior to conception, however, the opportunity to prevent innumerable negative outcomes closes (Sher, 2021).

Pregnancy intention has been equated with planning. Planned pregnancies have become the gold standard for measuring practitioners' collective effort (Dehlendorf et al., 2018). Interviews with practitioners and their patients make it clear that services currently emphasize contraception services and ignore the need to prepare for a healthy pregnancy. Patients report they experience this as their practitioner's judgment that they should not become pregnant and must choose the most effective contraceptive (Garbers et al., 2019).

There is an assumption that 'unintended' pregnancies are predominantly experienced by lower-income women. In 2020, 12.5 million (17.5%) babies were born into poverty in the United States. Babies born into financially stressed families were two-thirds more likely to have low birth weights, and their mothers were twice as likely to suffer from postpartum depression. Additionally, socioeconomic mobility is too often constrained by mistimed or inadequately prepared for pregnancies, and this contributes to intergenerational poverty and inequality across America (Venator & Reeves, 2015).

These risks are compounded by socioeconomic determinants of health at every age. No low-income adult needs to be told there is a connection between their wealth and their health, or the health of their children. However, 'low-income' is too often used to justify professional, political, and cultural norms that judge, shame, and blame the health practices of low-income populations. This framework assigns fault to the pregnant person for an unintended pregnancy. The system's responsibility for offering wellness care and education that includes preventative reproductive health services is ignored.

At the same time, some erroneously assume that unprepared for pregnancy is uncommon among middle class and wealthy people. This is both untrue and unjustifiably encourages the belief that the way to reduce unintended pregnancies is through targeting low-income people. The data show that a universal strategy encouraging people of all incomes to prepare for healthy pregnancies before conception will improve outcomes.

Others assert that good prenatal care is sufficient insurance for positive outcomes in 'surprise pregnancies'. However, an ample bank balance cannot magically restore the benefits of taking folic acid supplements for the three months prior to and the first month of a pregnancy (Sher, 2016). This is just one of dozens of examples of the added risks and lost opportunities when pregnancy preparation is ignored.

Consider this: On average, a woman in the United States is fertile for 39 years. She will, on average, have two children and therefore will have five years during which she is either pregnant or in the postpartum period. Except for women experiencing a fertility problem, that leaves 34 years to avoid or prepare for pregnancy. Health 'systems' inadvertently play a damaging role by ignoring preconception assessment. The traditional silos of reproductive care make little sense and do not bequeath the best outcomes (Shaw et al., 2020).

In the United States, two consistent realities are obvious. The first is that reproductive education, counseling, and care are seen as the 'business' of specialists, rather than of primary care providers. The second is that while prenatal care is 'part of the wallpaper' in America (for those with adequate health coverage), little pre-pregnancy information, preparatory counseling, or care are received or routinely accessible by everyone for whom pregnancy is a possibility. People are largely left on their own to understand the need for, seek out, and afford quality advice and assistance in preparing for a healthy pregnancy before conception. It is as if pregnancy does not begin until the first prenatal visit, late in the first trimester (Sher, 2021; Skogsdal et al, 2019; Stephenson et al., 2018).

Those two realities mean that most women simply do without the 'before the fact' conversations and do not have the knowledge or support to recognize a need to prepare for a healthy pregnancy before conception. This means the actual proportion of pregnancies not prepared for exceeds the 50% rate of 'unintended' pregnancies. The result is a strong alignment between an unprepared for pregnancy and subsequent pregnancy complications and poor birth outcomes (Bateson and Black, 2018).

## The Journey Begins

One Key Question® (OKQ) grew out of the search for a solution to reducing the number of unintended pregnancies. By evaluating the extent to which primary care and general practitioners proactively offer reproductive health services, through over 100 clinician interviews, we confirmed that the vast majority did not see themselves as first-line providers of reproductive health. Reproductive health was simply not on the radar within US primary care (Oregon Foundation of Reproductive Health, 2011).

My initial study was confirmed by other national data. The national studies revealed that US women received reproductive health advice in primary care only 14% of the time (Bello et al., 2015) and only 30% of reproductive age patients who could become pregnant went to a specialty provider (Lundsberg et al., 2014), such as a family planning clinic. When combined, the data demonstrated reproductive health advice was only being provided to 44% of reproductive age women. Most practitioners did not offer preventative reproductive health.

## From Here to Maternity (Or Not!)

According to Occam's Razor: When facing an intractable problem, the simplest solution is likely to be the best solution. With that in mind, the answer to how to reduce the proportion of pregnancies not prepared for is simplicity itself, ASK THE WOMAN WHAT SHE WANTS. Inquire if she wants children now, later, or never and then offer services supporting her choice.

Clearly needed was a strategy for proactive, patient-centered conversations about reproductive goals that could be integrated within general practice/ primary care services. Most needed was a screening question that when answered might change the treatment plan to include preventative services or referrals that support the patient's/client's reproductive goals.

Thus was born One Key Question® (OKQ). OKQ was created in 2010 by the Oregon Foundation for Reproductive Health with the aim of dramatically increasing the depth and breadth of women's opportunities to receive reproductive health advice within primary healthcare, and further, to encourage, assist, and support a person's own desires about parenthood.

In 2018, OKQ's registered trademark and associated intellectual property was transferred to Power to Decide, a national organization committed to reproductive autonomy to decide if, when, and under what circumstances to become pregnant. By 2019, OKQ had been implemented in 30 US states. Six states adopted OKQ as a state-wide strategy.

OKQ integrates proactive pregnancy desire screening by asking, 'Would you like to become pregnant in the next year?' as a routine part of primary care and other opportunistic health visits. Novel in its approach, OKQ asks what reproductive health information and services women need to be healthy and either avoid pregnancy or increase the chances of a successful one.

OKQ identifies pregnancy desire along a continuum by offering four response options: 'Yes', 'No', 'Unsure', or 'Okay Either Way'. Each answer warrants a specific practitioner response that may be implemented in a variety of care settings. OKQ is followed by contraception, preconception, or interconception counseling, education, and care, offered directly or through referral, based on the response (Stulberg et al., 2020).

OKQ therefore is an entry point to offer patient-centered, evidence-based contraception care for those who do not want to become pregnant and comprehensive preconception/inter-conception care for those who do.

OKQ steps away from the word 'plan' because 'planning to become pregnant' does not consistently resonate with some cultures or religions. OKQ advances the intent of 'reproductive life planning', but focuses on asking women what they want, rather than on what they plan. This may also be important for women whose lived experience is disapproval of 'planning pregnancy while poor' because this violates the taboo against having babies you can't afford. Research among low-income women has shown that 'planning was not a particularly salient concept', often because the context in which women felt planning should take place (a marital relationship and stable finances) was elusive (Borrero et al., 2015; Potter et al., 2019).

By including 'Unsure' or 'Okay Either Way' as options, women are offered a space to express (and normalize) ambivalent or neutral attitudes toward becoming pregnant. Identifying and acknowledging where each woman is on the continuum of pregnancy intentions is a mark of respect for her choices and a way of encouraging each woman's sense of agency (McQuillan et al., 2011).

From OKQ's first pilot to clinic-wide evaluations conducted, patients commented, 'I didn't know I could talk about that here' or 'Thank you for asking! No-one's ever asked me that before'. Providers reported a marked upturn in referrals for wrap-around services related to women answering the one key question and then adding a 'but' – for example, 'I want to get pregnant, but I've been feeling really depressed' or 'I don't want to get pregnant, but my boyfriend wants me to'.

## Practitioners' Words, Awareness, and Actions Matter

One Key Question® is simple, but implementing it properly requires significant 'behind the scenes' work with those asking. Using an iterative evaluation process, OKQ developed comprehensive practitioner training and guidance. The training was improved further by Power to Decide, and in 2020, offered an accredited on-line curriculum. Training includes how the question is asked – verbal/written; the timing/frequency; context; shared decision making and follow-up steps, all central to OKQ's success. The nature and quality of the practitioner's response, based on each person's answer, is critical. Not surprisingly, this works best when there is trust between the person asking and the person answering. Less obviously, such a relationship is not an essential pre-requisite for effective implementation.

It is not the role of the practitioner to be judgmental, resolve expressed ambivalence, or change any person's mind about their goal(s). OKQ is about offering information truly responsive to expressed needs, whether that means understanding the risk of pregnancy given contraceptive choices or preconception care needs based upon the individual's health status (Srinivasulu et al., 2019).

Practitioners report that the OKQ model structures an important conversation – one which they should have with those for whom pregnancy is a possibility. Research on OKQ has confirmed the acceptability of pregnancy desire screening and showed an increase in contraceptive counseling (Stulberg et al., 2019). Additional research has shown this screening is welcomed by patients and acceptable/feasible to practitioners. Post-implementation, clinicians have reported visit quality improved and visit length did not disrupt their schedule. Importantly, patient satisfaction has increased significantly (Song et al., 2021).

The question itself is straightforward, but the dilemmas revealed in the answers are not always easy to deal with well. In such situations, the main role of the initial provider is to make wise and practical referrals to other individuals, services, or agencies better equipped to take the next steps.

One Key Question is not the solution to all the vagaries of real life for both providers and the people they try to help. It is nothing more and nothing less than a model for universal screening of the desire to become pregnant among those of reproductive age at risk of pregnancy. A simple question can be the key that unlocks previously hidden goals, needs, and concerns around pregnancy.

## Conclusion

Most women already interact with the healthcare system through check-ups or visits for a variety of health issues. They have rarely been asked about their desire for pregnancy or encouraged to make choices in preparation for parenthood prior to conception. OKQ represents a crucial opportunity to lower the proportion of 'surprise' pregnancies by screening routinely for pregnancy goals, wherever and whenever women/those for whom pregnancy is a possibility may seek care (Boyd et al., 2016).

Asking the One Key Question offers a nudge to identify pregnancy desires. This then increases the chances that practitioners can help meet their patients'/ clients' (previously unstated) reproductive goals by dramatically increasing opportunities to receive critical information and services for preventing or supporting preparation to have as healthy a pregnancy as possible (Hammarberg et al., 2020).

When a person conceives while facing unresolved and unmanaged health and psychosocial challenges, prenatal care usually cannot undo already present adverse impacts on a developing fetus. To improve maternal and birth outcomes, our society, our practitioners, and the systems in which they work must promote optimal preconception health for every woman, recognizing that a significant proportion of all women will become pregnant not by choice but by chance (Moos et al., 2008).

Implemented properly, OKQ changes the conversation and the practice of mainstream healthcare for those of reproductive age for whom pregnancy is a possibility. It neither tries to make crucial choices for them, nor influence them toward or away from avoiding, accepting, or seeking pregnancy.

The dialogue and decisions after asking and answering the One Key Question® can profoundly and positively shape reproductive health outcomes and improve the wellbeing and life chances of both parents and the children they choose to have, whenever the time and circumstances are right for them.

## Practice Pointers

- Recognize that many pregnancy complications and poor birth outcomes are preventable. Most 'unintended' pregnancies are wanted but mistimed and therefore without preparation before conception.
- Integrate age-appropriate preventive reproductive healthcare into all routine visits by assessing reproductive health needs of all who can become pregnant.
- Be opportunistic, proactively ask those who can become pregnant about their desire to become pregnant in routine general health visits.
- Offer non-binary answers: 'Yes', 'Unsure', 'Ok either way', or 'No'.
- Ask permission to provide contraception, and/or pre/interconception information and services, directly or through referrals, based on the patient's/ client's answer.

## References

Aiken, A.R.A., Borrero, S., Callegari, L.S., Dehlendor, C. (2016) Rethinking the pregnancy planning paradigm: Unintended conceptions or unrepresentative concepts? Perspectives on Sexual and Reproductive Health, 48(3):147–151.

Bateson, D.J., Black, K.I. (2018) Pre-conception care: An important yet under-utilised preventive strategy. Medical Journal of Australia, 209(9):430.

Bello, J.K., Rao, G., Stulberg, D.B. (2015) Trends in contraceptive and preconception care in United States ambulatory practices. Family Medicine, 47(4):264–271.

Borrero, S., Nikolajski, C., Steinberg, J.R., Freedman, L., Akers, A.Y. et al. (2015) 'It just happens': A qualitative study exploring low-income women's perspectives on pregnancy intention and planning. Contraception, 91(2):150–156.

Boyd, M., Murphy, D., Bielak, D. Bridgespan Group (2016) 'Billion Dollar Bets' to reduce unintended pregnancies: Creating economic opportunity for every American. (Bridgespan Group). ERIC Number: ED606530.

Dehlendorf, C., Reed, R., Fox, E., Seidman, D., Hall, C. et al. (2018) Ensuring our research reflects our values: The role of family planning research in advancing reproductive autonomy. Contraception, 98:4–7.

Garbers S., Falletta K., Srinivasulu Y., et al. (2019) 'If you don't ask, I'm not going to tell you': Using community-based participatory research to inform pregnancy intention screening processes for Black and Latina women in primary care. Women's Health Issues, 30(1):25–34.

Goossens, J., DeRoose, M., Van Hecke, A., Goemaes, R., Verhaeghe, S. et al. (2018) Barriers and facilitators to the provision of preconception care by healthcare providers: A systemic review. International Journal of Nursing Studies, 87:113–130.

Hammarberg, J., Hassard, R., Johnson, L. (2020) Acceptability of screening for pregnancy intention in general practice: A population survey of people of reproductive age. BMC Family Practice, 21:40.

Lundsberg, L.S., Pal, L., Gariepy, A.M., Xu, X., Chu, M.C. et al. (2014) Knowledge, attitudes, and practices regarding conception and fertility: A population-based survey among reproductive-age United States women. Fertility and Sterility, 101(3):767–774.e2.

McQuillan, J., Greli, A.L., Sheffler, K.M. (2011) Pregnancy intention among women who do not try: Focusing on women who are okay either way. Maternal and Child Health Journal, 15:178–87.

Moos, M.K., Dunlop, A.L., Jack, B.W., Nelson, L., Coonrod, D.V. et al. (2008) Healthier women, healthier reproductive outcomes: Recommendations for the routine care of all women of reproductive age. American Journal of Obstetrics and Gynecology, 199(6):S280–289.

Oregon Foundation for Reproductive Health (2011) OKQ pilot study.

Potter, J.E., Stevenson, A.J., Coleman-Minahan, K., Hopkins, K., White, K. et al. (2019) Challenging unintended pregnancy as an indicator of reproductive autonomy. Contraception, 100(1):1–4.

Shaw, J., Steegers, E., Verbiest, S. (Eds.) (2020) Preconception Health and Care: A life course approach. Switzerland: Springer Nature.

Sher, J. (2016) Missed periods: Scotland's opportunities for better pregnancies, healthier parents and thriving babies the first time … and every time. Available at: http://www.nhsggc.org.uk/media/237840/missed-periods-j-sher-,ay-2016.pdf <accessed 10 June, 2017>

Sher, J. (2021) Editorial: Making preconception health, education and care real. International Journal of Birth and Parent Education, 4(4):4–8.

Skogsdal, Y., Fadl, H., Cao, Y., Karlsson, J., Tydén, T. (2019) An intervention in contraceptive counseling increased the knowledge about fertility and awareness of preconception health: A randomized controlled trial. Upsala Journal of Medical Sciences, 124(3):203–212.

Song, B., Van Gompel, E., Stulberg, D., Guzman, S., Carlock, F. et al. (2021) Effects of clinic-level implementation of One Key Question® on reproductive health counseling and patient satisfaction. Contraception, 103(1):6–12.

Srinivasulu, S., Falletta, K.A., Bermudez, D., Almonte, Y., Baum, R. et al. (2019) Primary care providers' responses to pregnancy intention screening challenges: Community-based participatory research at an urban community health centre. Family Practice, 36(6):797–803.

Stephenson, J., Heslehurst, N., Hall, J., Schoenaker, D.A.J.M., Hutchinson, J. et al, (2018) Before the beginning: Nutrition and lifestyle in the preconception period and its importance for future health. Lancet, 391(10132):1830–1841.

Stulberg, D.B., Dahlquist, I.H., Disterhoft, J., Bello, J.K., Hunter, M.S. et al. (2019) Increase in contraceptive counseling by primary care clinicians after implementation of One Key Question® at an urban community health center. Maternal and Child Health Journal, 23:996–1002.

Stulberg, D.B., Datta, A., White VanGompel, E., Schueler, K., Rocca, C.H. (2020) One Key Question and the Desire to Avoid Pregnancy Scale: A comparison of two approaches to asking about pregnancy preferences. Contraception, 101(4):231–236.

Venator, J., Reeves, R. (2015) The implications of inequalities in contraception and abortion. Brookings Institution. Available at: https://www.brookings.edu/blog/social-mobility-memos/2015/02/26/the-implications-of-inequalities-in-contraception-and-abortion/<accessed 10 June, 2017>

Verbiest, S., Malin, C.K., Drummonds, M., Kotelchuck, M. (2016) Catalyzing a re-productive health and social justice movement. Maternal and Child Health Journal, 20(4):741–748.

# 4

# BREASTFEEDING PROMOTION IN EARLY LEARNING SETTINGS

*Elizabeth Smith, Sarah Edwards and Amy Bryson*

NHS Ayrshire and Arran is a health board in the west of Scotland where breastfeeding rates are amongst the lowest in Scotland. The authors work there and decided to apply for a grant to undertake a partnership project which would introduce breastfeeding to nursery children (age three to five years) and promote it to young people in school (age 5–18 years). The bid was successful and the project was carried out from September 2017 until June 2018. The focus of this chapter will be the Early Learning work with children aged three to five years.

*

Breastfeeding rates in Scotland remain lower than we would wish them to be and there is a clear social gradient; younger mothers and those living in the most deprived areas are less likely to breastfeed (NHS National Services – Information Services Division). This results in a widening of inequalities as vulnerable infants are further disadvantaged. Levels of breastfeeding at six months nationally do not meet the WHO target of 50%. Policy at national and international level has sought to address these issues, and there is good evidence that interventions can improve breastfeeding rates. However, innovations to shift public attitudes have been limited and the growth and reach of the breast-milk substitute industry undermine efforts to improve breastfeeding (Victora et al., 2016).

## Messages from Breastfeeding Research

Midwifery and health visiting teams are tasked with encouraging mothers to breastfeed and to provide or to signpost to local services for advice and support

DOI: 10.4324/9781003223771-5

to enable mothers to continue breastfeeding. Yet, there is evidence that some professionals feel they have little influence on mothers' choice of feeding method; they also report anxiety around the tension between breastfeeding promotion and coercion and about making mothers who formula feed feel guilty (Marks & O'Connor, 2015).

Bartle and Harvey (2017) asked first-time mothers at an antenatal clinic in South East England to complete a questionnaire rating:

- Their infant feeding experiences (especially formula feeding)
- Self-efficacy (personal confidence in being able to breastfeed)
- Attitude to breastfeeding
- Subjective norm (if close family and friends had chosen to breastfeed or to formula feed).

Analysis of the data suggested that mothers who had experience of seeing babies formula feeding were more likely to give up breastfeeding when they experienced problems, as they already had more positive attitudes towards formula feeding. These mothers were living in an embedded formula feeding culture; formula feeding was the social norm and therefore the easy choice.

The 2010 infant feeding survey (McAndrew et al., 2012) gave an insight into the importance of role models. The results for the UK reported that 26% of mothers who were surrounded by friends who were formula feeding stopped breastfeeding in the first two weeks compared to only 6% of mothers who were surrounded by friends who were mainly breastfeeding.

The Scottish Infant Feeding Survey, 2017 (The Scottish Government, 2018) reported that around a quarter of mothers had not breastfed in a particular venue as they believed breastfeeding would not be welcomed there. This is despite the legislation in place to support breastfeeding in public (Breastfeeding etc. (Scotland) Act, 2005). Scottish mothers were found to be much less likely to breastfeed in public than Swedish mothers, where breastfeeding in public is the social norm. Scott et al. (2015) found an association between perception of acceptability of public breastfeeding and breastfeeding practice; mothers with a negative attitude towards breastfeeding in public were more likely to stop breastfeeding earlier.

There is little research around the portrayal of breastfeeding in the media, but representation of breastfeeding could affect social norms if women were repeatedly exposed to positive images of breastfeeding. Yet, whilst infant feeding is often mentioned in women's magazines, formula feeding is portrayed more often than breastfeeding (O'Brien et al., 2017).

The available evidence therefore suggests that:

- Midwives and health visitors need societal support to promote and support breastfeeding.

- Experience of formula feeding (that of the mother and those close to her) is highly influential. If formula feeding is the mother's primary experience, positive attitudes to formula feeding are formed.
- If there are no family/friends who have experience and knowledge of breastfeeding, mothers are more likely to stop breastfeeding if they experience problems.
- Positive breastfeeding role models are important and prolong breastfeeding practice.
- Mothers are concerned about breastfeeding when out and about, feeling they will meet with disapproval if they breastfeed in public.
- Breastfeeding is not well represented in the media; formula feeding receives more representation.

## Aims of the Early Years Project

The vision for our advocacy work is that Scotland becomes a society which values breastfeeding and supports mothers so they can feed their baby in the way that is best for their family. We recognise that one important aspect is to change perceptions of breastfeeding by starting before attitudes around infant feeding are firmly developed, especially in areas where breastfeeding rates are low. We therefore planned to introduce the concept of breastfeeding to children as soon as they started in education (aged three years) and to continue to broaden knowledge as they progressed through primary and secondary school.

Our project was delivered in an area of North Ayrshire where breastfeeding rates are critically low, with only 17% of women exclusively breastfeeding at six to eight weeks compared to the Scottish average of 26.8%.

## How We Approached the Early Learning and Childcare Staff

The Community Infant Feeding Nurse and Breastfeeding Network (BfN) Peer Supporters worked in partnership, and relationships were established with two schools. The schools were enthusiastic about the pilot project and staff welcomed the idea of early intervention to promote healthy lifestyles, positive attachment and responsive parenting and decrease the obesity rate in the area. Our work around breastfeeding complemented an existing project in the Primary School and Early Years Centre looking at healthy weight for children and their parents.

## Content of the Session

The breastfeeding session devised for the Early Years children was based on 'How Mammals Feed Their Young'. It followed the style of learning used in Early

Years settings: Interactive, learning through play and not as structured sessions delivered for older children. Children were welcome to play at the table where the Peer Supporter sat with toy animals and a matching jigsaw of mammals and their young.

## How the Children Were Engaged

Children were engaged through the use of toys and animals, familiar items in the Early Years setting. The Peer Supporter facilitated conversations about mammals and how humans are mammals and have a lot in common with other mammals, including feeding our young with our milk. The Peer Supporter had a jigsaw available for the children that involved pairing mum and baby mammals. The Peer Supporter talked about how one of the factors that links mammals is that they all produce milk to feed their babies. With older nursery children, we extended this work by talking about the correct names for each mum and baby animal, for example a vixen and a cub for the fox pair. We also asked the question, 'Where do all the mum animals get the milk to feed their babies?' We often got the answer from the children that milk to feed the baby came 'from a cow'. All of these discussions were led by the children, so they were different discussions every time, but with the same aim of getting across that all female mammals make milk specifically for their babies and that human mums are just the same.

We also used interesting facts about each mammal to engage the children; for example whales' milk is thick like toothpaste so that the calf can get every last drop if it escapes into the water. We demonstrated this by having two glasses of water and inviting the children to put small amounts of cow's milk into one and small amounts of toothpaste into the other to see how each behaved in the water. We also talked about how bats can breastfeed their babies whilst flying, which seemed to interest the boys especially! The children also interacted with a baby doll and wanted to put the baby in the sling (like a mother kangaroo); this prompted conversations about the importance of caring for babies and responding to their needs.

## Feedback from Parents/Carers

Staff were initially concerned that parents/carers might not see breastfeeding as an appropriate topic to discuss with young children. To help with this, it was suggested that an information stall be set up in the reception area during pick-up and drop-off times at the Early Years Centre so that parents/carers could be informed about the content of the sessions and reassured of the importance of talking about infant feeding at an early age. All parents/carers were positive and supportive, with some asking for support with their own breastfeeding experiences from the Peer Supporters.

## Raising Staff's Awareness of Breastfeeding

We were also keen to work with staff so that the simple activities around infant feeding that we were using could be embedded within the Early Years setting once the project had finished. To help with this, the Peer Supporters delivered a short (one hour) breastfeeding awareness session, developed by the Breastfeeding Network, a charity offering support and information for breastfeeding families and others, called 'First Milk Matters'. This is designed to raise knowledge and awareness around breastfeeding and can be tailored to the specific audience.

We used the accredited IOWA Infant Feeding Attitudes Assessment Scale to measure the change in attitudes in staff before and after the session. This scale measures [maternal] attitudes towards infant feeding methods (e.g. breastfeeding, formula feeding). It includes questions about the costs of infant feeding, nutrition, convenience and infant bonding. We saw a shift to staff being more positive about breastfeeding. During the session, there were lots of opportunities for staff to share their experiences and thoughts around breastfeeding, if they wished, giving them a chance to debrief their own experiences. There were lots of discussions about how staff could introduce the topic of breastfeeding with the children. Staff identified a theme that they already covered each year (Spring and Baby Animals) that could easily be adapted to include a discussion about mammals feeding their babies without adding extra work for staff. Some staff said that after the training, they felt confident to start conversations about breastfeeding with children in the 'home corner' when they were role playing feeding a baby. They said that before the training, they wouldn't have known how to start such a conversation.

## Conclusions

The Scottish Government has provided increased funding for breastfeeding and included in this are national advocacy and culture change activities. Since our initial project, two new programmes are being developed: Breastfeeding Friendly Scotland Early Learning and Breastfeeding Friendly Scotland Schools schemes which will be delivered across Scotland. This will ensure that children are introduced to breastfeeding at age three to four years and that this information can be built on as our children and young people progress through primary and secondary school. The consequent increase in breastfeeding knowledge will contribute to normalisation of breastfeeding, formation of more positive attitudes towards breastfeeding and increased initiation rates in the next generation.

## Practice Pointers

- Engagement with Early Learning practitioners is important – offering education to enable them to understand why breastfeeding is important, what their role is in delivering the breastfeeding sessions and to feel confident in talking to children about breastfeeding.
- Engaging with parents and carers is important to ensure they feel comfortable about and understand the purpose of the breastfeeding sessions and how they are delivered.
- The sessions should be child led, play-based and age appropriate; resources such as books with images of breastfeeding can be useful for starting conversations.
- Using interesting facts about mammals and how they feed their young engages the children and helps them to see the biological normality of breastfeeding.
- Talking about breastfeeding babies can include, or lead to, important conversation about wider aspects of nurturing and caring for babies.

## Acknowledgement

The authors wish to acknowledge funding from the Queen's Nursing Institute Scotland Catalyst for Change Programme, which allowed this project to take place.

## References

Bartle, N.C., Harvey, K. (2017) Explaining infant feeding: The role of previous personal and vicarious experience on attitudes, subjective norms, self-efficacy, and breastfeeding outcomes. British Journal of Health Psychology, 22(4):763–785.

de la Mora, A., Russell, D.W., Dungy, C.I., Losch, M., Dusdieker, L. (1999) The Iowa infant feeding attitude scale: Analysis of reliability and validity. Journal of Applied Social Psychology, 29(11):2362–2380.

Marks, D., O'Connor, R. (2015) Health professionals' attitudes towards the promotion of breastfeeding. British Journal of Midwifery, 23(1):50–58.

McAndrew, F., Thompson, J., Fellows, L., Large, A., Speed, M. et al. (2012) Infant feeding survey 2010. NHS: The Information Centre. Available at: https://sp. ukdataservice.ac.uk/doc/7281/mrdoc/pdf/7281_ifs-uk-2010_report.pdf <accessed 06 November, 2019>

NHS National Services Scotland - Information Services Division. Available at: https:// www.isdscotland.org/ <accessed 06 November, 2019>

O'Brien, E., Myles, P., Pritchard, C. (2017) The portrayal of infant feeding in British women's magazines: A qualitative and quantitative content analysis. Journal of Public Health, 39(2):221–226.

Scott, J.A., Kwok, Y.Y., Synnott, K., Bogue, J., Amarri, S. et al. (2015) A comparison of maternal attitudes to breastfeeding in public and the association with breastfeeding duration in four European countries: Results of a cohort study. Birth: Issues in Perinatal Care, 42(1):78–85.

The Scottish Government. (2005) Breastfeeding etc. (Scotland) Act. Available at: http://www.legislation.gov.uk/asp/2005/1/contents <accessed 06 November, 2019>

The Scottish Government (2018) Scottish Maternal and Infant Nutrition Survey 2017. Available at: https://www.gov.scot/publications/scottish-maternal-infant-nutrition-survey-2017/ <accessed 06 November, 2019>

Victora, C.G., Bahl, R., Barros, A.J.D., França, G.V.A., Horton, S. et al. (2016) Breastfeeding in the 21st century: Epidemiology, mechanisms, and lifelong effect. The Lancet, 387(10017):475–490.

# PART II
# Building Parents' Relationship with Their Infants from Pregnancy Onwards

## Introduction

As educators – and everyone who is trained in caring for and supporting families with very young children *is* an educator – we can't change people's lives, but nor should we underestimate the impact that we can have. It's important to steer a path between hopelessness in the face of the immense challenges that confront parents-to-be and accepting responsibility for the influence that we can certainly exert, if we are skilled and sensitive, on the transition to parenthood.

Over the last three decades, it has become ever more clear that maternal stress in pregnancy profoundly impacts the unborn baby, and that its effect can last throughout childhood and perhaps beyond. Yet, the problems that some parents face today – poverty, lack of education, violence, natural and man-made disasters – are often intractable and require national and international action to address. One of the chapters in this section looks at the situation of mothers and their unborn and newborn children who are living in war zones or are refugees. We may feel helpless and that there is little we can do. Yet, this chapter explains how support from concerned professionals and lay people can help women access immense reservoirs of strength for coping.

This section also examines how mothers and fathers and carers can build positive relationships with their babies from pregnancy onwards. From the start – from the womb – babies are sociable creatures; they are driven to make connections with other humans, connections that ensure their safety and wellbeing. Pregnant women may be stressed, but they can be encouraged to take time out to relax and connect with their babies; they can be taught relaxation skills and can be reassured that relaxing isn't an indulgence – it's an act of love which impacts their unborn baby today and for years to come.

DOI: 10.4324/9781003223771-6

Families can also be helped to understand attachment and how babies' sense of themselves and their trust in their environment stem from the way in which they are responded to during the first critical months of life – and especially whether and how they are responded to when they are distressed. The myriad daily and weekly sensitive interventions on the part of parents when they comfort their babies lay the foundations for a secure attachment that will stand the baby in good stead for the rest of his life.

Attachment also depends on joyful interactions – when parents talk to their babies and when they sing to them, rock them, play music to them and dance with them. The importance of 'chatting', music and playing is discussed in this section. Fathers' playfulness is given equal attention with mothers' because maternal and paternal playfulness are both important and unique. Fathers play with their babies and toddlers in a way that offers different challenges and stimulation to very young children.

What is current understanding on the relationship between LGBTQ+ parents and their children? Evidence from the last 40 years is clear that positive attachment is just as common on the part of young children who have LGBTQ+ parents as in the case of children of heterosexual parents.

All very young children depend on their parents to help them manage their emotions because the ability to do so predicts the success of their future relationships. At the heart of perinatal education is the aim of supporting parents to understand that babies and toddlers are driven to make social connections. Sharing with parents ways in which they can respond to that drive is one of the privileges and joys of being a perinatal educator.

# 5

# STRESSED PRE-BIRTH? HOW THE FOETUS IS AFFECTED BY A MOTHER'S STATE OF MIND

*Graham Music*

Parenting is a sufficiently guilt-laden process these days, and it might seem harsh to add to this burden by focussing on the powerful psychobiological impact of a mother's emotional states on her unborn child. However, recent research findings have described a range of powerful effects of prenatal experiences, particularly stress, on the growing foetus, many of which last well into the life-course. Armed with this information, we can try to ensure that robust services and support structures are in place to minimise some of the worst risks to the developing foetus and the future child and adult.

⋆

The foetus is, of course, not just a passive victim of influences and is very much its own being, with its own rhythms, urges and biological expectations. Its arrival transforms the mother's body into an effective host, and once plugged into the uterine wall, it basically fiddles with its mother's control mechanisms, leading some to liken it to a cosmonaut in charge of a spacecraft. The foetus determines which way it will lie in pregnancy, the timing of the birth and which way it will present for the birth. It has feeling, responds to painful stimuli by turning away (Goodlin & Schmidt, 1972) and has demonstrated a surprisingly clear capacity for choice. Indeed, observations using ultrasounds of foetuses have shown clear personality traits developing (Piontelli, 1992), such as one of a pair of twins being outgoing, another less so, traits which continue postnatally.

At 20 weeks, neurons in the cortex are already firing in response to events (Moore et al., 2011). As early as 1937, experiments showed that after adding saccharin to the amniotic fluid, foetuses swallowed more, whereas foetal drinking rates crashed after the injection of bitter substances (Bradley & Mistretta, 1975).

DOI: 10.4324/9781003223771-7

The foetus can learn to get used to unsettling stimuli. For example, the first time it encounters a vibrating stimulus, it might move, but on subsequent occasions, it pays less attention (Ogo et al., 2019). By eight to ten weeks, it is moving its limbs and rather than being an inert cell collection blissfully bathing in amniotic fluid, it is active and responsive.

The foetus is nonetheless profoundly influenced by its milieu. A foetus responds to musical signals, moving in synchrony to a rhythm and even continuing moving after the music has stopped (Sallenbach, 1993). As early as the first trimester, the foetus will jump if touched by an amniocentesis needle, turn away from the light of a doctor's foetal stethoscope (Goodlin & Schmidt, 1972), and foetal heart rates increase when pregnant mothers smoke cigarettes. Foetuses have been shown to respond to stimuli such as loud noises by making facial expressions such as grimacing, pain and what looks like crying (Bellieni, 2019). Already we see a nature/nurture interaction; the foetus is its own being but also is being socialised. It learns to recognise sounds and words that it later prefers after birth (Music, 2016), while culturally influenced tastes and flavour preferences are also being learnt.

## Perfect Harmony?

A mother's state of mind influences the prenatal environment via the release of hormones. When a small acoustic/vibrational sound stimulus is administered, ultrasounds reveal that foetuses of depressed and non-depressed mothers react differently. Heart rates of the foetuses of depressed mothers are higher than the norm anyway, and after the stimulus, they can take 3.5 times as long to return to their normal baseline. Foetuses of non-depressed mothers react more responsively and also calm down more quickly (Dieter et al., 2001). This is uncannily like chronically anxious or stressed older children and adults who tend to recover more slowly from alarming stimuli. Field presented research (2006) which showed not only that foetal movement is higher when a mother is depressed, but also that a foetus moves differently *in utero* depending on the *form* of the mother's depression. The foetuses of mothers whose later, postnatal, depression resulted in a more intrusive rather than withdrawn maternal style were the foetuses which moved around less than those of mothers who had a more withdrawn form of depression.

## Where Does Parental Influence Start? The Meeting of Biology and Psychology

It is interesting to think about when parental mental states begin to influence a baby's future. A pregnant mother's state of mind is, we know, predictive of an infant's behaviours a year or more after birth. In a famous experiment undertaken by Howard and Miriam Steele (Fonagy et al., 1991), pregnant first-time mothers were given the Adult Attachment Interview which asks about parents' own childhood memories. Their interviews predicted with surprising accuracy the future attachment status of their as yet unborn child. Such interviews reveal less about a mother's actual childhood and more about her ability to reflect on her own emotional experiences. Typically, an adult who produces a coherent narrative and self-reflective story tends to have a child who at a year is classified as securely attached. Mothers whose stories are more chaotic or inconsistent, or who are emotionally cut-off, tend to have insecurely attached children. Thus, extraordinarily, the psychological capacities of a pregnant mother predict how her unborn child will react to stressful situations such as separation a year after birth. It is a mother's sensitivity to emotional life, her own and others', which seems to lead to this effect. Presumably, such findings imply continuity between a mother's states of mind during and after pregnancy.

However, prenatal experiences have lasting influences in themselves, irrespective of a mother's state of mind after birth. A well-known example comes from the Second World War in Holland where a cohort of mothers did not have enough food to eat; many were starving and even resorted to eating tulips (Lumey et al., 2007). The foetuses of the starving mothers grew into children and adults with 'thrifty' metabolisms which stored more fat despite the food shortage disappearing after birth. Indeed, if nutrition is uncertain, the foetus 'decides' whether it needs to store more fat, adjusting the balance of blood flow to the liver and the brain accordingly. This kind of research describes what is called 'foetal programming', whereby unborn babies learn lessons to prepare for life later. In this case, such thrifty metabolisms led to difficulties such as heart disease and diabetes, as well as higher rates of psychiatric illness, in many of the starved babies who grew into adults living in a more plentiful world.

An extreme form of this might be seen from studies of pregnant women exposed to trauma where the stress has a profound effect. Women who happened to be present at the World Trade Center on 9/11, who later showed post-traumatic stress symptoms, also had children with altered stress responses and cortisol levels (Bowers & Yehuda, 2018). Being close to a hurricane in pregnancy hugely increases stress responses, as well as the likelihood of serious effects for the baby such as being on a ventilator or meconium aspiration syndrome after birth (Currie & Rossin-Slater, 2013), while exposure to stressors such as a rocket attack may lead to increased spontaneous abortions (Wainstock et al., 2013).

Obviously, there is little we can do in the face of huge unexpected calamities, but there are lessons to be learnt from them about the toxic effects of stress. Indeed, even stress preconception has been shown to have an effect on the developing foetus (Cissé et al., 2020). Generally, the social causes of stress, such as poverty or interpersonal trauma, are the most prevalent, and maternal stress levels might be best seen as the downstream effects of social, political, economic and cultural issues which are best tackled at a societal level, alongside offering increased support during pregnancy.

## Low Birth Weight

Low birth weight is often linked with prenatal stress and is also a predictor of illness decades later. Records of over 13,000 men born in Yorkshire showed that those with lower birth weight were more likely to suffer from conditions such as strokes, diabetes and heart disease as far ahead as 50 years of age (Barker et al., 2001). Indeed, if born less than 5.5 pounds, they had a 50% higher chance of developing heart disease, even accounting for socioeconomic circumstances.

In fact, birth weight often has psychological as well as physiological elements. There is consistent evidence that high stress levels in pregnancy increase the likelihood of birth complications and low birth weight and are linked with compromised immune functioning in the newborn (Denney et al., 2021). Cortisol, the best-known stress hormone, crosses the placental wall and affects the foetus, and there are correlations between maternal and foetal cortisol levels (Glover, 2020). When a mother becomes fearful, her heartbeat alters, often leading to reduced oxygen flow to the foetus, speeding up its heart rate and reducing nutrient flow. Mothers with bipolar disorder are far more likely for example to have premature and/or low birth-weight babies, irrespective of whether they are being treated (Bodén et al., 2012). Similarly, depressed mothers also tend to have smaller babies (El Marroun et al., 2012).

Low birth weight (less than 5.5 lbs) predicts a host of adult psychological problems from depression to mood disorders (Orri et al., 2021). Aggression and other behavioural problems are also more likely in low birth-weight children, and here the mediating factor seems to be poorer language skills (Vaske et al., 2012). We know that the size of a newborn's placenta is predictive of mental problems up until adolescence (Khalife et al., 2012), while the brains of adolescents born very prematurely tend to show a whole range of abnormalities (Taylor et al., 2011).

## Lasting Effects, Social Effects

Prenatal stress affects not only birth weight but also stress levels after birth. Severe antenatal stress affects hormones that regulate mood, such as dopamine and serotonin, and is linked to a range of childhood emotional and behavioural problems such as Attention-Deficit/Hyperactivity Disorder (ADHD). Such links hold firm after screening out factors such as gender, parental educational level, smoking in pregnancy, birth weight and postnatal maternal anxiety (Van den Bergh et al., 2007).

A big question is why we should see such profound effects. Many of the most rigorous researchers argue for an evolutionary perspective. Glover (2011) suggests that it makes sense to be more vigilant, hard to soothe and jumpy if the likelihood is that one will be born into a stressful or scary environment in which one has to be wary. Belsky suggests that our bodies 'choose' a different life-course, either a faster more stressful one or a slower more relaxed one, depending on the kinds of stressors we encounter as early as prenatal life (Pluess & Belsky, 2011). Stress hormones are in effect programming the developing foetus for later life.

Stress responses in the newborn might increase the likelihood of survival but they also have serious health consequences. Our immune systems are badly compromised by stress, and people exposed to high levels of prenatal stress tend to have premature cell ageing, or in other words, they get old faster. We are increasingly learning how such stressful experiences have profound effects at a cellular and indeed a genetic level. Adolescents of women exposed to violence in pregnancy have, for example, been found to have altered expression of genes central to behaviour and emotional regulation (Radtke et al., 2011). Women with high blood pressure and other signs of prenatal stress have children with less cognitive capacity in old age (Grainger et al., 2020).

Some stress can derive from one-off rather than chronic experiences, such as a mother experiencing bereavement during pregnancy. In such cases, if good support is available, the impact on the infant will be lessened by other more positive influences. More tragic are over-determined causative factors such as a highly stressed mother born into poverty, who is the victim of violence, and has little social support. She might be more likely to have a low birth-weight baby and have birth complications, which can lead to difficulties in bonding. If one then adds the likelihood of intrusive medical attention, a decreased likelihood of breastfeeding, less attuned interactions with the baby, poor housing and little support, then the baby's life chances exponentially worsen.

## Summary

On no account can stressed mothers be blamed for the physical and emotional health of their offspring. The research cited above takes us far beyond the responsibilities of the individual mother. Stress, anxiety, depression and other psychological issues are more likely in women who are socially and economically marginalised in an unequal society (Wilkinson, 2005).

Maternal stress and anxiety not only influence birth weight, but may be precipitating factors for birth complications and prematurity. High stress levels can alter the foetus' brain structure and functioning and contribute to later mood and anxiety disorders. Low birth-weight babies born to very anxious mothers are likely to have higher cortisol levels throughout their lifespan and a permanently altered stress response system. Adults who at birth are of low birth weight are more susceptible to the physiological effects of stress caused by factors such as poverty and unemployment (Barker et al., 2001).

Emotional support for mothers makes pregnancy and birth easier. Given the importance of psychological wellbeing from the very beginning of the lifecycle, research to date strongly supports the case for providing practical, psychological and social support for all pregnant mothers and especially those who are living with multiple challenges in their lives.

## Practice Pointers

- Develop a sensitivity to spotting potential depression or other stressors in the pregnant mother and learn to ask the right questions.
- Ensure services offer support before a baby is born, to the mother, a father if one is there and any other key family members.
- If possible, do informal or formal screening for potential issues such as anxiety, depression, major stress.
- Keep a close but sympathetic eye out for the use of substances in pregnancy, especially alcohol, but also recreational and prescription drugs.

## References

Barker, D.J.P., Forsén, T., Uutela, A., Osmond, C., Eriksson, J.G. (2001) Size at birth and resilience to effects of poor living conditions in adult life: A longitudinal study. British Medical Journal, 323(7324):1261–1262.

Bellieni, C.V. (2019) New insights into fetal pain. Seminars in Fetal and Neonatal Medicine, 24(4):101001.

Bodén, R., Lundgren, M., Brandt, L., Reutfors, J., Andersen, M. et al. (2012) Risks of adverse pregnancy and birth outcomes in women treated or not treated with mood stabilisers for bipolar disorder: Population based cohort study. British Medical Journal, 345:e7085.

Bowers, M.E., Yehuda, R. (2018) Intergenerational transfer of biological responses to trauma: Impact of psychosocial stress in fathers on offspring. In: Burggren, W., Dubansky, B. (Eds.) Development and Environment. Cham: Springer International Publishing: 421–433.

Bradley, R.M., Mistretta, C.M. (1975) Fetal sensory receptors. Psychological Reviews, 55(3):352–382.

Cissé, Y.M., Chan, J.C., Nugent, B.M., Banducci, C., Bale, T.L. (2020) Brain and placental transcriptional responses as a readout of maternal and paternal preconception stress are fetal sex specific. Placenta, 100:164–170.

Currie, J. Rossin-Slater, M. (2013) Weathering the storm: Hurricanes and birth outcomes. Journal of Health Economics, 32(3):487–503.

Denney, J.M., Nelson, E., Wadhwa, P., Waters, T., Mathew, L. et al. (2021) Cytokine profiling: Variation in immune modulation with preterm birth vs. uncomplicated term birth identifies pivotal signals in pathogenesis of preterm birth. Journal of Perinatal Medicine, 49(3):299–309.

Dieter, J.N.I., Field, T., Hernandez-Reif, M., Jones, N.A., Lecanuet, J.P. et al. (2001) Maternal depression and increased fetal activity. Journal of Obstetrics and Gynaecology, 21(5):468–473.

El Marroun, H., Jaddoe, V.W.V., Hudziak, J.J., Roza, S.J., Steegers, E.A.P. et al. (2012) Maternal use of selective serotonin reuptake inhibitors, fetal growth, and risk of adverse birth outcomes. Archives of General Psychiatry, 69(7):706–714.

Field, T., Diego, M., Hernandez-Reif, M. (2006) Prenatal depression effects on the fetus and newborn: A review. Infant Behavior and Development, 29(3):445–455.

Fonagy, P., Steele, H., Steele, M. (1991) Maternal representations of attachment during pregnancy predict the organization of infant-mother attachment at one year of age. Child Development, 62(5):891–905.

Glover, V. (2011) Annual Research Review: Prenatal stress and the origins of psychopathology - An evolutionary perspective. Journal of Child Psychology and Psychiatry, 52(4):356–367.

Glover, V. (2020) Prenatal mental health and the effects of stress on the foetus and the child. Should psychiatrists look beyond mental disorders? World Psychiatry, 19(3):331.

Goodlin, R., Schmidt, W. (1972) Human fetal arousal levels as indicated by heart rate recordings. American Journal of Obstetrics and Gynecology, 114(5):613–621.

Grainger, S.A., Crawford, J.D., Kochan, N.A., Mather, K.A., Chander, R.J. et al. (2020) An investigation into early-life stress and cognitive function in older age. International Psychogeriatrics, 32(11):1325–1329.

Khalife, N., Glover, V., Hartikainen, A-L., Taanila, A., Ebeling, H. et al. (2012) Placental size is associated with mental health in children and adolescents. PLoS One, 7(7):e40534.

Lumey, L.H., Stein, A.D., Kahn, H.S., van der Pal-de-bRuin, K.M., Blauw, G.J. et al. (2007) Cohort profile: The Dutch Hunger Winter families study. International Journal of Epidemiology, 36(6):1196–1204.

Moore, A.R., Zhou, W-L., Jakovcevski, I., Zecevic, N., Antic, S.D. (2011) Spontaneous electrical activity in the human fetal cortex in vitro. The Journal of Neuroscience, 31(7):2391–2398.

Music, G. (2016) Nurturing Natures: Attachment and children's emotional, social and brain development. London: Psychology Press.

Ogo, K., Kanenishi, K., Mori, N., AboEllail, M.A.M., Hata, T. (2019) Change in fetal behavior in response to vibroacoustic stimulation. Journal of Perinatal Medicine, 47(5):558–563.

Orri, M., Pingault, J-B., Turecki, G., Nuyt, A.-M., Tremblay, R.E. et al. (2021) Contribution of birth weight to mental health, cognitive, and socioeconomic outcomes: A two-sample Mendelian randomisation. British Journal of Psychiatry Open, 7 (S1):S44–S45.

Piontelli, A. (1992) From Fetus to Child: An observational and psychoanalytic study. London: Tavistock Publications.

Pluess, M., Belsky, J. (2011) Prenatal programming of postnatal plasticity? Development and Psychopathology, 23(01):29–38.

Radtke, K.M. et al. (2011) Transgenerational impact of intimate partner violence on methylation in the promoter of the glucocorticoid receptor. Translational Psychiatry, 1:e21. doi.org/10.1038/tp.2011.21.

Sallenbach, W.B. (1993) The intelligent prenate: Paradigms in prenatal learning and bonding. In: Blum, T.P. (Ed.) Prenatal Perception, Learning, and Bonding: Learning and bonding. Hong Kong: Leonardo: 61–106.

Taylor, H.G., Filipek, P.A., Juranek, J., Bangert, B., Minich, N. et al. (2011) Brain volumes in adolescents with very low birth weight: Effects on brain structure and associations with neuropsychological outcomes. Developmental Neuropsychology, 36(1):96–117.

Van den Bergh, B.R.H., Van Calster, B., Smits, T., Van Huffel, S., Lagae, L. (2007) Antenatal maternal anxiety is related to HPA-axis dysregulation and self-reported depressive symptoms in adolescence: A prospective study on the fetal origins of depressed mood. Neuropsychopharmacology, 33(3):536–545.

Vaske, J., Newsome, J., Boisvert, D. (2012) The mediating effects of verbal skills in the relationship between low birth weight and childhood aggressive behaviour. Infant and Child Development, 22(3):235–249.

Wainstock, T., Lerner-Geva, L., Glasser, S., Shoham-Vardi, I., Anteby, E.Y. (2013) Prenatal stress and risk of spontaneous abortion. Psychosomatic Medicine, 75(3):228–235.

Wilkinson, R. (2005) The Impact of Inequality: How to make sick societies healthier. London: Routledge.

# 6

# COMMENTARY

## Motherhood in Conditions of War – Biological and Psychosocial Routes to Infant Development

*Raija-Leena Punamäki*

Becoming a parent means a fundamental psychosocial reorganization of identities, roles, and preferences. These transformations happen in parallel with physiological, neuroendocrinological, and hormonal changes, thus together critically influencing mother and infant wellbeing. Research confirms that high maternal prenatal stress, as well as severe depression and anxiety, increases the risks for children's emotional and cognitive problems and future somatic and mental health disorders both in peaceful countries (Bergman et al., 2010; O'Donnell et al., 2014) and in war conditions (Glover et al., 2018; Punamäki et al., 2017a). Concerning fetal development, the cumulative stress model posits that maternal prenatal trauma produces a set of complex responses within the fetal neural circuitry of the brain and regulatory neuroendocrine pathways, interfering with optimal fetal growth and functioning (Glover, 2011). Evolutionary theories in turn posit that these neuroendocrinological alterations in fetal environment indicate adaptive preparation to fit the future dangerous postnatal environment (Del Giudice et al., 2011).

### Trauma and the Dyadic Relationship

Mothers create attachment to their future baby in pregnancy as the maternal caring system is activated (Laxton-Kane & Slade, 2002). War trauma with its life threats and losses can severely tax mothers' resources to care for the fetus and infant, as worry over survival interferes with optimal creation of early attachment.

During the first year of life, parents help infants regulate stress and overstimulation by aptly responding to their needs and arousal states. Dyadic regulation happens in day-to-day interactions where infants create inner models,

DOI: 10.4324/9781003223771-8

learn coping strategies, and experience physiological responses to both joy and distress (Beeghly et al., 2011). The quality of the mother–infant interaction is thus crucial in conditions of war or as refugees where challenges to emotional attunement owing to coping with fear and facing death are overwhelming. Interview studies have shown that Israeli mothers exposed to war trauma in pregnancy perceived themselves as damaged and inadequate because they could not provide safety for their infants and were overwhelmed by feelings of guilt. Giving birth evoked intrusive and horrific memories of traumatic scenes and made mothers feel helpless and fearful (Levy, 2006). Research among refugees has shown that mothers with post-traumatic stress disorder (PTSD) symptoms were more insensitive and hostile toward their infants and less able to structure encounters with them; in turn, their infants showed dysfunctional stress regulation and were less responsive and involved in dyadic interaction (Van Ee et al., 2012). Yet, importantly, another study has shown that maternal exposure to severe war trauma is associated with poor quality of mother–infant interaction *only* when there has been problematic maternal–fetal attachment, mental health difficulties, and lack of social support (Punamäki et al., 2017b).

## Maternal Resilience and War Trauma

Tailoring interventions to help mothers and infants in war conditions and who are refugees should focus on specific trauma impacts during pregnancy and infancy and on their biological and psychosocial underlying mechanisms. Pregnancy activates mothers' own attachment memories and is a period of unique openness to exploring strengths and vulnerabilities. Therapeutic tools involve alleviating maternal anxiety and distress, encouraging balanced fetal attachment, and facilitating preparation for labor and caregiving. In infancy, psychological help focuses on forming safe and sensitive close dyadic relationships, despite external dangers. The infant's neediness, crying, and distress may reactivate the mother's own trauma-related feelings of helplessness, and this should be considered in treatment. Psychosocial support is crucial for families in both the pre- and postnatal periods in order to prevent negative war impacts and promote resilience.

Pregnant women and mothers in war conditions also show great resourcefulness and mental openess. Their fundamental motivation relates to protecting, caring for, and investing in their infant's and whole family's safety. Although studies have focused on the negative and morally unsustainable impact of war trauma on dyadic wellbeing, nonetheless both biological and psychosocial theories emphasize human resilience, adaptation, survival skills, and capacity for mental thriving and growth (Beeghly et al., 2011; Cicchetti, 2015). Mothers aim to make sense of and construct meanings for their painful experiences in order to cherish self-worth and achieve psychological integration. These attempts reflect posttraumatic growth that involves gratitude for surviving, deepened appreciation of life, higher social affiliation, and spiritual, ideological, and philosophical enlightenment (Tedeschi & Calhoun, 2008). In a study by Diab et al. (2018), traumatic war events did not increase dysfunctional emotion regulation among infants whose mothers showed high cognitive resources (meaning making) and did not increase mothers' PTSD or dissociation symptoms if they showed posttraumatic growth. Learning about these protective factors among war-affected mothers and their infants is pivotal when tailoring effective help for them.

## Conclusion

International reports estimate that 29 million babies are born annually in life-endangering conditions of war, and 65 million war-affected people live as refugees, a third of them children under five (UN High Commissioner for Refugees, 2016; UNICEF, 2021). War trauma involves human and material losses, witnessing atrocities, and threats to life. Pregnant women, mothers, and infants are highly vulnerable because trauma impacts their wellbeing through multiple biological and psychosocial routes. Therefore, comprehensive preventive and treatment actions should be tailored for war-affected mothers and infants to prevent both pre- and postnatal harm.

## References

Beeghly, M., Fuertes, M., Liu, C. H., Delonis, M.S., Tronick, E. (2011) Maternal sensitivity in dyadic context: Mutual regulation, meaning-making, and reparation. In: Davis, D.W., Logsdon, M.C. (Eds.) Maternal Sensitivity: A scientific foundation for practice. New York: Nova Science Publishers: 45–69.

Bergman, K., Sarkar, P., Glover, V., O'Connor, T. G. (2010) Maternal prenatal cortisol and infant cognitive development: Moderation by infant-mother attachment. Biological Psychiatry, 67(11):1026–1032.

Cicchetti, D. (2015) Preventive intervention efficacy, development, and neural plasticity. Journal of American Academy of Child and Adolescence Psychiatry, 54(2):83–85.

Diab, S.Y., Isosävi, S., Qouta, S.R., Kuittinen, S., Punamäki, R.L. (2018) The protective role of maternal posttraumatic growth and cognitive trauma processing among Palestinian mothers and infants. Infant Behavior and Development, 50:284–299.

Del Giudice, M., Ellis, B.J., Shirtcliff, E.A. (2011) The adaptive calibration model of stress responsivity. Neuroscience & Biobehavioral Reviews, 35(7):1562–1592.

Glover, V. (2011) Annual research review: Prenatal stress and the origins of psychopathology: An evolutionary perspective. Journal of Child Psychology & Psychiatry, 52(4):356–367.

Glover, V., O'Donnell, K. J., O'Connor, T. G., Fisher, J. (2018) Prenatal maternal stress, fetal programming, and mechanisms underlying later psychopathology - A global perspective. Development and Psychopathology, 30(3):843–854.

Laxton-Kane, M., Slade, P. (2002) The role of maternal prenatal attachment in a woman's experience of pregnancy and implications for the process of care. Journal of Reproductive and Infant Psychology, 20(4):253–266.

Levy, M. (2006) Maternity in the wake of terrorism: Rebirth or retraumatization? Journal of Prenatal and Perinatal Psychology and Health, 20(3):221–248.

O'Donnell, K.J., Glover, V., Barker, E.D., O'Connor, T.G. (2014) The persisting effect of maternal mood in pregnancy on childhood psychopathology. Developmental Psychopathology, 26(2): 393–403.

Punamäki, R.L. Diab, S.Y., Isosävi, S., Kuittinen, S., Qouta, S.R. (2017a) Maternal pre- and postnatal mental health and infant wellbeing in conditions of war and military violence: The Gaza Infant Study. Psychological Trauma: Theory, Research, Practice, and Policy, 10(2): 144–153.

Punamäki, R.L. Isosävi, S., Qouta, S.R., Kuittinen, S., Diab, S.Y. (2017b) War trauma and maternal-fetal attachment predicting maternal mental health, infant development and dyadic interaction in Palestinian families. Attachment and Human Development, 18(4):391–417.

Tedeschi, R.G., Calhoun, L.G. (2008) Beyond the concept of recovery: Growth and the experience of loss. Death Studies, 32(1):27–39.

UN High Commissioner for Refugees (2016) Global Trends: Forced displacement in 2016. Available at: https://www.unhcr.org/statistics/unhcrstats/5943e8a34/global-trends-forced-displacement-2016.html <accessed 08 January, 2022>

UNICEF (2021) 29 million babies born into conflict in 2018 (Press Release). Available at: https://www.unicef.org/press-releases/29-million-babies-born-conflict-2018 <accessed 08 January, 2022>

van Ee, E., Kleber, R.J., Mooren, T. (2012) War trauma lingers on: Associations between maternal posttraumatic stress disorder, parent–child interaction, and child development. Infant Mental Health Journal, 33(5):459–468.

# 7

# ATTACHMENT

## A Play of Closeness and Distance

*Robin Balbernie*

All mammals inherit a motivational system that ensures that any perception of threat triggers firstly anxiety and then a sequence of search and approach behaviours in the very young in order to increase safety through nearness to a parent. Attachment theory is important as it provides a language that can be used to think about relationships, and relationships are central to human development and happiness.

*

There is more to attachment than initially meets the eye. Attachment starts from being a matter of closeness and protection. In humans, though, physical closeness coincides with mental closeness which in turn leads to language and personality development, making this synergistic evolutionary programming a power source for a wide swathe of human attributes and achievements. 'Our most distinctive and important human abilities – our capacities for learning, invention, and innovation, and for tradition, culture, and morality – are rooted in relationships between parents and children' (Gopnik, 2016:22). A major selective advantage that attachment conferred on homo sapiens was 'the opportunity it afforded for the development of social intelligence and meaning-making' (Fonagy et al., 2002:124) and thus the creation of culture that functions as a collective memory. Attachment dynamics have a far wider remit in humans than any other species. Just as the basic biological dynamic of attachment is behind wider aspects of personal and social awareness, so does attachment theory and research draw upon and lead into many different disciplines. Staying close to the one you love is the beginning of a lot of possibilities.

DOI: 10.4324/9781003223771-9

## The Scope and Purpose of Attachment in Humans

Bowlby defined attachment as 'any form of behaviour that results in a person attaining or maintaining a proximity to some other clearly identified individual, who is conceived as better able to cope with the world' (Bowlby, 1988:26). This nearness to a protective figure is the key to attachment; but in humans, with the ability to be self-reflective, this proximity implies an intersubjective overlap between child and parent with each party (in optimal circumstances) eventually having an awareness of just how important this relationship is for both. Early positive relationships get the infant off to a good start.

> When we have secure attachment to loving others, we are granted a lifelong gift. When attachment processes are impaired, the diverse manifestations of psychic pain within the higher mental apparatus can lead to chronic feelings of distress throughout life. This distress often encumbers the way in which we can relate to others.
>
> *(Panksepp & Biven, 2012:345)*

From the small child's point of view, the purpose of an attachment figure is to provide a sense of felt security, fulfil the role of a safe haven to return to in times of fear, and a secure base that holds the emotional supplies needed to set out and explore the world. This does not imply a single security figure; a cluster of kin-related caregivers was once the human norm (Hrdy, 2009), and the loss of support from the extended family is something practitioners meet every day.

Attachment behaviour is observed when the child is worried; most of the time, the attachment system should lie dormant until activated by threat. When attachment behaviour has not been switched on, the exploratory system remains online and children can leave parents and check out their wider environment through investigation, mischief, and play. This is how children develop cognitive flexibility and maintain curiosity, the foundations for many later achievements. Insecurity puts the brakes on.

The function of attachment behaviour is to ensure that the infant first of all remains safe by being protected and nurtured by his or her parents, leading to genetic survival. Next, as development proceeds, this automatic pull into the immediate group ensures that the growing child becomes dynamically embedded within those significant family relationships that structure both the internal and interpersonal worlds, and after that into their particular wider society.

> From all we know, every primate baby is designed to be physically attached to someone who will feed, protect, and care for it, and teach it about being human – they have been adapted over millions of years to expect nothing less.
>
> *(Small, 1998:40)*

We are an altricial species with an extended juvenile period of vulnerability and helplessness, so the early attachment dynamics have a protracted influence.

> Human infants have a profoundly undeveloped brain. Maintaining proximity to their caregivers is essential both for survival and for allowing their brains to use the mature states of the attachment figure to help them organize their own mental functioning.

> *(Siegel, 1999:149)*

The growing child's mind is sculpted by these close relationships, psychologically and neurologically, as she adapts to the family's emotional environment.

## The Move from Watching to Listening

Attachment theory has its own vocabulary derived from a number of seminal studies; this is no more than a coded communication of expertise, although to begin with it may be a bit off-putting. Following the creation by Ainsworth and colleagues (1978) of a laboratory method for differentiating distinct patterns of attachment, called the Strange Situation Procedure, attachment behaviour was initially split into three observable patterns. The Strange Situation is a graded series of separations and reunions between caregiver (usually the mother) and toddler with the occasional presence and departure of a stranger. This standardised paradigm demonstrates within a comparatively short period of time how small children expect and accept comfort as well as their preferred strategy for regulating their own emotions, with or without the help of their caregiver, when under mild stress. The majority of children (about 65%) demonstrate secure attachment, to be contrasted with anxious-avoidant, anxious-resistant (or ambivalent) and, a later conceptualisation, disorganised patterns of attachment. All children need access to someone more competent, and they automatically adapt to the quality of care available. The Strange Situation reveals a child's particular stratagem, not a quantified score, and each attachment pattern is fit for purpose. These are descriptions not diagnoses or value-judgements.

   A pattern of attachment behaviour can be thought of as a cluster of goal-directed activity whose aim is to maintain the best available emotional and physical connection, as the child sees it, with the caregiver. These are strategies for enlisting the caregiver in the service of alleviating stress; with the disorganised being the least successful, leaving the child trapped in a state of constant stress and high alert. The secure infant explores freely and seeks contact with the attachment figure as necessary. Avoidant infants de-activate attachment behaviour and repress emotional awareness (but still register anxiety physiologically) while focusing on exploration. They monitor and maintain proximity to the attachment figure, but do not express attachment needs in order to avoid risking rejection. Resistant children are preoccupied with the availability of an inconsistent caregiver, making repeated exaggerated demands to ensure that at least some elicit attention. They have hyperactivated their attachment system in their unsureness about a consistent calming response. The disorganised child struggles in survival mode, attempting to create safety rather than finding it on offer while adapting to stress and unsafety on a psychological and neurological level. Without intervention, this may prove a disadvantage in the future. Disorganised attachment does not invariably stem from maltreatment, as some assume, nor is it always a reason to remove a child from their family (Granqvist, et al., 2017); it is always a reason to offer help.

The different attachment patterns, once in place, demonstrate the child's 'chosen' method of emotional control created by a process of responding within the family's relationship-based environment. The different categories of attachment behaviour do not just help the child acclimatise to immediate parenting, they also give them the skills for negotiating their likely future in so far as 'patterns of attachment represent nascent facultative reproductive strategies that evolved to promote reproductive fitness in particular reproductive niches' (Belsky, 1999:150). Thus, a rough infancy leads to a rough adult. Such software of intimacy can be long lasting, as shown by a longitudinal study of high-risk infants where infant security was 'associated with the observed quality of participants' romantic relationships in young adulthood' (Roisman et al., 2005).

Although it is fair to state that secure attachment is the most auspicious, insecure attachment is not a form of psychopathology and, apart from disorganised attachment, cannot be assumed to indicate a severe emotional disturbance, although it may well be an emotional disadvantage in later life. Attachment is a quality of a relationship; it is created by two people, so if the relationship changes then (especially if early enough) so will the quality of attachment. What is called 'attachment disorder' is relatively rare – only found in extreme cases such as early institutionalisation (and not always then). Also, although secure attachment is an emotional asset, it does not invariably confer psychological immunity. There is a danger that the findings of attachment research can be hijacked in a naïve way and used to rationalise draconian 'therapy' or even unnecessary removal of a child from their primary caregiver – a traumatic experience even when this is an abusive relationship, as strength and quality of attachment are not the same thing.

The patterns of behaviour associated with the different categories of insecure attachment are only maladaptive outside of the relational context in which they were constructed. These are unconscious ruses for achieving the best version of felt security that is available within a particular family context. However, all forms of insecure attachment can be viewed as risk factors that may have an adverse effect on development when combined with other stresses, or outright traumas, that may be encountered in the course of life.

## The Influence of Early Experiences

In order to explain how interpersonal experience could become a mental construct that then stamps its mark on future relationships and development in general, Bowlby utilised the concept of internal working models, unconscious structures within procedural (implicit) memory whose function is 'to transmit, store and manipulate information that helps in making predictions as to how set goals can be achieved' (Bowlby, 1969:111). If Bowlby were writing today, the analogy of computer software might be appealing. These dynamic representations function within close relationships as an anticipatory and interpretive framework that takes the strain out of everyday interactions while at the same time modulating the experience and expression of emotional states.

Internal working models are as much a product of the pressures of evolution as is basic attachment behaviour and are an example of categorical thinking held in procedural memory. The ability to respond to a new situation on the basis that it roughly fits a pre-constructed class of experience saves a vast amount of mental effort; the alternative would involve having to puzzle out every surprise anew – by which time 'the surprise' would probably have eaten or bopped you. The human brain is an anticipatory instrument. Internal working models carry information on how close relationships will be handled and what will be expected of them; they are not a blueprint that can never be deviated from so that all subsequent relationships are fated to be a facsimile of some prototype. Secure attachment confers the most adaptability (resilience or flexible emotional regulation), and this lessens with each increase in insecurity.

A dramatic example of an internal working model that must have remained dormant in procedural memory concerns a young mother urgently referred to me by her health visitor just after the birth of her baby. She was having fantasies of harming her baby, avoided handling him and was getting very frightened of her own impulses whenever the baby cried. After a few home visits, the tension lessened so we could begin to think about a possible 'ghost in the nursery'. I suggested that we ask her mother to tell us about her babyhood to see if there were any clues to the current difficulties. It turned out that she had not been held for over two weeks after she was born. This information began the improvement in the relationship between her and her baby (although there were other issues that needed addressing). She realised that her negative feelings were both a consequence and an 'explanation' of a pattern of behaviour she was trapped within. On a follow up nearly three years later, mother and baby were fine.

## Emotional Health from the Outside In

Attachment research has examined the influence of early parenting on both current and later development.

The patterning or organisation of attachment relationships during infancy is associated with characteristic processes of emotional regulation, social relatedness, access to autobiographical memory, and the development of self-reflection and narrative.

*(Siegel, 1999:67)*

A child has a sense of confidence and self-esteem derived from internal (felt) security, if, when he was an infant, his parents appreciated how he felt and responded appropriately in a way that communicated a sense of being understood and thus held or contained in a safe way. The development of secure attachment depends more upon parental attitudes, empathy, and self-awareness than on any catalogue of 'correct' parenting techniques. Internal working models of relationships are built upon the general quality of day-to-day emotional contact with all its usual ups and downs – certainly not on short bursts of 'quality time'.

The foundations of a later secure attachment are laid down by an atmosphere of sensitive and appropriately responsive parenting in the first six months of life.

Emotional regulation is accomplished through built-in regulatory capacities of the infant and a responsive caregiving environment. The caregiver reads the infant's signs of distress and other affective communications, imbues them with meaning, and responds to them – dyadic regulation being accomplished without intentionality on behalf of the infant.

*(Sroufe, 1995:172)*

It takes two to tango at the beginning of life, and this is a dance babies are eager to join once they feel felt by their parents and become held in mind. The newborn will pull the parent in by mimicking facial expressions and even simple hand gestures, and in return, the sensitive parent responds as if the baby had intentionality. Babies from the start are active promoters of their own point of view since, as Trevarthen (1980:336) stresses, 'they also possess rudimentary personal powers that affect their caregivers intimately so that within a short time of birth, a subtle infant-caretaker relationship is established'. Mothers are uniquely placed and motivated to encourage and pick up on their baby's first communication, and the baby is born already acclimatised to the interesting mother.

Intrinsically prompted developments have profound effects on the behavior of an affectionate, firmly 'attached' parent, binding him or her to the life experiences of the child. The child 'educates' the adult how to discover meanings that make sense and bring joy to both of them.

*(Trevarthen, 2005:61)*

These proto conversations based on mutual adoration have a 'serve and respond' rhythm and structure when they are going well. It does not have to be anyway near perfect; recognising and sorting a glitch is what counts.

## Conclusion

Attachment theory has become an important paradigm that integrates many branches of social and biological science with the insights of psychoanalysis. It is no longer easy to ignore just how important relationships are throughout life, especially during the first few years when the unconscious foundations of our emotional responses are put in place. An attachment perspective on individual development, backed up by data from research, confirms how the events that occur between very young children and their caregivers in the context of intimate family life can have a lifelong influence. The secure child is naturally confident and socially responsible, able to get along with others while appreciating their feelings and point of view, and is generally busy checking out what the world has to offer and learning through play; the insecure child, on the other hand, misses out here and may as an adult struggle with relationships – including with their own children in turn.

## Practice Pointers

- Attachment theory allows us to consider relationships, not to judge them.
- Attachment begins as a characteristic of a relationship, *not* a characteristic of the child. Two people are involved. If relationships change, so too will the quality of the child's attachment.
- Attachment is a biological motivational system that has most influence in the first two or three years of life. After that, both interpersonal behaviour and relationships are increasingly open to other influences.
- Behaviour stemming from the attachment system is only observed when the child is anxious. However, a lack of an attachment response when the child would be expected to be fearful may be significant. A practitioner visiting a family, as a stranger, is a legitimate source of horror.
- What theory labels as 'insecure attachments' are appropriate adaptations to specific family environments. These behaviours may be transitory depending on circumstances, but if the emotional habitat remains unchanged, they may become more fixed and colour all subsequent relationships to a certain degree.
- Practitioners should hold in mind that the behaviours associated with the different categories of insecure attachment are never, by themselves, a justification to remove a child; this includes the 'worst case' of disorganised attachment.
- The 'gold standard' of attachment evaluation is the Strange Situation Procedure. This is a highly specialised skill that calls for a lot of training;

it is time-consuming and generally only done as part of University-based research. It is usually applied in the child's second year.

- If a practitioner wishes to gain a rough understanding of a child's attachment pattern (at that point in time), s/he could make detailed observations of their behaviour under different conditions where the child's felt security might have an influence. Examples are: The child's capacity to learn and play creatively; for children under age three, the mutual responsiveness when they greet a parent after a separation; their confidence in using adults appropriately as a source of information or reassurance; the manner in which they adapt to new situations; and their capacity to regulate their own emotions (for the younger child, this will naturally involve the help of a parent).

## References

Ainsworth, M.D., Blehar, M.C., Waters, E., Wall, S.N. (1978) Patterns of Attachment: A psychological study of the Strange Situation. Hillsdale, NJ: Erlbaum.

Belsky, J. (1999) Modern evolutionary theory and patterns of attachment. In: Cassidy J., Shaver, P.R. (Eds.) Handbook of Attachment. New York: The Guilford Press: 141–161.

Bowlby, J. (1969) Attachment. London: The Hogarth Press & Institute of Psychoanalysis.

Bowlby, J. (1988) A Secure Base. London: Routledge.

Fonagy, P., Gergely, G., Jurist, E.L., Target, M. (2002) Affect Regulation, Mentalization, and the Development of the Self. New York: Routledge.

Gopnik, A. (2016) The Gardener and the Carpenter. London: The Bodley Head.

Granqvist, P., Sroufe, A.L., Dozier, M., Hesse, E., Steele, M. et al. (2017) Disorganized attachment in infancy: A review of the phenomenon and its implications for clinicians and policy-makers. Attachment & Human Development, 19(6):534–558.

Hrdy, S.B. (2009) Mothers and Others: The evolutionary origins of human understanding. Cambridge, MA: The Belknap Press of Harvard University Press.

Panksepp, J., Biven, L. (2012) The Archaeology of Mind. New York: W. W. Norton & Co.

Roisman, G.I., Collins, W.A., Sroufe, L.A., Egeland, B. (2005) Predictors of young adults' representations of and behaviour in their current romantic relationship: Prospective tests of the prototype hypothesis. Attachment & Human Development, 7(2):105–121.

Siegel, D.J. (1999) The Developing Mind: Towards a neurobiology of interpersonal experience. New York: The Guilford Press.

Small, M.F. (1998) Our Babies, Ourselves. New York: Anchor Books.

Sroufe, L.A. (1995) Emotional Development: The organization of emotional life in the early years. Cambridge: Cambridge University Press.

Trevarthen, C. (1980) The foundations of intersubjectivity: Development of interpersonal and co-operative understanding in infants. In: Olsen D.R. (Ed.) The Social Foundation of Language. New York: W.W. Norton and Company: 316–342.

Trevarthen, C. (2005) Stepping away from the mirror: Pride and shame in adventures of companionship. In: Carter C. S., Ahnert L., Grossmann K. E. et al. (Eds.) Attachment and Bonding: A new synthesis. Cambridge, MA: The MIT Press: 56–84.

# 8

# JUST CHATTING WITH A BABY IS MORE THAN YOU MIGHT THINK

*Robin Balbernie*

Newborn babies are biologically primed to make social connections, a survival mechanism that paves the way to the later attachment relationship. Parents and babies communicate with each other, acknowledge and encourage each other even before birth, and the lilt of language is important from the beginning – which is not to say that deaf babies fail to form good relationships; there are many other sensory channels that can be used. Occasionally, a parent may find it hard to chat with their baby. Appreciating the effects of this everyday act shows how important it is to listen whenever we observe babies and parents interacting.

★

Babies are all set to converse and interact from birth. The neonate's capacity to mimic facial and hand movements tells parents, 'I can see and respond to you', winding them in and softening them up for the next six or so months of sleepless nights and anxious days. Most babies respond almost immediately to speech directed to them by their parents if this is done in the right way. Simply put, they like listening to people speaking to them in a certain heartfelt fashion, preferring this above all other complex sounds and are soon quite capable of soliciting, reciprocating or ignoring adult communications as they feel fit. This intuitive style of talking to babies, whose acoustic properties seem to be universal across most cultures (Broesch & Bryant, 2014), is called by many names: 'parentese', 'motherese' (common in the past), 'infant-directed speech' or just 'baby talk'. Interestingly, the contours of stress, intonation and the patterns of rhythm and sound (prosody) vary in similar ways according to the parent's intentions. Thus, across different languages, similar contours convey the same types of meaning such as arousing/soothing, turn opening and closing, approving/disapproving

DOI: 10.4324/9781003223771-10

and didactic modelling (Papoušek et al., 1991). Chatting to a baby joins parents across the world.

## Parentese

There is a delightful theory that the language ability of homo sapiens has its evolutionary roots in our remote hominid ancestors where new foraging strategies, concurrent with less time in the trees and bipedalism, less furry mums, more helpless babies, larger brains and a change of habitat, called for the maternal silencing, reassuring and controlling of physically separate infants who had lost the ability to cling on and so needed to be stashed occasionally to free up mum's hands and energy to search for food (Falk, 2004). Parentese, the only universal language, thus stands in direct line with the soothing prosody, facial signals and gestures that ensured our ancestors' reproductive success through calming babies when necessary, a prelinguistic selective factor that eventually led to the use of words. Chatting to a baby is time travel.

Parentese seems to be most effective on a one-to-one basis. It has arousing properties and helps capture attention. This is also how many people speak to their pets (Burnham et al., 2002), but whether this is because the pet is a child-substitute or the unconscious wish to teach the beast to speak is unclear. Compared to normal adult speech, infant-directed speech is marked by a heightened pitch which has a wider range and exaggerated undulating contours. It has a slower tempo with longer pauses and tends to be composed of repetitive vocalizations and is associated with exaggerated gestures.

> The prosodic patterns of Infant Directed Speech are more informative than those of Adult Directed Speech, and they provide infants with reliable cues about a speaker's communicative intent.

> *(Saint-Georges et al., 2013:3)*

There is a slight difference between mothers and fathers here, with the latter tending to use a narrower frequency range. Most importantly, though, infant-directed speech has a fascinating melody to it: What Malloch (1999) calls 'communicative musicality', an inherent organizing principle in parent–baby interactions that facilitates turn-taking and influences the pitch and musical timbre of their vocalizations to each other.

> Communicative musicality consists of the elements pulse, quality and narrative – those attributes of human communication, which are particularly exploited in music - that allow co-ordinated companionship to arise.

> *(Malloch, 1999:32)*

Infant and parent are partners in a musical dialogue. This style of exaggerated speech elongates vowel sounds, thus making them easier to tell apart within their native language's linguistic structure. Chatting to a baby is a mutual melody of love.

## Musical Mind-Sharing

That the communication between parent and baby can be seen as music is hardly surprising given that the baby's right hemisphere, the place where the neural networks for both relationships and music are mostly located, is the part of the brain that is developing at the greatest rate in the first two years of life; the left hemisphere, where speech processing largely sits, is mostly nascent up until about 18–24 months when there is the vocabulary spurt.

> The inborn responsive musicality of infants is a rich manifestation of the representation of purposes and emotions evoked by one individual's brain in the brain of another.

> (Trevarthen, 2008:17)

All parents instinctively sing to their babies and the distinctive style of infant-directed song is also recognizable across different cultures (Trehub et al., 1993), although the proportion of rousing or soothing songs does vary, perhaps reflecting differences in caregiving practices. Babies are universally entranced by lullabies, matching bodily movements to the rhythms. Look closely and you will see them conduct. Chatting to a baby is musical mind-sharing.

When a baby arrives in a family, all changes for everyone concerned, so it is fortunate that the new arrival can make herself known.

> [Babies] possess rudimentary personal powers that affect their caregivers intimately so that within a short time of birth, a subtle infant-caretaker relationship is established.

> (Trevarthen, 1980:336)

Babies selectively reward parental signalling behaviour. Newborns prefer communications that signal a readiness to interact (direct gaze, baby-directed speech, smiling, etc.); they can appreciate intention. This applies to pre-term births as well, and baby-directed speech and singing enhance premature babies' physiological stability (Filippa et al., 2013) and can be used for pain management in a neonatal intensive care unit (Ullsten et al., 2018), especially if parents are coached by a specialized music therapist. After only a couple of weeks of life, babies show a distinct preference for parentese over adult-directed speech, and this is clearly established by four months. So begins the cunning and subtle plan of how to train parents through the process of choosing whether to respond or not.

## 'Desired' Parental Behaviour

Babies cannot understand the literal meaning of words, of course, but they usually respond to the exaggerated rhythm, tone, prosody, gestures, facial expressions and postural messages of an attentive adult; this is the act not necessarily the message. They have arrived in the world familiar with their mother's voice (and that of any siblings at bump height); they can hear muffled noise from about 24 weeks in utero and recognize the tunes inflicted on them. Familiar sounds become attractive; they help to organize the post-partum confusion and from then on language will be a key feature of their interpersonal world and a conduit for culture. Intentions expressed in parentese appear to be understood across different languages (Bryant & Barrett, 2007). By about four and a half months, babies can recognize their own name, and by six months, they can recognize the word in their family that designates mother – mum, mummy, Alice, etc. – depending on family use.

Parentese will usually capture an alert and relaxed baby's attention. Eye contact is a central element here, although having a blind parent does not affect the development of normal social communication skills and actually benefits visual memory and attention (Senju et al., 2013). Building on prenatal experiences, neonates can recognize communication and show sensitivity to temporal sequence and pattern with expectations of social contingency (sharing experiences) and turn-taking appearing at eight weeks.

The engagement involved in 'serve and return' communication becomes alluring, and by four months, babies show a clear preference for adults who do this with them, an aspect of attunement. They have picked up the trick of social smiling during the first three months, and this is another reinforcer of 'desired' parental behaviour. Chatting to babies creates a feedback that has a dynamic effect on the quality of infant-directed speech with the parent intuitively adapting to the infant's abilities, emotional state and immediate needs. (If the parent is troubled in any way, this may be hard.) The preference for contingent communication extends to the toddler, and a child who has learned to take this for granted (a part of the 'goal-corrected partnership' of attachment theory) is more likely to show pro-social behaviour (Thompson & Newton, 2013). There is no getting away from the fact that mothers talk more to their young children than fathers and more to their girls than boys. They also use more supportive speech, while fathers are more directive and informing (Leaper et al., 1998), but these may be contextual effects based more on access and role within the family than gender. Chatting to a baby gives him or her felt security.

## Native Language Development

To begin with, babies can respond to every language in the world. Unlike adults, they can discriminate among virtually all phonetic units, but as they grow and are increasingly exposed to the phonetics of their native language, this capacity soon becomes narrowed down. By the first birthday, the ability to selectively distinguish the different sounds of their native language has been pretty well wired in (Kuhl et al., 2006) based on the selective cues offered by parents, although they will continue to learn to differentiate between these as they grow older concurrent with a decline in non-native speech perception. In an experiment, one group of nine-month-old babies was exposed to a native Mandarin speaker who sang, read to and played with them for 12 sessions of 25 minutes over one month. At age one, they were just as good at discriminating sounds in Mandarin Chinese as infants raised in Taiwan, so exposure had reversed the usual decline in foreign language speech perception, whereas the two control groups who had only either watched or heard recordings of the same sessions (rather than being present with the Mandarin speaker) were just as duff at this as those infants with no exposure at all (Kuhl et al., 2003). Bilingual families give their children a distinct advantage (Garcia-Sierra et al., 2011). Chatting to a baby is the scaffolding for language.

## Neuroplasticity

Neuroplasticity plays a large part here – neurons that fire together wire together – and the theory of 'native language neural commitment' proposes that the baby forms dedicated neural networks that code the sounds and patterns of their home language while also pruning the circuits potentially sensitive to other sounds – use it or lose it (Kuhl, 2004). But for this to occur, babies must be directly addressed; neural networks for speech recognition are chosen by chatting. This is supported by experimental data showing significant increase in native language performance over the first year coupled with a decline in non-native perception (Kuhl et al., 2006). Also, as babies listen to speech, Broca's area and the cerebellum, the brain areas that coordinate and plan the motor movements for speaking, become activated (Kuhl et al., 2014), suggesting that babies are rehearsing motor movements for speaking well before expressive language begins and again neuroplasticity will narrow down alternatives.

Babies who are not chatted with will fall behind here, with some aspects of language facility perhaps compromised in the long term as babies only learn language through social interaction and their experiences at home are critical for this (Tamis-LeMonda & Rodriguez, 2014). As an extreme, children who have experienced the deprivation of social isolation as infants never acquire normal language skills (Fromkin et al., 1974). However, in normal development, infants between ages six to eight and ten to twelve months whose mothers used more parentese become better at discriminating the sounds of speech (Liu et al., 2003), and at age two, these infants have larger productive vocabularies (Ramírez-Esparza et al., 2014). Productive vocabulary is the words the child regularly uses as opposed to those she can understand when used by others.

This advantage continues up to age 33 months (Ramírez-Esparza et al., 2017) by which time the use of parentese is fading. By age three, in all cultures, children can use full sentences to communicate, although their skill and vocabulary will vary depending on the early experience they have had. Chatting to a baby changes her mind.

## Emotional Attunement in Action

The process of communication is a process of containment, where the parent lets the baby know that they are prepared to do their best to work out what the baby is feeling and respond appropriately: this may range from comfort and calming to rousing and excitement. The emotional bond between baby and parent is created and reinforced by this mutually pleasurable interaction that serves to coordinate and communicate what each is feeling at any one time, paving the way towards secure attachment. When a baby and parent chat, each partner in the dialogue acknowledges that the other has a mind with something on it that can be shared (not that the baby can conceptualize a mind; she just experiences its working). An attuned parent is able to share experiences with the baby. When doing so, they are the partner who takes most responsibility to shape and hold what is going on since the baby has yet to develop the neurological capacity to do this for herself.

Speaking to a baby, enlisting the 'proto-musical features' (Dissanayake, 2008) of mother–baby interaction, is emotional attunement in action. By this means, the parent acknowledges and regulates the baby's internal state as part of the everyday reciprocal exchanges found in chatting and playfulness. The factual meaning of the parent's words can have little effect much before the age of two, but the gist of this right brain to right brain communication is connection and concern. Like the ever-enjoyable conjointly improvised playful and physical interactions between mother and baby, chatting provides an experience of regulation through intimacy. It would be fair to say that, 'language is simply a subset of music from a child's view' (Brandt et al., 2012) that has multiple functions.

> The prosodic and melodic contours emitted in lullabies and motherese cause corresponding neural activation contours in the recipient listener [i.e. the baby], experienced as shifts between tension and relaxation.
>
> *(Volgsten, 2016:202)*

Chatting to a baby, with mutual interest and appreciation, is regulation within a relationship, the fundamental basis of secure attachment. Truly, the medium is the message here (McLuhen, 1965) and the medium is musical.

## Good Communication and Healthy Relationships

Chatting, affect attunement and just having fun together are forms of regulatory dialogue that go hand in glove with each other and, when the parent gets it roughly right, these exchanges bring a sense of stability and relief to the infant while building communication skills that will last a lifetime. Relief in the sense that tension or stress is reduced while ennui is met with appropriate stimulation since:

> Infants respond strongly to the different moods of action games and soothing lullabies, allowing the vital rhythms of their minds and bodies to be excited or slowed into peaceful states.

> *(Trevarthen, 2008:18)*

Healthy relationships are built on good communication. In this intersubjective overlap, the engaged parent who is communicating directly with the child does not always get it right in terms of the infant's need for regulation; but this is OK as the inevitable mistakes provide a chance for interactive repair which in itself is an act of emotional connection and containment. It is important to remember that the neural networks of the baby's right hemisphere develop first, before those of the left hemisphere where language functions and verbally organized logical thought are predominantly located, and the emotional connection between mother and baby is a right brain to right brain flow of energy and information. That is why all over the world, parents predominantly cradle and nurse while holding the baby in the left arm, thus setting up mutual left eye to-and-from right hemisphere communication. Interestingly, mothers tend to swop sides when baby is bored and needs a healthy prod. Babies are hardwired to seek a social and emotional partner and communicate from birth. The neuroplasticity that corresponds to the period of infancy, when many areas of the child's brain are forming connections that may last a lifetime as they adapt to the family environment, means that the emotional communication that flows through the musicality of parentese will lay the foundation for the developing personality.

## Practice Pointers

- The two-way flow of communication between a baby and parent is central to many facets of development, not just language. Thus, all early years' practitioners should consciously tune into this aspect of the baby/parent relationship.
- A parent who struggles consistently to hold her or his baby in mind may find it hard to slip into the lilt of parentese; the baby may then appear less engaged and this may lead to a negative cycle if the parent feels rejected or inadequate. Sensitive help may well be called for to prevent this from happening.

- In these digital days, many parents have lost touch with traditional lullabies. Simply setting up a group to re-connect with the musicality of babyhood will be beneficial (see: https://www.rockabye.org.uk).
- Six principles of language learning are laid out in the article by Hirsch-Pasek and Golinkoff (2018). They are:
  1 Children learn what they hear most.
  2 Children learn words for things and events that interest them.
  3 Interactive and responsive environments build language learning.
  4 Children learn best in meaningful contexts.
  5 Children need to hear diverse examples of words and language structures.
  6 Vocabulary and grammatical development are reciprocal processes.

## References

Brandt, A., Gebrian, M., Slevc, L.R. (2012) Music and early language acquisition. Frontiers in Psychology, 3, Article 327:1–17.

Broesch, T.L., Bryant, G.A. (2014) Prosody in infant-directed speech is similar across Western and traditional cultures. Journal of Cognition and Development, 16(1). Available at: https://doi.org/10. 1080/15248372.2013.833923 <accessed 1 April, 2020>

Bryant, G.A., Barrett, H.C. (2007) Recognizing intonations in infant-directed speech: Evidence for universals. Psychological Science, 18:746–751.

Burnham, D., Kitamura, C., Vollmer-Conna, U. (2002) What's new, pussycat? On talking to babies and animals. Science, 296:1435.

Dissanayake, E. (2008) If music is the food of love, what about survival and reproductive success? Musicae Scientiae (special issue):169–195.

Falk, D. (2004) Prelinguistic evolution in early hominins: Whence motherese? Behavioral and Brain Sciences, 27:491–541.

Filippa, M., Devouche, E., Arioni, C., Imberty, M., Gratier, M. (2013) Live maternal speech and singing have beneficial effects on hospitalized preterm infants. Acta Paediatrica, 102(10):1017–1020.

Fromkin, V., Krashen, S., Curtiss, S., Rigler, D., Rigler, M. (1974) The development of language in Genie: A case of language acquisition beyond the 'critical period'. Brain and Language, 1:81–107.

Garcia-Sierra, A., Rivera-Gaxiola, M., Conboy, B.T., Romo, H., Klarman, L. et al. (2011) Bilingual language learning: An ERP study relating early brain responses to speech, language input, and later word production. Journal of Phonetics, 39:556–557.

Hirsch-Pasek, K., Golinkoff, R.M. (2018) 'Languagizing' their world: Why talking, reading, and singing are so important. Zero to Three, 38(3):12–18.

Kuhl, P. (2004) Early language acquisition: Cracking the speech code. Nature Reviews Neuroscience, 5:831–834.

Kuhl, P.K., Ramírez, R.R., Bosseler, A., Lin, J.F.L., Imada, T. (2014) Infants' brain responses to speech suggest analysis by synthesis. Proceedings of the National Academy of Sciences, 111:11238–11245.

Kuhl, P.K., Stevens, E., Hayashi, A., Deguchi, T., Kiritani, S. et al. (2006) Infants show a facilitation effect for native language phonetic perception between 6 and 12 months. Developmental Science, 9(2):F13-F21.

Kuhl, P.K., Tsao. F.-M., Liu, H.M. (2003) Foreign-language experience in infancy: Effects of short-term exposure and social interaction on phonetic learning. Proceedings of the National Academy of Sciences, 100:9096–9101.

Leaper, C., Anderson, K.J., Sanders, P. (1998) Moderators of gender effects on parents' talk to their children: A meta-analysis. Developmental Psychology, 34(1):3–27.

Liu, H.M., Kuhl, P.K., Tsao, F.M. (2003) An association between mothers' speech clarity and infants' speech discrimination skills. Developmental Science, 6:F1–F10.

Malloch, S.N. (1999) Mothers and infants and communicative musicality. Musicae Scientiae, Special issue, 1999–2000:29–57.

McLuhen, M. (1965) The medium is the message. In: Durham, M.G. & Kellner, D.M. (Eds.) (2006) Media and Cultural Studies. Oxford: Blackwell Publishing: 107–116.

Papoušek, M. Papoušek, H., Symmes, D. (1991) The meaning of melodies in motherese in tone and stress languages. Infant Behavior and Development, 14(4):415–440.

Ramírez-Esparza, N., García-Sierra, A., Kuhl, P. (2014) Look who's talking: Speech style and social context in language input to infants are linked to concurrent and future speech development. Developmental Science, 17:880–891.

Ramírez-Esparza, N., García-Sierra, A., Kuhl, P.K. (2017) Look who's talking NOW!: Parentese speech, social context, and language development across time. Frontiers in Psychology, 8:Article 1008.

Saint-Georges, C., Chetouani, M., Cassel, R., Apicella, F., Mahdhaoui, A., et al. (2013) Motherese in interaction: At the cross-road of emotion and cognition? PLoS one, 8(10):1–17.

Senju, A., Tucker, L., Pasco, G., Hudry, K., Elsabbagh, M. et al. (2013) The importance of the eyes: Communication skills in infants of blind parents. Proceedings of the Royal Society B, Biological Sciences, 280(1760):20130436.

Tamis-LeMonda, C., Rodriguez, E.T. (2014) Parents' role in fostering young children's learning and language development. Downloaded from: Encyclopedia on Early Child Development. New York: New York University.

Thompson, R.A., Newton, E.K. (2013) Baby altruists? Examining the complexity of prosocial motivation in young children. Infancy, 18:120–133.

Trehub, S.E., Unyk, A.M., Trainor, L.J. (1993) Maternal singing in cross-cultural perspective. Infant Behavior and Development, 16:285–295.

Trevarthen, C. (1980) The foundations of intersubjectivity: Development of interpersonal and cooperative understanding in infants. In: Olsen, D.R. (Ed.) The Social Foundation of Language and Thought. New York: W.W. Norton and Company: 316–342.

Trevarthen, C. (2008) The musical art of infant conversation: Narrating in the time of sympathetic experience, without rational interpretation, before words. Musicae Scientifiae, Special Issue:15–46.

Ullsten, A., Eriksson, M., Klässbo, M., Volgsten, U. (2018) Singing, sharing, soothing – biopsychosocial rationales for parental infant-directed singing in neonatal pain management: A theoretical approach. Music & Science, 1:1–13.

Volgsten, U. (2016) The roots of music: Emotional expression, dialogue and affect attunement in the psychogenesis of music. Musicae Scientiae, 16(2):200–216.

# 9

# THE MUSICAL KEY TO BABIES' COGNITIVE AND SOCIAL DEVELOPMENT

*Graham F. Welch*

(This chapter was originally published as Henriksson-Macaulay, L., Welch, G.F. (2015) The musical key to babies cognitive and social development. *International Journal of Birth and Parent Education*, 2(2):21–25. It has been updated by Graham Welch.)

In today's world, filled with myriad parenting methods and high-tech toys that promise to enhance infant development, it is easy to overlook how fundamental is the time-honoured practice of music for all children – starting pre-birth. Music is crucial for babies in every developmental sense: with regards to communication and language, emotional and social well-being, and even motor skills. But it is only relatively recently that science has begun to elaborate in more detail the true extent of its significance.

*

Over the past decade or so, neuroscientific studies have established that babies are born with all the key components of musical understanding, such as recognizing intervals (Stefanics et al., 2009) and consonance (i.e. whether a piece of music is 'in tune' or not, Perani et al., 2010); identifying where the beat of a song lies (Winkler et al., 2009); whether a chord is in a major or minor key, based on Western musical harmonic conventions (Virtala et al., 2013), and soon demonstrating implicit knowledge of complex harmonic music–syntactic regularities (Jentschke et al., 2014).

Being musical is part of our human design (Mithen, 2009; Welch, 2005) and our musical development begins pre-birth (Woodward, 2019). Hearing is normally functioning before birth in the final trimester of pregnancy (Lecanuet, 1996), and the newborn enters the world already having experienced sounds from the maternal culture and able to perceive and discriminate tiny differences

DOI: 10.4324/9781003223771-11

in voiced sound (Eimas et al., 1971). The human brain has specialist areas whose prime functions are networked for a wide variety of musical processing, but also linked into other areas of the brain related to major areas of functioning, such as movement, language and emotional experience (Patel, 2012).

Therefore, a child at birth already responds to music. Contrast this to other methods of communication, such as language and pictures: These are not in the range of comprehension of a newborn. A baby's caregivers instinctively understand this, which is why all around the world, it is found that adults spontaneously adapt their 'infant-directed speech' into a higher-pitched, more melodic and more emotionally expressive form of communication (also known as 'motherese' and 'parentese') (Saint-Georges et al., 2013; Trehub & Gudmundsdottir, 2019). In other words, as humans, we already know intuitively to emphasize the musical elements of speech (i.e. using expressive prosodic contours, pitch glides and a prevalence of basic harmonic intervals – 3rds, 4ths, 5ths, octaves) because these are sounds to which babies universally respond.

## Babies, Music and Language Development

There is strong evidence that babies, in fact, develop their language skills and vocabulary in a way that is mediated by the musical aspects of speech (Brandt et al., 2019; Chen-Hafteck, 1997; Cross, 1999). In this manner, music paves a way for linguistic development. It is also found that when babies engage in weekly, age-appropriate music lessons, they develop communication skills to a much higher degree than infants of the same age who undertake other activities (Gerry et al., 2012). Passive music listening alone does not produce the same effect. Moreover, active music making is a form of relationship-building in which parents and other caregivers engage to a degree spontaneously: singing to a baby, bouncing them on your lap to a rhythmic jingle and clapping to them – these are all common and beneficial forms of musical engagement between a caregiver and a small child (Pitt & Welch, 2022; Trehub & Gudmundsdottir, 2019).

In the ancestral environment, where most of human neurobiological development took place, music-type behaviours were likely to have played a much larger part in everyday activities than they do in twenty-first century Western society. Leading evolutionary researcher, Robin Dunbar from the University of Oxford, concludes, based on existing evidence, that pre-humans already made music (sang and engaged in making rhythms) 500,000 years ago, whereas our species only developed language 200,000 years ago (Dunbar et al., 2007). The baby's linguistic development mimics this progress from music to language in microcosm. These days, our parenting culture is very focused on words; a baby's first words are often recorded and talked about to anyone who is willing to listen, and milestones of vocabulary development are keenly watched. Consequently, it is relatively easy to ignore the fact that it is musical features of the maternal sound culture that pave the way for optimizing this aspect of development.

On the other hand, it is possible to argue that music has been alienated from everyday use, with the invention of recording technology. It is a common misconception for people, even music teachers, to believe that only a small minority of people are 'musical' in the first place (Sloboda, 2000; Sloboda et al., 1994; Welch, 2001). In general, the neuroscientific findings on the musical abilities of newborns have not attracted wide media coverage.

## Music and Emotional Development

But it is not just language and communication for which music is useful; engaging with music is also an emotional experience, and babies and young children are no exception. A striking example of this is the finding by the Italian music educator and early childhood specialist, Johannella Tafuri. Parents and caregivers commonly struggle with trying to comfort a distressed baby, but Tafuri reported that when babies were sung to, they calmed down, with a 94.5% success rate (Tafuri, 2009). This is linked to the moderation of cortisol (the stress hormone), with maternal singing either arousing the infant by raising cortisol or reducing distress by lowering cortisol (Shenfield et al., 2001). Similar effects are reported in studies of choral singing and emotion (e.g., Kreutz et al., 2004). Tafuri reported that playing recorded music was also relatively successful in 78.4% of instances, but it is notable how much better a baby was likely to respond when the music that they encountered was presented live by the adult in front of them.

Studies have shown that music is a crucial way to help a small, pre-verbal child manage their emotions. As mentioned above, not only can a distressed baby be stopped from crying via soothing singing, but, likewise, a placid baby can be actively engaged via music (Robb, 2000; Saarikallio, 2009). The emotional benefits also extend to social benefits. Scientists have measured the 'helpfulness' of 14-month-old babies after two conditions, one where they were bounced to a regular beat of music, compared to another where they were bounced asynchronously while listening to unpredictable beats. After the two types of bouncing experiences, babies had the opportunity to help the experimenter by handing over desired objects. It was found that when babies experienced predictable beat bouncing, they tended to exhibit 'helpful' behaviour 61% of the time, compared to only 25% after non-rhythmic bouncing (Cirelli et al., 2012). This implies that music making can build empathy and social cohesion and also that social facilitation as a fundamental component of musical behaviour is found early in development.

## 'The Mozart Effect'

When discussing the power of music to effect other kinds of behavioural benefit, it is necessary to account for the media storm that followed publication of the so-called 'Mozart Effect' in the 1990s when it was claimed that listening to Mozart before taking an IQ test raised the test scores of adult participants for the duration of 15 minutes (Rauscher et al., 1995). The Mozart Effect has remained as a popular notion about music and babies, despite the fact that many studies since have moderated and, in some cases, challenged its existence. Even its original researcher, Francis Rauscher, has stated that there is no evidence to support the claim that listening to classical music CDs improves children's spatial–temporal reasoning – or any other aspect of intelligence (Rauscher, 2002). Nevertheless, there is evidence that this type of music can have a positive effect on human physiology and pathophysiology, such as on cardiovascular parameters (Trappe, 2012) and that exposure can improve weight gain in preterm infants by reducing resting energy expenditure (Lubetzky et al., 2010).

So, did something go wrong with The Mozart Effect? With regards to the original study, it was discovered that the short-term IQ increase had nothing to do with Mozart or music, but was due to the relative advantage that the music-listening group had in relation to the control group who had to sit in uncomfortable silence before taking their test (Nantais & Schellenberg, 1999; Thompson et al., 2001). Yet, the appeal of The Mozart Effect is easy to see: In our society focused on the prestige of experts and the effectiveness of passive consumption, what would be better than to be able to press a button and make your child a genius simply by listening to a famous composer? Unfortunately, this is unlikely to happen, just as if you sat a child in front of a video to watch sports, you could expect them to get fitter. To develop physically, a child needs to move; to develop musically, a child needs to be actively making music in some form.

## Encouraging Music Making

How is it possible, then, to encourage active music making in babies and small children? There are many ways to do so. Singing to a child and playing musical games with them is crucial, because not only are you engaging the child in a way that is – at the same time – musical, social and personal, but you are also leading by example, demonstrating that it is socially acceptable to sing and make music. It is important not to worry about being musically 'expert'. The important thing is to explore sounds and sound patterns with the child, using the voice and anything else that comes to hand, and to share musical items from the maternal music culture, such as nursery rhymes (e.g., using web-based materials, including YouTube, for support as necessary). Remember that rhythm is equally as important as pitch, so rhythmic chanting, exploring lyrics and making up rhymes will engage the child musically, especially if they can be encouraged to imitate and join in as they get older. The key to success is exploration and repetition; these will build knowledge and understanding through practice and by recognizing that – as adults – we are senior learners (cf. Jerome Bruner) and able to share in and learn from the infant's musical learning journey (see Trehub & Gundmundsdottir, 2019). For example, data analyses of a longitudinal study of Australian children found higher frequency of shared home music activities contributed small but unique variance to measures of children's vocabulary, numeracy, attentional and emotional regulation and prosocial skills (Williams et al., 2015).

In recent years, an additional approach that has been acquiring more and more confirmation for its nurturing potential is quality music education for babies and toddlers. Child-centred, age-appropriate methods (such as the Hungarian Kodaly, the Finnish Musiikkileikkikoulu and the Japanese Suzuki, and many others) have been successful in helping babies to develop communication skills and increase their emotional well-being, even above and beyond babies who only get exposure to music at home (Gerry et al., 2012). For example, a longitudinal German study of one- and two-year olds compared the musical behaviours and development of a group of children participating with their parents in a special weekly music programme to an equivalent 'control' group in a day care setting (Gruhn, 2002). After 40 weeks, there were marked differences between the two groups (notwithstanding individual differences) with higher ratings for the special programme infants in the quality of their physical movements to music and in their imitation of rhythmic patterns.

These are not the only benefits when a parent and their baby or toddler go to a regular music class together: the parent–child relationship also improves (Nicholson et al., 2008; Walworth, 2009). This benefit has important implications for the healthy psychological development of babies and implies that, in an ideal world, every baby should have the opportunity to engage in a weekly musical class and be supported towards longer-term, positive health effects.

Yet, another way to enhance the musical development of babies and very young children is to expose them to a wide variety of music and musical vocabularies on a regular basis. 'Musical vocabulary' refers to musical concepts at an experiential level, not in terms of naming them. A child need not learn to name different elements, but it is suggested that their musical development would be optimized if they could get to experience these through songs and other musical activities. It is worthwhile, therefore, to develop a suitably varied music collection for an infant. New recording technology has made this kind of endeavour easier than ever before, as long as listening to music is not passive, but active, such as involving movement as part of the listening activity or taking the musical example as a starting point for improvisation.

Babies are curious and are likely to be open to all types of music. For example, very young babies appear to make sense of complex time signatures (underlying rhythmic structures) better than babies aged one year or older (Hannon et al., 2011) unless the one-year olds have experienced such rhythmic complexity throughout their first year of life; in which case, they retain this early ability. This is comparable to the development of the mother tongue (Eimas et al., 1971). A newborn is open to learning any language that they are exposed to, but by the time a baby is one year old, they have already learned to be selective: they direct their attention only to sounds of their mother tongue and away from sounds of other (non-native) languages, unless the home is multi-lingual (Christophe & Morton, 1998).

Babies are able to process music, therefore, at a much deeper level than had been previously thought. For example, they remember tunes that they have heard regularly, even after a long break (Saffran et al., 2000; Trainor et al., 2004). Also, young babies will engage in attempts at singing. Johannella Tafuri, who studied the musical development of babies given regular 'InCanto' music classes with their caregivers at the local conservatoire in Bologna, writes:

> The various musical skills developed by the children in the 'InCanto' project are not in fact 'precocious', in the sense that nature has jumped ahead, but in the sense that they were developed earlier than would normally happen to children that do not live in a stimulating environment. Therefore, they should be considered as 'normal', because they show that nature is ready. These considerations allow us to conclude that if the children in the first year of our elementary schools cannot sing in tune, do not keep in tempo, do not respect the rhythm of a song etc., this means that they have been kept in a state of 'musical deprivation'.
>
> *(Tafuri, 2009:87)*

## The Musical Journey from the Womb Onwards

The musical prerequisites with which babies are born are key markers of an inherent musicality. When these are nurtured appropriately through musical encounters, exploration and play, children will develop musically and also be supported in other aspects of their physical, cognitive, emotional and social development (Hallam, 2014; Welch, 2006; Welch et al., 2014). What better time to encourage a child's musical journey than from the final months of foetal development onwards?

## Practice Pointers

- Being musical is integral to human design. We are all musical, but we can have unequal access to the development of our innate musicality. So? Music should be an integral part of activities in the home and wider community, from the final weeks of pregnancy into infancy and toddlerhood. Exploring sound and music will enhance musical and other-than-musical development – social, emotional, cognitive (such as language) and physical.
- Encourage parents and caregivers to sing and share songs from the maternal culture, improvise, make up songs for parts of the daily routine, explore vocal and instrumental timbres (tone colours), rhythmic patterns and pulse,

and find space to encourage children's imitation, creativity and exploration in sound. Each of these will enrich a child's all-round development.

- Musical behaviours can be classified into three main groups: Pro-active (initiating sounds), re-active (responding to sounds) and inter-active (making sounds with others, sound 'conversations'). Help parents explore how each of these can be part of daily routines with their babies, infants and toddlers.

## References

Brandt, A., Slevc, L.R., Gebrian, M. (2019) The role of musical development in early language acquisition. In: Thaut, M.H., Hodges, D.A. (Eds.) The Oxford Handbook of Music and the Brain. New York: Oxford University Press: 566–591.

Chen-Hafteck, L. (1997) Music and language development in early childhood: Integrating past research in the two domains. Early Child Development and Care, 130(1):85–97.

Christophe, A., Morton, J. (1998) Is Dutch native English? Linguistic analysis by 2-month-olds. Developmental Science, 1(2):215–219.

Cirelli, L.K., Einarson, K., Trainor, L.J. (2012) Bouncing babies to the beat: Music and helping behaviour in infancy. Proceedings of the 12th International Conference on Music Perception and Cognition and the 8th Triennial Conference of the European Society for the Cognitive Sciences of Music: 224.

Cross, I. (1999) Is music the most important thing we ever did? Music, development and evolution. In: Suk Won Yi, (Ed.) Music, Mind and Science. Seoul: Seoul National University Press: 10–39.

Dunbar, R.I., Barrett, L., Lycett, J. (2007) Evolutionary Psychology, a Beginner's Guide: Human behaviour, evolution, and the mind. Oxford: Oneworld Publications.

Eimas, P.D., Siqueland, E.R., Jusczyk, P.W., Vigorito, J. (1971) Speech perception in infants. Science, 171:303–306.

Gerry, D., Unrau, A., Trainor, L. J. (2012) Active music classes in infancy enhance musical, communicative and social development. Developmental Science, 15(3):398–407.

Gruhn, W. (2002) Phases and stages in early music learning. A longitudinal study on the development of young children's musical potential. Music Education Research, 4(1):51–71.

Hallam, S. (2014) The Impact of Actively Making Music on the Intellectual, Social and Personal Development of Children and Young People: A research synthesis. London: UCL Institute of Education.

Hannon, E.E., Soley, G., Levine, R.S. (2011) Constraints on infants' musical rhythm perception: Effects of interval ratio complexity and enculturation. Developmental Science, 14(4):865–872.

Jentschke, S., Friederici, A.D., Koelsch, S. (2014) Neural correlates of music-syntactic processing in two-year-old children. Developmental Cognitive Neuroscience, 9:200–208.

Kreutz, G., Bongard, S., Rohrmann, S., Hodapp, V., Grebe, D. (2004) Effects of choir singing or listening on secretory immunoglobin A, cortisol, and emotional state. Journal of Behavioural Medicine, 27(6): 623–635.

Lecanuet, J.P. (1996) Prenatal auditory experience. In: Deliege, I., Sloboda, J. (Eds.) Musical Beginnings. Oxford: Oxford University Press: 3–34.

Lubetzky, R., Mimouni, F.B., Shaul Dollberg, M.D., Reifen, R., Ashbel, G. et al. (2010) Effect of music by Mozart on energy expenditure in growing preterm infants. Pediatrics, 125(1):e24–e28.

Mithen, S. (2009) The music instinct. The evolutionary basis of musicality. Annals of the New York Academy of Sciences, 1169:3–12.

Nantais, K.M., Schellenberg, E.G. (1999) The Mozart Effect: An artifact of preference. Psychological Science, 10(4):370–373.

Nicholson, J.M., Berthelsen, D., Abad, V., Williams, K., Bradley, J. (2008) Impact of music therapy to promote positive parenting and child development. Journal of Health Psychology, 13(2):226–238.

Patel, A.D. (2012) Language, music, and the brain: A resource-sharing framework. In: Rebuschat, P., Rohrmeier, M., Hawkins, I., Cross, J.A. (Eds.) Language and Music as Cognitive Systems. Oxford: Oxford University Press: 204–223.

Perani, D., Saccuman, M.C., Scifo, P., Spada, D., Andreolli, G. et al. (2010) Functional specializations for music processing in the human newborn brain. Proceedings of the National Academy of Sciences, 107(10):4758–4763.

Pitt, J., Welch, G.F. (2022) Music in early education and care settings for communication and language support. In: Barrett, M., Welch, G.F. (Eds.) The Oxford Handbook of Early Childhood Music Learning and Development. New York: Oxford University Press (in press). See pre-print: https://www.researchgate.net/publication/341219685_Music_in_early_education_and_care_settings_for_communication_and_language_support_1

Rauscher, F.H. (2002) Mozart and the mind: Factual and fictional effects of musical enrichment. In Aronsen, J. (Ed.) Improving Academic Achievement: Impact of psychological factors on education. San Diego, CA: Academic Press: 267–278.

Rauscher, F.H., Shaw, G.L., Ky, K.N. (1995) Listening to Mozart enhances spatial-temporal reasoning: Towards a neurophysiological basis. Neuroscience Letters, 185(1):44–47.

Robb, L. (2000) Emotional musicality in mother-infant vocal affect, and an acoustic study of postnatal depression. Musicae Scientiae, 3(1 suppl):123–154.

Saarikallio, S. (2009) Emotional self-regulation through music in 3–8-year-old children. Proceedings of the 7thTriennial Conference of European Society for the Cognitive Sciences of Music (ESCOM 2009). Jyväskylä, Finland: August 12th–16th.

Saffran, J.R., Loman, M.M., Robertson, R.R. (2000) Infant memory for musical experiences. Cognition, 77(1):B15–B23.

Saint-Georges, C., Chetouani, M., Cassel, R., Apicella, F., Mahdhaoui, A. et al. (2013) Motherese in interaction: At the cross-road of emotion and cognition? (A Systematic Review). PLoS One, 8(10): e78103.

Shenfield, T., Trehub, S.E., Nakata, T. (2001) Maternal singing modulates infant arousal. Psychology of Music, 31(4):365–375.

Sloboda, J. (2000) Individual differences in music performance. Trends in Cognitive Sciences, 4(10):397–403.

Sloboda, J.A., Davidson, J.W., Howe, M.J.A. (1994) Is everyone musical? The Psychologist, 7(7):349–354.

Stefanics, G., Háden, G.P., Sziller, I., Balázs, L., Beke, A. et al. (2009) Newborn infants process pitch intervals. Clinical Neurophysiology, 120(2):304–308.

Tafuri, J. (2009) Infant Musicality: New research for educators and parents [Edited by Graham Welch and translated by Elizabeth Hawkins]. Farnham: Ashgate.

Thompson, W.F., Schellenberg, E.G., Husain, G. (2001) Arousal, mood, and The Mozart Effect. Psychological Science, 12(3):248–251.

Trainor, L.J., Wu, L., Tsang, C.D. (2004) Long-term memory for music: Infants remember tempo and timbre. Developmental Science, 7(3):289–296.

Trappe, H.-J. (2012) The effect of music on human physiology and pathophysiology. Music and Medicine, 4(2):100–105.

Trehub, S., Gudmundsdottir, H.R. (2019) Mothers as singing mentors. In: Welch, G.F., Howard, D.M., Nix, J. (Eds.) The Oxford Handbook of Singing. New York: Oxford University Press: 455–470.

Virtala, P., Huotilainen, M., Partanen, E., Fellman, V., Tervaniemi, M. (2013) Newborn infants' auditory system is sensitive to Western music chord categories. Frontiers in Psychology, 4. doi:10.3389/fpsyg.2013.00492.

Walworth, D.D. (2009) Effects of developmental music groups for parents and premature or typical infants under two years on parental responsiveness and infant social development. Journal of Music Therapy, 46(1):32–52.

Welch, G. (2001) The Misunderstanding of Music. London: Institute of Education, University of London.

Welch, G.F. (2005) We are musical. International Journal of Music Education, 23(2):117–120.

Welch, G.F. (2006) The musical development and education of young children. In: Spodek, B., Saracho, O. (Eds.) Handbook of Research on the Education of Young Children. Mahwah, NJ: Lawrence Erlbaum Associates Inc.: 251–267.

Welch, G.F., Himonides, E., Saunders, J., Papageorgi, I., Sarazin, M. (2014) Singing and social inclusion. Frontiers in Psychology, 5:803. doi:10.3389/fpsyg.2014.00803

Williams, K.E., Barrett, M.S., Welch, G.F., Abad, V., Broughton, M. (2015) Associations between early shared music activities in the home and later child outcomes: Findings from the Longitudinal Study of Australian Children. Early Childhood Research Quarterly, 31:113–124.

Winkler, I., Háden, G.P., Ladinig, O., Sziller, I., Honing, H. (2009) Newborn infants detect the beat in music. Proceedings of the National Academy of Sciences, 106(7):2468–2471.

Woodward, S. (2019) Fetal, neonatal, and early infant experiences of maternal singing. In: Welch, G.F., Howard, D.M., Nix, J. (Eds.) The Oxford Handbook of Singing. New York: Oxford University Press: 431–453.

# 10

# "DADDY'S FUNNY!" FATHERS' PLAYFULNESS WITH YOUNG CHILDREN

*Jennifer St George and Richard Fletcher*

Children's play with fathers can be raucous, vigorous and stimulating. In this chapter, we tease out the specificities of fathers' play with infants and young children and suggest some developmental benefits for children. An understanding of how fathers' playfulness facilitates children's attachment and development may help parent educators find more opportunities to include fathers in their practice.

*

Although it is relatively easy to identify play, it is harder to define. Simply, it can be described as behaviours that elevate arousal (Ellis, 1973:107). More specifically, play is not fully functional behaviour; it resembles real life but does not have its consequences; it is spontaneous, pleasurable, rewarding, and it is exaggerated, patterned, and repetitive (Miller, 2017). For humans, play that occurs in relationships has the most profound influence. Beginning in infancy, stimulating, playful interactions with adult carers shape children's identity and their ability to regulate emotions and behaviours (Nagy, 2011).

An important condition for play is that the child feels safe. Infants and children need to be sure that any uncertainty or anxiety they experience will elicit from their most proximate caregiver, protection from harm and comfort when in distress. As the attachment system described by Bowlby (1988) posits, a child will explore only to the extent that they have this sense of security. When this is in place, then children's innate curiosity primes them to explore their world, and increasing amounts of research show that fathers are key figures in play support and guidance (Amodia-Bidakowska et al., 2020; Robinson et al., 2021).

DOI: 10.4324/9781003223771-12

Fathers' play interactions vary widely. Physical play with toddlers and children, activities such as tickling, wrestling, hugging, and other big body contact are typical (MacDonald & Parke, 1986). Much of this vigorous physical play has important emotional characteristics. Fathers laugh and tussle with the child at the same time as encouraging them to be strong and to persevere (Kazura, 2000). An exemplar of this type of play is rough and tumble. In high-quality rough and tumble, the father is attentive and playful, encouraging effortful, competitive play, and children respond with joy and motivation. The father succeeds in keeping a good balance between actively challenging the child on the one hand and 'letting the child win' on the other. The father actively focuses on what the child is doing, watching him or her carefully and being ready to follow the child's lead. The interaction invites, creates, and maintains trust and affection (Fletcher et al., 2012).

However, there is more to fathers' playfulness than physical, tactile stimulation. While both mothers and fathers play conventional games and use toys with their children, it seems that when fathers are involved in interactions, their play can be more stimulating than mothers' (Labrell, 1996; Roggman et al., 2004). While mothers' interactions with infants tend to be smooth and regulated, fathers' play often involves bursts of high energy that increase as playtime extends (Feldman, 2003). Fathers' energy, expressed as teasing, humour, or incongruity, brings novelty, surprise, and complexity to the child. Under the wing of a warm connection with the father, these cognitive stimulations are highly arousing and engaging (Zaouche-Gaudron et al., 1998). This sort of stimulating, contradictory, and challenging behaviour between fathers and their children has been documented in numerous studies (Keltner et al., 2001; Yogman, 2001). When fathers sing to their infants, for example, they are likely to choose unconventional songs or make up their own rather than sing traditional nursery songs (Trehub et al., 1997), their exuberant singing being highly engaging (O'Neill & Trainor, 2001). Similarly, they tend to use longer and more abstract words than mothers (Pancsofar & Vernon-Feagans, 2010). Teasing is another example of fathers' playfulness. When men tease their child, the smooth flow of cooperative play is interrupted by ambiguity or uncertainty because the father deliberately provokes a reaction from the child in one way or another. Blocking play moves, sudden changes of routine to provoke surprise or pretending to fight are all examples of this type of teasing (Labrell, 1994). Importantly, these actions are not antagonistic, they are 'pretend', just as rough and tumble is 'play'-fighting.

Evidence now suggests that the effects of fathers' contribution to their child's development are different from mothers' and that some of this may even be unique (Dumont & Paquette, 2013; Majdandžić et al., 2014). Over time, myriad playful moments generate joy and mutual warmth, intensifying the bond between father and child. As this attachment grows stronger, the child gains confidence to explore. At the same time, the father's play and interaction style can improve the child's emotional regulation (Hagman, 2014), mastery motivation (Lang et al., 2014), and nascent academic skills, such as language, reading, and numeracy (Cook et al., 2011). Rough and tumble play, for example, is linked to children' social competence, such as positive peer relationships (Fletcher et al., 2012), regulation of aggression (Peterson & Flanders, 2005), and social anxiety (Bögels & Perotti, 2011). Fathers' impact can be lasting – one longitudinal study showed that sensitive and challenging father–child play at two years predicted teenagers who were more comfortable with uncertainties and complexities, were less likely to seek reassurance from others, and less likely to withdraw in the face of frustration and adversity (Grossmann et al., 2002).

It is important to note, however, that play as experienced by children in Western societies is not a universal template. Cultural differences exist in respect to parents' beliefs about the purpose and value of child play – parents may be less involved, 'fun' is not necessarily a concomitant for example (see detail in Roopnarine et al., 2018). Individual differences in fathers also have an effect on quality of play. Fathers' parenting style may not be optimal – less warmth, more negativity (Davis et al., 2011) – and other factors such as depression, role identity, and parenting-efficacy can impact upon play style (Harvey et al., 2011; Zaouche-Gaudron et al., 1998).

Given the importance of playfulness to child attachment and developmental trajectories therefore, infants and young children need interaction with someone who is willing to extend, reach out, and have fun (Nakano et al., 2007). While security and parent responsiveness remain the a priori conditions for play, when this is in place, stimulation and arousal through fathers' sensitive and challenging play will help shape children's brain structures and processes, and ultimately, their intellectual and emotional capacities (Collins et al., 2000).

Play is an outstanding leverage point for clinicians and birth and parenting educators to include fathers in their work. Practitioners' beliefs in fathers' capacity to contribute to children's development will be an important resource for families. Interactions with families that demonstrate a value for fathers and support them in developing positive father–child relationships will help men to activate their own knowledge and strengths.

## Practice Pointers

- Play is spontaneous, pleasurable, and rewarding.
- Play is a child's way of learning about their world.
- Children need to feel safe and relaxed to play.
- Fathers are often available and willing to enable play.
- Playful interactions with any responsive adult will help children grow.
- A father's play can improve the child's emotional regulation, mastery motivation, and nascent academic skills.

## References

Amodia-Bidakowska, A., Laverty, C., Ramchandani, P.G. (2020) Father-child play: A systematic review of its frequency, characteristics and potential impact on children's development. Developmental Review, 57:100924.

Bögels, S.M., Perotti, E.C. (2011) Does father know best? A formal model of the paternal influence on childhood social anxiety. Journal of Child and Family Studies, 20(2):171–181.

Bowlby, J. (1988) A Secure Base: Clinical applications of attachment theory. East Sussex: Brunner-Routledge.

Collins, W.A., Maccoby, E.E., Steinberg, L., Hetherington, E.M., Bornstein, M.H. (2000) Contemporary research on parenting: The case for nature and nurture. American Psychologist, 55(2):218–232.

Cook, C., Goodman, N.D., Schulz, L.E. (2011) Where science starts: Spontaneous experiments in preschoolers' exploratory play. Cognition, 120(3):341–349.

Davis, R., Davis, M.M., Freed, G.L., Clark, S.J. (2011) Fathers' depression related to positive and negative parenting behaviors with 1-year-old children. Pediatrics, 127(4):612–618.

Dumont, C., Paquette, D. (2013) What about the child's tie to the father? A new insight into fathering, father–child attachment, children's socio-emotional development and the activation relationship theory. Early Child Development & Care, 183(3–4):430–446.

Ellis, M.J. (1973) Why People Play. Englewood Cliffs, NJ: Prentice-Hall.

Feldman, R. (2003) Infant–mother and infant–father synchrony: The co-regulation of positive arousal. Infant Mental Health Journal, 24(1):1–23.

Fletcher, R., StGeorge, J., Freeman, E. (2012) Rough and tumble play quality: Theoretical foundations for a new measure of father–child interaction. Early Child Development and Care, 183(6):746–759.

Grossmann, K., Grossmann, K.E., Fremmer-Bombik, E., Kindler, H., Scheuerer-Englisch, H. (2002) The uniqueness of the child–father attachment relationship: Fathers' sensitive and challenging play as a pivotal variable in a 16-year longitudinal study. Social Development, 11(3):301–337.

Hagman, A. (2014). Father-child play behaviors and child emotion regulation. Master of Science Thesis. Utah State University.

Harvey, E., Stoessel, B., Herbert, S. (2011) Psychopathology and parenting practices of parents of preschool children with behavior problems. Parenting, 11(4):239–263.

Kazura, K. (2000) Fathers' qualitative and quantitative involvement: An investigation of attachment, play, and social interactions. Journal of Men's Studies, 9(1):41–57.

Keltner, D., Capps, L., Kring, A.M., Young, R.C., Heerey, E.A. (2001) Just teasing: A conceptual analysis and empirical review. Psychological Bulletin, 127(2):229–248.

Labrell, F. (1994) A typical interaction behaviour between fathers and toddlers: Teasing. Early Development and Parenting, 3(2):125–130.

Labrell, F. (1996) Paternal play with toddlers: Recreation and creation. European Journal of Psychology of Education, 11(1):43–54.

Lang, S.N., Schoppe-Sullivan, S.J., Kotila, L.E., Feng, X., Kamp Dush, C.M. et al. (2014) Relations between fathers' and mothers' infant engagement patterns in dual-earner families and toddler competence. Journal of Family Issues, 35(8):1107–1127.

MacDonald, K., Parke, R.D. (1986) Parent-child physical play: The effects of sex and age of children and parents. Sex Roles, 15(7):367–378.

Majdandži, M., Möller, E., de Vente W., Bögels S., van den Boom D. (2014) Fathers' challenging parenting behavior prevents social anxiety development in their 4-year-old children: A longitudinal observational study. Journal of Abnormal Child Psychology, 42(2):301–310.

Miller, L.J. (2017) Creating a common terminology for play behavior to increase cross-disciplinary research. Learning & Behavior, 45:330–334.

Nagy, E. (2011) The newborn infant: A missing stage in developmental psychology. Infant and Child Development, 20(1):3–19.

Nakano, S., Kondo-Ikemura, K., Kusanagi, E. (2007) Perturbation of Japanese mother-infant habitual interactions in the double video paradigm and relationship to maternal playfulness. Infant Behavior and Development, 30(2):213–231.

O'Neill, C., Trainor, L.J. (2001) Infants' responsiveness to fathers' singing. Music Perception, 18(4):409–425.

Pancsofar, N., Vernon-Feagans, L. (2010) Fathers' early contributions to children's language development in families from low-income rural communities. Early Childhood Research Quarterly, 25(4):450–463.

Peterson, J.B., Flanders, J.L. (2005) Play and the regulation of aggression. In: Tremblay, R.E., Hartup, W., Archer, J. (Eds.) The Developmental Origins of Aggression. New York: Guildford Press: 133–159.

Robinson, E.L., StGeorge, J., Freeman, E.E. (2021) A systematic review of father–child play interactions and the impacts on child development. Children, 8(5):389.

Roggman, L.A., Boyce, L.K., Cook, G.A., Christiansen, K., Jones, D. (2004) Playing with Daddy: Social toy play, Early Head Start, and developmental outcomes. Fathering, 2(1):83–108.

Roopnarine, J.L., Yildirim, E.D. (2018) Paternal and maternal engagement in play, story telling, and reading in five Caribbean countries: Associations with preschoolers' literacy skills. International Journal of Play, 7(2):132–145.

Trehub, S.E., Unyk, A.M., Kamenetsky, S.B., Hill, D.S., Trainor, L.J., et al. (1997) Mothers' and fathers' singing to infants. Developmental Psychology, 33(3):500–507.

Yogman, M.W. (2001) Games fathers and mothers play with their infants. Infant Mental Health Journal, 2(4):241–248.

Zaouche-Gaudron, C., Ricaud, H., Beaumatin, A. (1998) Father-child play interaction and subjectivity. European Journal of Psychology of Education, 13(4):447–460.

# 11

# CREATIVE PLAY SPACES

## Finding the Space for Play

*Frances Brett*

At a time when it seems that creativity is demanded more and more as a desirable attribute in the working world, there is an increasing emphasis on creativity within curricula and a demand for creative play. Play and creativity are terms that we use freely but may mean different things to different people, dependent on context or the phase of life we are experiencing. As adults, we are apt to define play as the opposite to work – so it becomes the gamut of freely chosen activities that we seek out as leisure. Play may be viewed as non-serious, frivolous, and ephemeral, and so consequently without inherent value. However, for a child, play may be their predominant mode of engaging with the world.

*

Here's a picture: a parent – mother or father – holds the gaze of their very young baby. They are close to each other, the baby in the parent's arms, or simply near – lying on the floor perhaps. The baby opens their mouth wide, and after a moment, the parent responds, opening their mouth wide too, copying that face. The baby continues to make the face and the parent continues to reflect it back…until the baby's expression changes and the parent's changes too. A small moment, an endless game. But already, a relationship is being established in which playfulness is key and the place for play – the play space, if you like – is defined by that relationship. The actual space is very small – as small as the field of their shared gaze – but it is the connection between the two people involved that makes play possible, that creates the space for play to begin.

At its simplest, perhaps play can be delineated as an approach that is characterised by the impulse to discover, 'What if?' What will happen if I drop this bottle, open this door, step in that mud, tickle my dad's nose? If you like, play begins with a question, an openness, however deep in our consciousness, and it

DOI: 10.4324/9781003223771-13

develops in an atmosphere that sustains the asking of questions, an environment where possibility is recognised and honoured: A place for possibility thinking, as Craft describes it (see Burnard et al., 2006). This confers a seriousness and sense of purpose that should not be underestimated, and along with this, a respect for children's play as their means of questioning and thinking.

To reduce creativity to its most fundamental aspect is to view it as the process of making connections, of recombining separate elements in numerous varying (and possibly surprising) ways. Inevitably, a playful approach that embraces the possibility of thinking described above leads to making connections, and not necessarily the most obvious ones: What will happen if I mix this thick blue paint with spaghetti? Tie these spoons together? Press this brick into the mud? In the act of making connections, new discoveries occur allowing for transformation in thinking and the concrete expression of this as realised objects, plans, or conceptions. Connection allows ideas to flow forward and find new forms of expression.

The facial communication between parent and child described above is rooted in 'What if?' and grows into an exchange if there is the time for this to unfold and if there is a developing bond. This bond, of course, has its basis in trust, and without this emotional security, it is hard to find the freedom to be open – in order to play!

Here's another picture: A group of children, all under five, playing in the river on a summer's day. The water level is low and their initial freely chosen engagement is with collecting stones – beautiful rounded white pebbles that fit comfortably and pleasingly into the palm of the hand, and hurling these into the water as far or as high as possible to make the biggest or the quietest splash. Then, subtly, the activity changes into several different preoccupations: Gathering stones, organising them by size or colour, piling them, making structures. Towers and walls start to emerge and then sorties are made to find things to put around or within these structures: Twigs, leaves, flowers, or more stones. For some of the children, the focus is simply the water: Capturing it in their hands, buckets, or nets, releasing it, pouring it....the children work together, in pairs or small groups, or apart, as their interest takes them, in the water or at its margins. As the afternoon wears on, stories begin to emerge of fish heroes, underwater princesses, tiny people who live in the stone castle that has been constructed, and pictures develop in the mud, drawn with sticks or made from assemblages of whatever has been found, including pieces of twine and a piece of fallen branch.

In this example, the field of play is much larger, more diffuse, involving more people, but there are similarities with the example of the parent and child gazing at each other. In both cases, there is a relationship between those involved; there are freely available materials – whether the parent's face, as a kind of mirror, or the naturally occurring playthings of the riverbank; and there is the freedom to try things out to see what might emerge. The play unfolds and develops in the luxury of time just to be, and imagination, artistry, and construction are elicited naturally as a consequence.

The examples above support the identification of some defining features of a creative play space, and it is clear that these do not apply simply to the physicality of the area, but also to the emotional atmosphere and the attitudes brought to bear. What is key appears to be a space which is open, both literally and metaphorically: That is, a space which is not pre-defined in terms of its use but is the 'whatever you want it to be' space that Broadhead and Burt (2012) examine through numerous vibrant examples. Such a space is potent, open to improvisation, suggestion and change, leading directly to the possibility of and opportunities for making connections. Alongside this, the attitudes of those within the space (parents, practitioners, key or family support workers, other children) foster this spirit directly through their own responses and by supporting a prevailing atmosphere of security and trust – leading to openness once again!

Defining the creative play space in this way means it is much less important to be concerned with the kind of space that is offered, its size, or even what you put into it; instead, the emphasis is on the feelings and attitudes that surround it. In a sense, these become the play boundaries, so that it doesn't matter whether the space is as small as a kitchen table or as large as an open field. In the examples above, the play and creativity arise from materials immediately to hand, whether the face of a trusted other or the elements of the natural world. The constants that release the play and creativity are a sense of trust and safety, establishing an open space in which the 'What if?' question can be asked again and again.

In one setting where I have worked, a pre-school for two- to five-year olds in which the age groups were not separate, we adopted the practice of clearing the main play room ready for the start of each session, so that it was simply an empty carpeted space: A blank slate. Into this the children brought their own starting points for exploration, whether a loved toy from home, a snail shell found in the garden, or an idea in their heads. Our role was to listen and respond and support the children's ideas as they emerged. So, on one particular day, these ideas were a lullaby for Ellen's baby doll, spiral patterns copied from the shape of the back of the snail Ben had found, and how to make a rucksack – Nila's key question on arrival that morning. The lullaby developed by playing (and so experimenting) with instruments and sounds, trying to find 'whispery' music, as Ellen put it. Ben's experimental, spiral patterns were found everywhere, in sand, paint, chalk on the ground outside, and a pattern of books laid out on the floor – as if he were leaving his own snail trails. As the day went on, it was possible to see Ben's development in the control of the shape he was making – he was also experimenting with making an 's' shape alongside the spirals. Nila drew her ideas for rucksack design and discussed these at length with her closest friend and her key person, before trying out different materials to see which would be strongest but also easiest to cut.

All the above, from the lullaby to the rucksack, were creative products if you like, but were arrived at through the child's own mode – play – and developed through a playful process that is the essence of creativity. The process was driven by 'What if?' and the possibility of making connections in terms of materials and ideas. The creative process was supported by a potentiating environment offering space (both physical and temporal) and access to a range of open-ended materials that enabled expression and had the ability to be transformed into something new.

The other element that supported the creative process was the opportunity for dialogue, child to child (or children), or child to adult, enabling ideas to be articulated, questioned, examined, and so further developed. Again, such dialogue is only comfortable in an atmosphere of trust where thoughts can be aired in safety. In recent years, Ephgrave (2018) has promoted 'in the moment' planning in early years environments in England, rooted in these principles.

An extended UK project that explored the nature of creativity and how this might be supported in children's and adults' lives involved collaborative work between educational settings, artists, and cultural centres and led to the establishment of the arts-based action research organisation, 5x5x5=creativity. The original research, captured by Bancroft et al. (2008), offers excellent examples of a varied range of environments in which creativity was fostered through a playful approach. Here, Deborah Jones, one of the artists involved, outlines the kind of environment that supports her own creative work and that she sought to recreate with children and adults:

> I had in mind a model of an imaginary studio – fairly empty with work spaces, lots of light, almost formless materials which can take on any shape, for example, Plaster of Paris, stone. It will have openness and spaciousness. A space in which I can be there and leave other things aside; in that space I can make anything.

> *(Jones quoted in Bancroft, 2008)*

Here, then, is a simple formula for a creative play space:

- Open space
- Open minds
- Open-ended materials

And taking the 'O' of 'open' as a circle, a useful symbol is created: An empty space bounded by a sense of safety, security, and trust, in which things can happen!

## Practice Pointers

- Demonstrate playful interactions with babies and young children.
- Give new parents confidence in their ability to be playful.
- Encourage new parents to see themselves as their babies' first point of play.

## References

Bancroft, S., Fawcett, M., Hay, P. (2008) Researching Children Researching the World: 5x5x5=creativity. Stoke-on-Trent: Trentham Books.

Broadhead, P., Burt, A. (2012) Understanding Young Children's Learning Through Play: Building playful pedagogies. London: Routledge.

Burnard, P., Craft, A., Duffy, B., Hanson, R., Keene, J. et al. (2006) Documenting 'possibility thinking': A journey of collaborative inquiry. International Journal of Early Years Education, 14(3):243–262.

Elders, L., Aguirre Jones, D., Fawcett, M. (2008) Case study a) Kinder Garden Nursery. In: Bancroft, S., Fawcett, M., Hay, P. (Eds.) Researching Children Researching the World 5x5x5=Creativity. Stoke-on-Trent: Trentham Books Ltd: 76.

Ephgrave, A. (2018) Planning in the Moment with Young Children: A practical guide for early years practitioners and parents. London: Routledge.

# 12

# SUPPORTING THE DEVELOPMENT OF EMOTION REGULATION IN YOUNG CHILDREN

## Role of the Parent–Child Attachment Relationship

*Shauna L. Tominey, Svea G. Olsen and Megan M. McClelland*

For infants and toddlers, emotions play an important role in enabling them to communicate their needs to their parents and caregivers. Although we don't like to see children upset or having unpleasant feelings like anger, disappointment, or sadness, these emotions and others give us helpful information. Helping children learn to effectively express and manage their many emotions is an important part of development and grounded in the parent–child attachment relationship.

*

Happy. Sad. Frustrated. Excited. Angry. Disappointed. Calm. These are just a few of the many emotions that play a role in shaping our daily lives. Emotions influence our behaviour and are foundational to the human experience. We all experience a range of emotions, and from birth, emotions play a critical role in our lives. Starting in infancy, we express a core set of emotions, including happiness, sadness, anger, surprise, and disgust (Berk, 2011). We continue to experience these emotions throughout our childhood and adult lives, developing more complex and subtle emotions as we grow, including shame, hope, and guilt (Tangney & Fischer, 1995). Parents and caregivers can learn to read young children's emotional cues to figure out a child's likes, dislikes, wants, and needs. If sensitive and responsive to these cues, parents and caregivers can help regulate a child's emotions (Thompson & Meyer, 2007). For example, a parent might soothe a crying infant with feeding and rocking or calm a frustrated toddler by hugging and using a calm voice. Regulating a child's emotions in this way is referred to as 'external regulation' (Bernier et al., 2010). As children progress through early childhood, they begin to shift from relying solely on external regulation (a caregiver giving them a hug) to a combination of co-regulation and self-regulation (e.g. taking a deep breath to calm themselves down on their

DOI: 10.4324/9781003223771-14

own), also called 'internal regulation'. The term 'emotion regulation' refers to the external and internal processes that help an individual monitor, evaluate, and modify their reactions to emotions (Thompson & Meyer, 2007). Developing emotion regulation (and in particular, internal regulation abilities) is an important milestone for children. In fact, research shows that children who have strong emotion regulation skills are more likely to have positive relationships with peers, do better academically in the short- and long-term, and transition more easily into later grades than peers with weaker emotion regulation skills (Blair & Diamond, 2008).

There are many different factors that affect the development of emotion regulation, including a child's temperament and personality, physiological processes (brain development and maturation), and the role of the parent–child attachment relationship (Calkins & Hill, 2007; Thompson & Meyer, 2007). In this chapter, we focus on the role of the parent–child attachment relationship as it relates to emotion regulation development and share specific ways that parents and caregivers can lay a foundation for children's emotion regulation during the early childhood years.

## Importance of Parent–Child Attachment for Emotion Regulation

The development of a secure and trusting relationship (a secure attachment) between a child and at least one parent or caregiver lays the foundation for many positive outcomes, including emotion regulation (Calkins & Hill, 2007). A secure attachment is formed when a caregiver provides consistent sensitive care, adapting their caregiving to fit their child's needs (Bowlby, 1998). Although most infants have the same basic needs (attention, food, diapering, sleep, comfort, and love), the emotional cues they show through facial expressions, body language, crying, and cooing may be drastically different. Some children rarely cry and soothe quickly. Other children are highly reactive, cry easily, and take more effort to calm down. Most children fall somewhere in between these extremes. How reactive children are and how easily they calm down is related to their temperament – the individual differences that serve as the foundation for a child's personality (Eisenberg et al., 2009). Whether we are aware of it or not, a child's temperament and personality can affect the way that we respond to them, too. The match between a child and the adults in their life (parents or caregivers) can be thought of in terms of a 'goodness of fit' (Rothbart et al., 2006). Adults who can adjust their caregiving style to meet the temperament and personality of their infant are likely to develop a strong goodness of fit, sending a message to children that they can be trusted and relied on. This relationship helps children feel secure and safe. By two to three years, children develop expectations for the important people in their lives (Ainsworth et al., 1978; Bowlby, 1998). If children learn that the adults in their lives will consistently respond with warmth and support, they are more likely to seek comfort from them and to look to them for support. The shift of emotion regulation from a primarily external process to a primarily internal process relies on the foundation laid by this early attachment relationship. With a secure attachment relationship in place, there are many things parents and caregivers can do to further promote the development of strong emotion regulation skills in young children. The early childhood years are an important time to promote these skills because this is the time that children's brains are growing most rapidly in areas related to emotion regulation, especially the prefrontal cortex (Couperus & Nelson, 2006).

What can parents and caregivers do to promote emotion regulation during early childhood? We provide six recommendations that professionals and others working in the very early years can offer for specific strategies to try at home to foster a secure attachment relationship and to support the development of emotion regulation in children.

## Spend Time Actively Engaging with Your Child

Spending time with children, engaging in face-to-face activities such as talking, cuddling, and playing is one way to strengthen your relationship with your child. To make the most of this time together, remove potential distractions, including cell phones, the television, or other digital devices which could divide attention and detract from the connection that you are building with your child. Talk to your child about your day, your likes and dislikes, and what you appreciate about them. You can ask questions about your child's likes, dislikes, and interests as well. Quality time can occur as part of everyday errands, including going to the grocery store or preparing dinner. Time spent actively engaging with children helps you get to know your child better and supports the development of a secure attachment and a trusting relationship.

## Get to Know Your Child's Cues

Every child expresses emotions in different ways. Paying careful attention to emotional cues will help you understand how your child is feeling, enabling you to better support your child's needs. What does your child's face look like when she is feeling upset? How does your child express feelings like excitement or anger? What signs does your child show when tired? Identifying your child's emotional cues helps you to better anticipate emotional frustrations and either prevent them or prepare for them effectively, thus providing external emotion regulation. Getting to know your child's cues will also aid in the development of strong connections.

## Model Strong Emotion Regulation Abilities

A powerful and effective way to teach children new skills, including emotion regulation, is through modelling of the target behaviour. When children see skills modelled by people they trust, they are more likely to replicate and practice those skills themselves (Bandura, 1973). You can provide your child with a framework of 'what to do' rather than 'what not to do' by modelling positive emotion regulation skills. Throughout the day, take time to demonstrate ways that you regulate your emotions, describing what you are doing and why (e.g. 'When that happened, I felt very upset so I took a few deep breaths to calm myself down before I said anything so that I would not yell'). Describing actions can not only help you become more intentional about the strategies you use to regulate your emotions, but can also help children understand why you are doing what you are doing so that they can make these choices themselves in the future.

## Use Words to Help Your Child Identify and Express Their Emotions and Feelings

Helping children develop a rich vocabulary of emotion words and words related to the expression and regulation of emotions is important. During early childhood, the number of words children know and use grows exponentially. Making sure children have the words they need to talk about their emotional experiences can help them describe how they are feeling, ask for help when needed and ultimately, regulate their emotions. Talk about how you are feeling throughout the day and describe your child's emotional experiences (e.g. 'I'm feeling disappointed because I really wanted to visit my friend today and I did not have a chance' or 'I see you are frowning and stomping your feet. You look like you might be feeling angry or frustrated. How are you feeling?') Additionally, it's important to point out to children when they demonstrate strong emotion regulation skills and to acknowledge their efforts (e.g. 'It looks like you are really excited to play, but are waiting patiently to have a turn'). Integrating discussion of emotions that you and your child experience into daily interactions lets children know that everyone has emotions (children and adults alike), both positive and negative.

## Teach Your Child Specific Emotion Regulation Strategies

There are many things that you can do to teach children specific emotion regulation strategies. First, you can share personal stories with your child about your own experiences with emotions (e.g. 'I remember a time when I felt disappointed'). As part of these stories, you can share things that you thought, said, or did to help manage your emotions well. Second, you can integrate conversations about emotions into shared reading of storybooks with children, pointing out how characters look when they are expressing different emotions or asking your child questions about characters' experiences with emotions. Third, playing games with children gives them the opportunity to practice regulation and impulse control outside of emotionally charged moments. Children's games such as 'Simon Says' and 'Red Light, Green Light' that encourage children to stop and think before acting can strengthen their self-regulation (McClelland et al., 2019; Schmitt et al., 2015; Tominey & McClelland, 2011). Practicing emotion regulation strategies outside of emotionally charged moments increases the likelihood that children will be able to call upon these strategies during emotionally challenging moments. Finally, taking time to discuss with your child effective ways to express and regulate their emotions is important; for example, what do you want your child to do when feeling angry? How can they let you know they are feeling this way? Is it okay to hit a family member? No. What about stomping feet? Probably. What are the rules about expressing emotions at home? Just like other household rules, it is important to discuss what the rules are so that children and adults can work on following them together.

## Realize That Emotion Regulation Development Is a Process

Just like any skill, developing emotion regulation takes significant time and practice and, for most people, these skills continue to develop throughout life. As you strive to model strong emotion regulation abilities for your child, it is important to realize that we all may have difficulty managing emotions, particularly when we are tired or stressed. We need to be forgiving of ourselves and of our child in these moments and reinforce the notion that emotion regulation is a skill that needs to be practiced and developed and that everyone makes mistakes. After experiencing a breakdown in regulation skills (e.g. yelling back at your child instead of remaining calm), you can think about what you would like your child to do in a similar situation. If you would like to see your child apologize and make amends once they are calm, you can model these actions in your interactions with your child (e.g. 'I'm sorry. I should not have shouted in that way. I was very upset and had a hard time calming down. Next time, I'm going to take a few deep breaths and calm down before I say anything'). When your child has difficulty regulating their emotions (e.g. throwing a temper tantrum), you can have a conversation once your child has calmed down about what happened and what they can do next time the trigger arises in order to respond more effectively (e.g. 'What do you think you can do next time your brother takes your toy? What about saying, "That's mine. Please give it back." Let's practice that together').

## Conclusion

Emotions are an integral part of our lives. Fostering a secure parent–child attachment relationship lays an important foundation for helping children manage their own emotions. There are many things that parents and caregivers can do to help children practice managing their emotional experiences effectively, and, in doing so, support children to learn skills that will help them socially and academically from birth through adulthood.

## Practice Pointers

*Below are prompts practitioners can share with parents and caregivers to help children practice emotion regulation skills.*

- Spend Time Actively Engaging with Your Child
  - What parts of your day can you reserve for connecting with your child while putting away other distractions?
  - What are some questions you can ask to connect with your child? For example, 'What is something that made you laugh today?' Or, 'Tell me about a time today that you felt calm.'
- Get to Know Your Child's Cues
  - How do you know when your child is expressing a certain emotion? For example, what do their face and body look like when they are feeling excited, scared, angry, or calm?
  - What cues do you recognize in yourself when you experience these different emotions? How are your cues similar to and different from your child's emotions?
- Model Strong Emotion Regulation Abilities
  - What strategies do you use to regulate your own emotions effectively?
  - What happens when you can't manage your emotions well?
  - When you are not able to regulate your emotions well, what is something you wish you could have done differently?
- Use Words to Help Your Child Identify and Express Their Emotions and Feelings
  - Point out the feelings of characters in storybooks. What new feeling words can you introduce into your child's vocabulary through stories and in everyday moments?
  - When describing your own or another's feelings to your child, how can you use more nuanced emotion words? For example, was the character in the storybook feeling scared, or just a little nervous?
- Teach Your Child Emotion Regulation Strategies
  - How do you want your child to express big feelings such as frustration or anger? Talk about your family emotion rules together.
  - What stories can you share with your child about a time you felt really good about the way you managed an emotion?
  - What storybooks can you read with your child that involve a character managing (or not being able to manage) an emotion they experience?
  - When reading together, what questions can you ask your child about the way characters are regulating their emotions? For example, 'What could they do to help themselves feel better?' Or, 'When you feel that way, what is something that makes you feel better?'
  - What games can you play with your child that involve stopping and starting (impulse control)?

- Recognize That Emotion Regulation Development Is a Learning Process
  - What can you do to show yourself patience and forgiveness when you do not regulate your emotions in a way that you feel good about?
  - What can you say to your child to show patience and forgiveness when they are not able to regulate their emotions?

## References

Ainsworth, M.D.S., Blehar, M.C., Waters, E., Wall, S. (1978) Patterns of Attachment: A psychological study of the Strange Situation. Oxford: Lawrence Erlbaum.

Bandura, A. (1973) Social Learning Theory. New York: General Learning Press.

Berk, L.E. (2011) Infants and Children: Prenatal through middle childhood (7th ed.) New York: Pearson.

Bernier, A., Carlson, S.M., Whipple, N. (2010) From external regulation to self-regulation: Early parenting precursors of young children's executive functioning. Child Development, 81(1):326–339.

Blair, C., Diamond, A. (2008) Biological processes in prevention and intervention: The promotion of self-regulation as a means of preventing school failure. Development and Psychopathology, 20(03):899–911.

Bowlby, J. (1998) A Secure Base: Parent-child attachment and healthy human development. London: Basic Books.

Calkins, S., Hill, A. (2007) Caregiver influences on emerging emotion regulation. In: Gross, J.J. (Ed.) Handbook of Emotion Regulation. New York: Guilford Press: 229–248.

Couperus, J.W., Nelson, C.A. (2006) Early brain development and plasticity. In: McCartney, K., Phillip, D. (Eds.) Blackwell Handbook of Early Childhood Development. Malden, MA: Blackwell Publishing: 85–105.

Eisenberg, N., Vaughan, J., Hofer, C. (2009) Temperament, self-regulation, and peer social competence. In: Rubin, K.H., Bukowski, W.M., Laursen, B. (Eds.) Handbook of Peer Interactions, Relationships and Groups. New York: Guilford Press: 473–489.

McClelland, M.M., Tominey, S.L., Schmitt, S.A., Hatfield, B.E., Purpura, D.J. et al. (2019) Red Light, Purple Light! Results of an intervention to promote school readiness for children from low-income backgrounds. Frontiers in Psychology, 10:2365.

Rothbart, M.K., Posner, M.I., Kieras, J. (2006) Temperament, attention, and the development of self-regulation. In: McCartney, K., Phillip, D. (Eds.) Blackwell Handbook of Early Childhood Development. Malden, MA: Blackwell Publishing: 338–357.

Schmitt, S.A., McClelland, M.M., Tominey, S.L., Acock, A.C. (2015) Strengthening school readiness for Head Start children: Evaluation of a self-regulation intervention. Early Childhood Research Quarterly, 30:20–31.

Tangney, J.P., Fischer, K.W. (Eds.) (1995) Self-conscious Emotions: The psychology of shame, guilt, embarrassment, and pride. New York: Guilford Press.

Thompson, R.A., Meyer, S. (2007) Socialization of emotion regulation in the family. In: Gross, J.J. (Ed.) Handbook of Emotion Regulation. New York: Guilford Press: 249–268.

Tominey, S.L., McClelland, M.M. (2011) Red Light, Purple Light: Findings from a randomized trial using circle time games to improve behavioral self-regulation in preschool. Early Education and Development, 22(3):489–519.

# 13

# THE TRANSITION TO PARENTHOOD AND EARLY CHILD DEVELOPMENT IN FAMILIES WITH LGBTQ+ PARENTS

*Rachel H. Farr and Samantha L. Tornello*

*

The numbers and visibility of LGBTQ+ parents are increasing around the world. In the United States, as many as 6 million individuals have an LGBTQ+ parent, including 2–3 million under age 18, with LGBTQ+ people of color (POC) being more likely to be a parent (American Psychological Association [APA], 2020; Patterson et al., 2021). Of note, very little research has accounted for intersectionality among LGBTQ+ parents with multiple identities such as LGBTQ+ POC (Tornello, 2020). LGBTQ+ adults become parents through many pathways, including adoption and foster care, co-parenting with other adults, and assisted reproductive technologies (ART) (Cao et al., 2016; Patterson et al., 2021; Tornello et al., 2019). Thus, as the diversity of families grows, there is an increased need for new parents and their service providers to have accessible information about parenthood and early child development in LGBTQ+ parent families (Goldberg & Allen, 2020; National Academies of Science, Engineering and Medicine [NASEM], 2020).

---

**BOX 13.1: KEY QUESTIONS RELEVANT TO LGBTQ+ PRO-SPECTIVE PARENTS AND SERVICE PROVIDERS:**

1 What can LGBTQ+ parents and their partners expect during the transition to parenthood?
2 How are young children (birth to four years) with LGBTQ+ parents developing?

---

DOI: 10.4324/9781003223771-15

## Transition to Parenthood for LGBTQ+ Parents and Their Partners

Although becoming a parent is wonderful, it can put great stress on individuals and relationships. Among cisgender, heterosexual (cis-het) adults, the transition to parenthood has been associated with decreases in marital quality and relationship functioning (e.g. Cowan & Cowan, 2000). Becoming parents as LGBTQ+ partners can present similar challenges. For example, the transition to parenthood brings changes in individual roles within the family. Among cis-het partners, roles are often differentiated by gender, with mothers performing more childcare (e.g. Farr & Patterson, 2013). For LGBTQ+ parents, there are unique factors that should be considered when thinking about the transition to parenthood (Cao et al., 2016; Rubio et al., 2020).

How LGBTQ+ people become parents can vary greatly. The majority of older LGBTQ+ parents formed their families within the context of a former cis-het identity and/or relationship; in contrast, younger LGBTQ+ people are more likely to become parents within the context of their LGBTQ+ identities and relationships (NASEM, 2020; Tornello et al., 2015, 2019). Some common pathways to parenthood for LGBTQ+ people include adoption or foster care, donor insemination, sexual intercourse, as well as the use of ART, including embryo donation, in vitro fertilization, and surrogacy. These pathways each involve different challenges that LGBTQ+ people must weigh against their personal desires and reproductive abilities (Cao et al., 2016; Park et al., 2020), along with variations in opportunity, access, and obstacles based on socioeconomic status and additional minoritized identities (Carpenter & Niesen, 2021; NASEM, 2020). In the context of barriers related to stigma, cost, and access to services, LGBTQ+ people pursuing parenthood face numerous practical and emotionally laden decisions regarding reproductive health and finances (Carpenter & Niesen, 2021; Levitt et al., 2020; Park et al., 2020; Tornello & Bos, 2017). For example, among two LGBTQ+ partners who both have a uterus and ovaries and want to pursue donor insemination, decisions must be made about who will carry the child, which individual's eggs will be used, who will be the sperm donor, and what role (if any) the donor(s) will have in the child's life (Carpenter & Niesen, 2021; Goldberg & Allen, 2020). These decisions can be compounded by additional challenges; for example, donor sperm representing racial/ethnic minority backgrounds are often very limited. These choices (or lack of) about their family and the role other individuals may play in the child's life are important among LGBTQ+ people becoming parents.

Becoming a parent brings tremendous changes to an individual's life, partner relationships, and the overall family system, regardless of sexual orientation and gender identity (NASEM, 2020). Much of the research comparing LGBTQ+ to cis-het adults during the transition to parenthood has revealed similar experiences (Goldberg & Allen, 2020). All parents of newborn babies and young children experience sleep deprivation and time spent as partners is decreased (Goldberg & Allen, 2020; Saxbe et al., 2018). Thus, it is unsurprising that partners becoming parents typically experience changes in relationship quality (Cao et al., 2016) and satisfaction (Baiocco et al., 2015). For LGBTQ+ and cis-het partners across the transition to parenthood, there are, on average, declines in relationship quality, intimacy, love, and satisfaction, as well as increases in ambivalence, stress, and conflict (Goldberg & Allen, 2020; NASEM, 2020). Changes in partner relationship functioning occur, but these are due to becoming parents, not parental sexual or gender identity.

Beyond changes in relationship functioning, the transition to parenthood can impact parents' mental and physical health (Saxbe et al., 2018). Becoming a parent is typically seen as a positive experience, yet it also involves many individual stressors. LGBTQ+ and cis-het parents can experience increases in depression, anxiety, and parenting-related stress, across the transition to parenthood (Goldberg & Allen, 2020). Some of the expected or experienced changes among new parents regard job and careers (Simon et al., 2018, 2019). LGBTQ+ parents, like cis-het parents, report changes in paid employment or work hours, as well as in living arrangements related to childcare and new parenting (Goldberg & Allen, 2020).

## Bonding

In two-parent LGBTQ+ families, research has indicated that children bond with both parents. However, for many LGBTQ+ families, biological relatedness can create legal hurdles or social invisibility (Goldberg & Allen, 2020). Legal invisibility can result when only one parent is able to be a legal parent based on biological ties (Cao et al., 2016; Farr & Goldberg, 2018). Social invisibility may result when biological relatedness becomes linked with the legitimacy of being a parent, which can fuel feelings of anxiety or jealousy among partners (Cao et al., 2016). Anxious feelings are commonly reported among LGBTQ+ partners who do not share a biological or genetic link to their children, or for whom the genetic ties are discrepant (i.e. one partner is biologically related to their child while the other is not), such as among those who pursue surrogacy, donor insemination, or other ART (Carpenter & Niesen, 2021; Goldberg & Allen, 2020). Anxiety about biological connection and feelings of rejection and tension resulting from children's parental preferences have also been described among LGBTQ+ adoptive parents (Goldberg & Allen, 2020). These challenges can be associated with relationship issues among partners, but they are not necessarily unique to LGBTQ+ parents.

## Who Does What?

One area that has varied consistently across sexual orientation is how couples divide their household (cleaning, laundry) and childcare (feeding, bathing) tasks. Typically, heterosexual couples divide chores based on gender norms, with women doing more of the housework and childcare and men working more in outside paid employment (Farr & Patterson, 2013). The research on LGBTQ+ partners (with and without children) has uncovered that they tend to divide labor in an egalitarian fashion (NASEM, 2020). There have been some interesting exceptions to these findings, with some research uncovering that parents biologically related to the child perform more childcare, especially early in the child's life (Farr et al., 2019; NASEM, 2020). Biological relatedness, however, is not always a factor – preferences for certain tasks and other practical considerations driven by hours in paid employment may be more influential (Farr et al., 2019; NASEM, 2020; Tornello, 2020). Among gay surrogate fathers, biological fathers did not do more household or childcare-related tasks, although biological fathers in stepfamilies were providing more childcare labor (Tornello et al., 2015). These same patterns have been found among transgender and non-binary parents (Tornello, 2020). Among LGBTQ+ parents, division of labor is designed differently compared to cis-het parents, but regardless of sexual and gender identity, partners who are less satisfied with how labor is divided report poorer relationship quality and well-being (Goldberg & Allen, 2020; Tornello, 2020).

## Discrimination and Stigma

LGBTQ+ parents experience discrimination and stigma related to sexuality and/ or gender, which can impact every individual in the family system, both during the transition to parenthood and after becoming parents. This can come from many sources: Professionals who interact with LGBTQ+ people, other interpersonal interactions, institutional policies or practices, and state or federal laws (Levitt et al., 2020; Patterson et al., 2021; Perrin et al., 2016).

LGBTQ+ adults pursuing parenthood commonly report discrimination from medical professionals or adoption agencies who will not assist them in trying to have children due to religious beliefs (Goldberg & Allen, 2020; NASEM, 2020). LGBTQ+ prospective parents overall may be ignored or treated poorly, which may result in part from implicit bias (i.e. unconscious preferences) favoring cis-het individuals among medical and adoption agency staff (Goldberg & Allen, 2020; NASEM, 2020; Sabin et al., 2015). Prospective LGBTQ+ parents describe concerns about raising children in a cis/heterosexist, discriminating society as well as facing stigma from service providers working with these families (Cao et al., 2016; Carpenter & Niesen, 2021; Levitt et al., 2020; Park et al., 2020). LGBTQ+ parents also experience or have fears of potential discrimination from pediatricians, day care providers, lawyers, religious institutions, family, and friends (Goldberg & Allen, 2020; NASEM, 2020; Park et al., 2020; Perrin et al., 2016; Simon et al., 2019). Friendships with childfree LGBTQ+ adults, as well as other parents, are described as important to LGBTQ+ parents and are known to change when becoming a parent (Goldberg & Allen, 2020; Simon et al., 2019). Given that 'mothers' are often viewed and culturally valued as superior, natural, or 'default' parents, LGBTQ+ parents who are not perceived as being a 'real' parent may also be particularly vulnerable to discrimination (Cao et al., 2016;

Carone et al., 2018; Perrin et al., 2016). Stigmatization negatively impacts the health of LGBTQ+ parents, although good social support can counteract these negative experiences (Goldberg & Allen, 2020; NASEM, 2020).

## Social Support

Changes in social networks and family relationships can occur during the transition to parenthood, and for all new parents, social support is an important component of well-being (Goldberg & Allen, 2020; NASEM, 2020). One challenge is that LGBTQ+ parents are often less close, on average, to their families of origin compared to cis-het parents (APA, 2020; NASEM, 2020). Some LGBTQ+ adults, however, report closer relationships with their family of origin after a (biologically related) child joins the family (Goldberg & Allen, 2020). Many LGBTQ+ parents describe wanting to have social support from other LGBTQ+ parents or those who have become parents through similar pathways (e.g. other adoptive parents) regardless of sexual orientation or gender (Simon et al., 2019). Indeed, social support – from partner relationships, chosen family (i.e. close relationships not based on biological ties) – can buffer negative impacts on mental health (e.g. depressive symptoms), including across the transition to parenthood (Goldberg & Allen, 2020; NASEM, 2020).

## The Development of Young Children with LGBTQ+ Parents

Public debate about LGBTQ+ parenting has focused on how children fare (APA, 2020). Over 40 years of research has consistently demonstrated the healthy development of children with LGBTQ+ parents from infancy to adulthood across many developmental domains, including academic achievement, socio-emotional development, peer relationships, behavioral adjustment, sexual identity, gender development, and so on (APA, 2020; Patterson et al., 2021). Many studies have examined outcomes for children's later development (in middle childhood, adolescence, and adulthood) rather than during the first few years of life, specifically among LGBTQ+ parents who created their family within the context of a former cis-het relationship, often including parental divorce/ separation. Studies examining school-age, adolescent, and young people's development in planned LGBTQ+ parent families (formed through different pathways) have been conducted across the United States, Europe, and Australia (APA, 2020; Patterson et al., 2021).

Of the research examining the outcomes for children with LGBTQ+ parents, many have focused on children's early development – infancy to four years. This research has explored children's attachment to parents, parent–child relationship quality, gender development, and mental health, as well as outside factors that may be associated with children's outcomes (e.g. stigmatization) (APA, 2020; Patterson et al., 2021). For instance, in a study of 97 adoptive families in the United Kingdom, children with gay fathers showed higher levels of secure-autonomous attachment than those with heterosexual parents (McConnachie et al., 2020). Available evidence indicates healthy attachment to parents among young children in LGBTQ+ parent families.

The gender development of children with LGBTQ+ parents has been a particular area of interest. In studies of toddlers and preschoolers with LGBTQ+ parents, few differences in overall gender typicality as compared to peers with cis-het parents have been uncovered, yet some point to greater flexibility in gendered play (APA, 2020; Bruun & Farr, 2021; Carone et al., 2020; NASEM, 2020). Thus, parental sexual and gender identity may play a role in more child-directed gender development. More research could identify the ways, the degree, and which mechanisms are involved.

Much of the existing research regarding children's development with LGBTQ+ parents has targeted behavioral adjustment. Across different family constellations and among samples around the world, the theme is consistent: children raised by LGBTQ+ parents do not show elevated behavior problems early in life. In the United States, Goldberg and Smith (2013) found that the externalizing and internalizing behavior problems of two-year-old children from 120 lesbian, gay, and heterosexual parent adoptive families did not vary by parental sexual orientation. Using a similar US sample, Farr et al. (2010) found no differences by parental sexual orientation in behavioral adjustment of 106 three-year-old children adopted as infants.

Studies outside the United States have also investigated early behavioral outcomes for children in LGBTQ+ parent families. In Australia, Crouch et al. (2014) found that among 500 children (median age, four years old) with same-sex parents, general health and behavioral adjustment were reported as being significantly better than population norms. Same-sex parents were more likely to immunize their children, and same-sex mothers were more likely to breastfeed (Crouch et al., 2014). Among 80 Italian lesbian (donor insemination), gay (surrogacy), and heterosexual parent families with toddlers, children's psychological well-being, emotional regulation, and peer relationships were indistinguishable based on parental sexual orientation (Baiocco et al., 2015). Using a similar sample, Baiocco et al. (2018) found that 3- to 11-year-old children with same-gender parents had fewer psychological problems than did those with heterosexual parents. Among 40 gay surrogate father families in the United Kingdom, three- to nine-year-old children had few behavior problems and were no different from those in lesbian mother families (through donor insemination) (Golombok et al., 2018). Similarly, Carone et al. (2018) found that three- to nine-year-old children (n=80) with gay fathers (via surrogacy) and lesbian mothers (via donor insemination) in Italy showed internalizing and externalizing behavior problems in the typical population range.

Research on early child development indicates that family processes matter more to child outcomes than family structure. In Farr and colleagues' research (2010), parenting stress, parenting approaches, and couple relationship were associated with preschool children's behavioral adjustment in their sample of 106 lesbian, gay, and heterosexual parent adoptive families. Farr and Patterson's (2013) study with the same sample demonstrated that parents who were more supportive of their partners in their parenting roles were more likely to have children with fewer behavior problems, regardless of whether parents were lesbian, gay, or heterosexual. Similarly, Goldberg and Smith (2013) found that among 120 adoptive lesbian, gay, and heterosexual parents, relationship conflict was significantly associated with their two-year-old children's internalizing behaviors. Greater depressive symptoms among parents were significantly associated with more internalizing and externalizing child behavior problems. Specifically related to adoption, parents' lack of adoption preparation was significantly related to greater internalizing and externalizing problems among children (Goldberg & Smith, 2013).

Stigma and discrimination appear particularly impactful to parenting and children's outcomes in LGBTQ+ parent families (Patterson et al., 2021; Perrin et al., 2016). In Crouch et al.'s (2014) study of 500 Australian children with same-sex parents, negative outcomes (e.g. less physical activity, poorer mental health, and family cohesion) were all significantly associated with increased stigma. Among Italian gay fathers (through surrogacy) with three- to ten-year-old children, homophobic microaggressions were linked with lower parental sensitivity (Carone et al., 2021). Greater behavior problems among three- to nine-year-old children through surrogacy were also reported among LG parents in the United Kingdom as well as in Italy who had experienced more stigma (Carone et al., 2018; Golombok et al., 2018). Thus, early child development in LGBTQ+ parent families appears to relate more strongly to parent adjustment, family relationships, and experiences of stigma, rather than parental sexual or gender identity.

## Conclusion

Many LGBTQ+ people are parents or want to become parents in the future (NASEM, 2020; Tasker & Gato, 2020; Tornello et al., 2019). Thus, knowledge about relationship dynamics as LGBTQ+ partners become parents is key for supporting healthy family relationships and strong parenting. Research that prioritizes the intersectional experiences of LGBTQ+ (prospective) POC, of lower-income backgrounds, and represents other marginalized identities is particularly under-represented and critical for future practice (Carpenter & Niesen, 2021; Tornello, 2020). Understanding factors that contribute to positive child development in LGBTQ+ parent families is essential for supporting new parents striving to provide their young children with the best possible foundation for a happy and healthy life.

## Practice Pointers

- Understand the different pathways to parenthood, along with the strengths/ challenges of each method.

- Encourage partners to discuss parenting and relationship expectations (including role divisions).
- Understand relevant laws and policies (at country, state/province/region, or local levels) that could impact LGBTQ+ parents.
- Support LGBTQ+ parents, partners, and their children in coping with discrimination and stigma.
- From an intersectional perspective, account for multiple identities (e.g. racial, cultural, or socioeconomic class) of every individual and the impact that those identities have on the experiences of all LGBTQ+ people.
- Encourage partners to develop strong and affirmative social support networks.
- Support relationship partners to engage in self-care activities that promote stress reduction.

## References

American Psychological Association (APA) (2020) Resolution on sexual orientation, gender identity (SOGI), parents, and their children. Available at: www.apa.org/pi/lgbt/resources/policy/sexual-orientation <accessed 09 Nov, 2021>

Baiocco, R., Carone, N., Loverno, S., Lingiardi, V. (2018) Same-sex and different-sex parent families in Italy: Is parents' sexual orientation associated with child health outcomes and parental dimensions? Journal of Developmental & Behavioral Pediatrics, 39:555–563.

Baiocco, R., Santamaria, F., Loverno, S., Fontanesi, L., Baumgartner, E. et al. (2015) Lesbian mother families and gay father families in Italy: Family functioning, dyadic satisfaction, and child well-being. Sexuality Research and Social Policy, 12:1–11.

Bruun, S.T., Farr, R.H. (2021) Longitudinal gender presentation and associated outcomes among adopted children with lesbian, gay, and heterosexual parents. Journal of GLBT Family Studies, 17:231–250.

Cao, H., Mills-Koonce, W.R., Wood, C., Fine, M.A. (2016) Identity transformation during the transition to parenthood among same-sex couples: An ecological, stress-strategy-adaptation perspective. Journal of Family Theory & Review, 8:30–59.

Carone, N., Lingiardi, V., Baiocco, R., Barone, L. (2021) Sensitivity and rough-and-tumble play in gay and heterosexual single-father families through surrogacy: The role of microaggressions and fathers' rumination. Psychology of Men & Masculinities, 22:476–487.

Carone, N., Lingiardi, V., Chirumbolo, A., Baiocco, R. (2018) Italian gay father families formed by surrogacy: Parenting, stigmatization, and children's psychological adjustment. Developmental Psychology, 54:1904–1916.

Carone, N., Lingiardi, V., Tanzilli, A., Bos, H.M.W., Baiocco, R. (2020) Gender development in children with gay, lesbian, and heterosexual parents: Associations with family type and child gender. Journal of Developmental & Behavioral Pediatrics, 41:38–47.

Carpenter, E., Niesen, R. (2021) 'It's just constantly having to make a ton of decisions that other people take for granted': Pregnancy and parenting desires for queer cisgender women and non-binary individuals assigned female at birth. Journal of GLBT Family Studies, 7:87–101.

Cowan, C.P., Cowan, P.A. (2000) When Partners Become Parents: The big life change for couples. Mahwah, NJ: Lawrence Erlbaum Associates Publishers.

Crouch, S.R., Waters, E., McNair, R., Power, J., Davis, E. (2014) Parent-reported measures of child health and wellbeing in same-sex parent families: A cross-sectional survey. BMC Public Health, 14:635–646.

Farr, R.H., Bruun, S.T., Patterson, C.J. (2019) Longitudinal associations between coparenting and child adjustment among lesbian, gay, and heterosexual adoptive parent families. Developmental Psychology, 55:2547–2560.

Farr, R.H., Forssell, S.L., Patterson, C.L. (2010) Parenting and child development in adoptive families: Does parental sexual orientation matter? Applied Developmental Science, 14:164–178.

Farr, R.H., Goldberg, A.E. (2018) Sexual orientation, gender identity, and adoption law. Family Court Review, 56:374–383.

Farr, R.H., Patterson, C.J. (2013) Coparenting among lesbian, gay, and heterosexual couples: Associations with adopted children's outcomes. Child Development, 84:1226–1240.

Goldberg, A.E., Allen, K.R. (Eds.) (2020) LGBTQ-parent Families: Innovations in research and implications for practice (2nd ed.). New York: Springer.

Goldberg, A.E., Smith, J.Z. (2013) Predictors of psychological adjustment in early placed adopted children with lesbian, gay, and heterosexual parents. Journal of Family Psychology, 27:431–442.

Golombok, S., Blake, L., Slutsky, J., Raffanello, E., Roman, G.D. et al. (2018) Parenting and the adjustment of children born to gay fathers through surrogacy. Child Development, 89:1223–1233.

Levitt, H.M., Schuyler, S.W., Chickerella, R., Elber, A., White, L. et al. (2020) How discrimination in adoptive, foster, and medical systems harms LGBTQ+ families: Research on the experiences of prospective parents. Journal of Gay & Lesbian Social Services, 32:261–282.

McConnachie, A.L., Ayed, N., Jadva, V., Lamb, M., Tasker, F. et al. (2020) Father-child attachment in adoptive gay father families. Attachment & Human Development, 22:110–123.

National Academies of Science, Engineering, and Medicine (NASEM) (2020) Understanding the well-being of LGBTQ+ populations. Washington: The National Academies Press.

Park, N., Schmitz, R.M., Slauson-Blevins, K. (2020) "It takes a lot of planning": Sexual minority young adult perceptions of gay and lesbian parenthood. Journal of Family Issues, 41:1785–1809.

Patterson, C.J., Farr, R.H., Goldberg, A.E. (2021) LGBTQ+ parents and their children. National Council on Family Relations: Policy Brief, 6:1–8.

Perrin, E.C., Pinderhughes, E.E., Mattern, K., Hurley, S.M., Newman, R.A. (2016) Experiences of children with gay fathers. Clinical Pediatrics, 55:1305–1317.

Rubio, B., Vecho, O., Gross, M., van Rijn-van Gelderen, L., Bos, H. et al. (2020) Transition to parenthood and quality of parenting among gay, lesbian and heterosexual couples who conceived through assisted reproduction. Journal of Family Studies, 26:422–440.

Sabin, J.A., Riskind, R.G., Nosek, B.A. (2015) Health care providers' implicit and explicit attitudes toward lesbian women and gay men. American Journal of Public Health, 105:1831–1841.

Saxbe, D., Rossin-Slater, M., Goldenberg, D. (2018) The transition to parenthood as a critical window for adult health. American Psychologist, 73:1190–1200.

Simon, K.A., Tornello, S.L., Bos, H.M.W. (2019) Sexual minority women and parenthood: Perceptions of friendship among childfree and new parents. Journal of Lesbian Studies, 23:476–489.

Simon, K.A., Tornello, S.L., Farr, R.H., Bos, H.M.W. (2018) Envisioning future parenthood among bisexual, lesbian, and heterosexual women. Psychology of Sexual Orientation and Gender Diversity, 5:253–259.

Tasker, F., Gato, J. (2020) Gender identity and future thinking about parenthood: A qualitative analysis of focus group data with transgender and non-binary people in the United Kingdom. Frontiers in Psychology, 11:865.

Tornello, S.L. (2020) Division of labor among transgender and gender non-binary parents: Associations with individual, couple, and children's behavioral outcomes. Frontiers in Psychology, 11. doi:10.3389/fpsyg.2020.00015

Tornello, S.L., Bos, H.M.W (2017) Parenting intentions among transgender individuals. LGBT Health, 4:115–120.

Tornello, S.L., Kruczkowski, S.M., Patterson, C.J. (2015) Division of labor and relationship quality among male same-sex couples who became fathers via surrogacy. Journal of GLBT Family Studies, 11:375–394.

Tornello, S.L., Riskind, R.G., Babíc, A. (2019) Transgender and gender non-binary parents' pathways to parenthood. Psychology of Sexual Orientation & Gender Diversity, 6:232–241.

Tornello, S.L., Sonnenberg, B., Patterson, C.J. (2015) Division of labor among gay fathers: Associations with parent, couple, and child adjustment. Journal of Psychology of Sexual Orientation and Gender Diversity, 2:365–375.

# PART III

# Preparation for Labour and Birth

## Introduction

This section of the book comprises three chapters inviting educators to reflect on how we prepare women and their partners for labour and birth, and why we prepare them in the way we do. In a profoundly personal piece of writing, one author examines the contribution mindfulness can make to childbirth preparation and explains how positively pregnant parents respond to new information about the way in which emotions (fear, hopefulness, excitement, calm) trigger hormones that in turn affect the way in which the body behaves during labour.

A midwife working in a Home Birth team looks at informed decision-making in relation to place of birth – how do we respond to couples' concerns and questions? She asks us to dig deep within ourselves and acknowledge and understand our perhaps unconscious biases about place of birth, and then with an open mind, seek the latest evidence on safety. She also asks us to listen to women's stories and, with humility, seek to understand what makes their experiences of giving birth positive and what leaves them emotionally damaged so that we can truly confront and understand the influence of different environments of care.

Taking up themes implicit in the previous two chapters, the final author in this section argues that a woman's preparation for birth needs to be experiential and body-centred, and that antenatal preparation should be minimally information-based, but instead focus on the pelvis and seek to awaken the birthing instinct.

All three authors would agree that women have an instinct for giving birth. If we are to challenge increasing rates of intervention in labour and birth across the world, we need to be part of an educational project that promotes birth as an event with a defined 'default' position that sits within the parameters of normal instinctual physiology.

DOI: 10.4324/9781003223771-16

# 14

# COMMENTARY

## A Mindful Approach to Childbirth Education and Preparation for Childbirth

*Lorna Davies*

In a world of increasing complexity, the pressures and expectations imposed upon pregnant women and their partners are great. For many, the notion of childbirth as a normal physiological process has been replaced by paradigms related to choice, risk, safety and fear (Scamell et al., 2019). The belief that we can prevent, manage and control risk is a potent, pervasive and persuasive one in birthing territory, an area of life that is in many ways fraught with uncertainty. Thus, safety has been turned into a commodity within the techno-rational healthcare setting, and healthcare professionals are expected to provide 'safety' for patients/clients (Skinner & Maude, 2016) often in the shape of technological intervention ranging from antenatal screening through to surgical childbirth. Fear results in women having greater reliance on technology in order to reduce any element of risk and to seek reassurance that the pregnancy or labour and birth are progressing normally (Scamell, 2014). It is hardly surprising, therefore, that many expectant parents enter what should be a time of excitement and hopeful anticipation in a state of anxiety and stress, and this can have significant effects on how they grow, birth and parent their babies (Zietlow et al., 2019).

This leaves those of us in the field of childbirth and parenting education in what feels to be a precarious position. We may find ourselves asking how we can justifiably promote a confident and positive attitude towards labour and birth with such a backdrop of risk, fear and blame.

In 2011, a significant life event changed everything about the way that I view the world. I live in Christchurch in New Zealand and in February that year, I was caught up in the might of the significant earthquakes here. Following the trauma of the earthquake and the subsequent aftershocks, I felt that I was coping well on a day-to-day basis even though our house was seriously damaged and our city broken. However, I went almost immediately into menopause following the seismic event and, within a couple of months, found myself feeling cold,

DOI: 10.4324/9781003223771-17

fatigued and generally under par. I sought medical advice and was diagnosed with hypothyroidism. I learned that adrenal depletion was almost certainly at the root of my menopausal 'crisis' and my thyroid issues. I researched what I could do myself to address this condition, not wanting to be at the mercy of medication for the rest of my days. And I discovered the practice of mindfulness as a means of calming my sympathetic nervous system and activating my parasympathetic system to create a sense of equilibrium within both my mind and body. I found that I could control my own neuro-hormonal responses to some extent at least. By focusing on the present rather than worrying about things that have happened or might happen, I could alter my heart and respiratory rate and lower my blood pressure as well as achieving a state of calm. I began to study the science behind mindfulness and was impressed by the number of studies I generated (e.g. Arch & Landy, 2015; Donald et al., 2016; Keng et al., 2011; Schreiner & Malcolm, 2008; Verplanken & Fisher, 2014) that reported a raft of benefits in using a practice built around a focus on the present moment. I found that the studies included a respectable number that had looked at mindfulness in relation to pregnancy and childbirth. Gaining insight into what happens when hormonal equilibrium is affected by shock, trauma and even sadness, and into how it can be countered by a relatively simple activity, opened my mind to the value of using mindfulness within childbirth and parenting education.

The continuum of pregnancy, birth and parenting is an extraordinary and yet normal part of life and the attitudinal foundations of a mindful approach can provide numerous benefits throughout this continuum. Pregnancy is for some, the first time in life where there is a requirement to be selfless. It is also a time when control needs to be relinquished to a large extent and we must learn to trust the process. This can be very challenging for some in a world where being in control is a virtue and may prevent prospective parents from developing an attitude of curiosity about their state of being during pregnancy (Scamell, 2014). A mindful birth requires self-compassion, acceptance, confidence, patience, and these qualities are enhanced when the individual is actively practising mind-fulness (Bardacke, 2012). Parenting requires us to be present in the moment with our children, just as they are (Keller & Bard., 2017). The need for social connection is a fundamental human motive that increases psychological and physical well-being (Hutcherson et al., 2008). Children allow us to view the world through fresh-eyes. 'Children, if they're fortunate enough to be brought up lovingly, are the greatest mindfulness teachers in the world!' (Alidina, 2014). However, it can be argued that this will only happen if the parents themselves are mindful.

In terms of antenatal education, a good starting point for introducing mindfulness as the foundation for learning is an acceptance that our bodies and minds connect to create the world that we experience physically, emotionally and psychologically. In many areas of healthcare, we remain enmeshed in a dualistic Cartesian model where mind and body are viewed as separate entities. A belief prevails that the body as 'machine' can be fixed without any consideration being given to the part that the mind plays (Martins, 2018). Exercises such as mindful eating and mindful movement can be used as a trigger for discussion around this fundamental connection. The basic tenets of neuro-hormonal physiology can then be unpacked in order to help those attending our antenatal sessions to understand the effect that excessive production of catecholamines has on the body; how a hormone like cortisol can go from being a healing element to a destructive element when the balance of endocrine activity is out of kilter; how oxytocin can open the door to love and trust and how melatonin can heal deep emotional wounds as well as helping us to achieve good quality sleep (Davies, 2017). Ensuring that parents understand this hormonal activity fosters an appreciation that mindfulness is underpinned by science and is not something esoteric or alternative.

An interesting observation in the mindfulness courses that I have facilitated to date has been the enthusiastic involvement of men. Early introduction to the hard science of neuro-hormonal activity seems to encourage engagement on the part of men and stirs enthusiasm that I have rarely seen in nearly 30 years as a childbirth educator. Information such as the fact that vasopressin, described as a 'sibling of oxytocin', enhances protective behaviours in men and encourages them to hold the space for their new family (Uvnäs Moberg, 2013) is a powerful invitation into the birthing environment. Another mechanism of engagement is the use of the concept of the 'default position'. Normal physiological pregnancy, labour and birth and the puerperium are viewed in the course as the default position. However, it is acknowledged that not all women will be able to stay at default, and so we explore ways of moving closer to that position by adopting strategies to enable this. For example, if someone is having an elective caesarean section, they can request deferred cord clamping and skin-to-skin contact in theatre. This discussion seems to have a profound effect on how the women view their birthing experience as they move from a position of fear to one of empowerment, enabling the potential for a positive transition to motherhood regardless of modality of birth. This is not a passive acceptance of intervention, but an honouring of the sanctity of birth and motherhood, and research may eventually validate this approach as a means of reducing intervention.

There are already research studies that indicate that the inclusion of mindfulness in childbirth education makes a difference to birth outcomes, including a reduction in the use of epidural anaesthesia (Levett et al., 2016) and a trend towards reduced systemic opioid administration (Duncan et al., 2017). A systematic review published in 2017 analysed the pooled results of a number of studies, including randomised controlled trials (RCTs), and concluded that anxiety, depression and perceived stress were less prevalent in the mindfulness groups (Dhillon et al., 2017). These findings are encouraging. However, more research is required, including a large scale RCT exploring the antenatal introduction of mindfulness and the resulting outcomes relating to labour, birth and beyond.

It is broadly acknowledged that the increase in rates of intervention in labour and birth in western style healthcare systems in recent decades is unacceptable and needs to be addressed as a matter of urgency. This will call for a paradigm shift of magnitude, requiring support from many factions within the networks of childbirth. Facilitators of childbirth education need to promote birth as an event with a defined 'default position' that sits within the parameters of normal physiology. This is critical if we are to reduce interventions in birth and optimise the neuro-hormonal environment of the mother/baby dyad, thus offering a woman and her significant others the best possible start for their new family. If a simple non-invasive intervention measure such as mindfulness can help to temper the risk-focussed culture that fosters a climate of fear and blame, then it needs to be given a platform for serious discussion and consideration.

## References

Alidina, S. (2014) Mindfulness for Dummies (2nd Ed.). New York: Wiley.

Arch, J.J., Landy, L.N. (2015) Emotional benefits of mindfulness. In: Brown, K.W., Creswell, J.D., Ryan, R.M. (Eds.) Handbook of Mindfulness: Theory, research, and practice. New York: The Guilford Press: 208–224.

Bardacke, N. (2012) Mindful Birthing: Training the mind, body and heart for childbirth and beyond. New York: Harper Collins.

Davies, L. (2017) Biobehavioural aspects of parenting. In: Rankin, J. (Ed.) Physiology in childbearing (4th Ed.) Edinburgh, GB: Elsevier: 597–603.

Dhillon, A., Sparkes, E., Duarte, R.V. (2017) Mindfulness-based interventions during pregnancy: A systematic review and meta-analysis. Mindfulness, 8(6):1421–1437.

Donald, J.N., Atkins, P.W., Parker, P.D., Christie, A.M., Ryan, R.M. (2016) Daily stress and the benefits of mindfulness: Examining the daily and longitudinal relations between present-moment awareness and stress responses. Journal of Research in Personality, 65:30–37.

Duncan, L.G., Cohn, M.A., Chao, M.T., Cook, J.G., Riccobono, J. et al. (2017) Benefits of preparing for childbirth with mindfulness training: A randomized controlled trial with active comparison. BMC Pregnancy & Childbirth, 17: article no.:140.

Hutcherson, C.A., Seppala, E.M., Gross, J.J. (2008) Loving-kindness meditation increases social connectedness. Emotion, 8(5):720–724.

Keller, H., Bard, K.A. (2017) The Cultural Nature of Attachment: Contextualising relationships and development. Cambridge: MIT Press.

Keng, S.L., Smoski, M.J., Robins, C.J. (2011) Effects of mindfulness on psychological health: A review of empirical studies. Clinical Psychology Review, 31(6):1041–1056.

Levett, K.M., Smith, C.A., Bensoussan, A., Dahlen, H.G. (2016) Complementary therapies for labour and birth study: A randomised controlled trial of antenatal integrative medicine for pain management in labour. BMJ Open, 6:e010691.

MacKenzie, B., van Teijlingen, E. (2010) Risk, theory, social and medical models: A critical analysis of the concept of risk in maternity care. Midwifery, Safety in Maternity Care, 26(5):488–96.

Martins, P.N. (2018) Descartes and the paradigm of Western medicine: An essay. International Journal of Recent Advances in Science and Technology, 5(3):32–34.

Scamell, M. (2014) Childbirth within the risk society. Sociology Compass, 8(7):917–928.

Scamell, M., Stone, N., Dahlen, H.G. (2019) Risk, safety, fear and trust in childbirth. In: Downe, S., Byrom, S. (Eds.) Squaring the Circle: Normal birth research, theory and practice in a technological age. London: Pinter and Martin:100–110.

Schreiner, I., Malcolm, J.P. (2008) The benefits of mindfulness meditation: Changes in emotional states of depression, anxiety, and stress. Behaviour Change, 25(3):156–168.

Skinner, J., Maude, R. (2016) The tension of uncertainty: Midwives managing risk in and of their practice. Midwifery, 35–41.

Uvnäs Moberg, K. (2013) The Hormone of Closeness: The role of oxytocin in relationships (1st Ed.) London: Pinter and Martin.

Verplanken, B., Fisher, N. (2014) Habitual worrying and benefits of mindfulness. Mindfulness, 5(5): 566–573.

Zietlow, A.L., Nonnenmacher, N., Reck, C., et al. (2019) Emotional stress during pregnancy – associations with maternal anxiety disorders, infant cortisol reactivity, and mother–child interaction at pre-school age. Frontiers in Psychology, 10. doi:10.3389/fpsyg.2019.02179.

# 15

# PREPARING WOMEN FOR HOMEBIRTH

*Cathy Green*

This chapter outlines some of the issues involved in deciding whether or not to plan a homebirth. It is intended as a practical tool to enable those working with women and their partners to begin or take up the place of birth discussion. It outlines and offers responses to some frequently asked questions and concerns of couples and provides practical tips on preparing for a homebirth that may be helpful when discussing plans for the birth of a woman's current or subsequent baby.

★

Homebirth accounts for approximately 2.1% of all births in England (Office for National Statistics [ONS], 2019), with pockets of the country having significantly lower as well as higher levels. We know many more women would like a homebirth – 10% of those surveyed in the UK National Maternity Review (2016). The Homebirth Team at the Birmingham Women's Hospital has used a variety of techniques to take our homebirth rate from 0.3% in 2013 to 3% in 2020. As a former National Childbirth Trust (NCT) antenatal teacher and now as a midwife, I have had the opportunity to meet many couples making the decision about where to have their baby. There are various issues involved in this decision.

## Key Concerns about Choosing Homebirth

Safety is voiced as one of the key concerns by women and their partners when homebirth is suggested. The Birthplace Study (Birthplace in England Collaborative Group, 2011) provided England-wide evidence on safety, and this evidence has been strengthened more recently by a larger international

DOI: 10.4324/9781003223771-18

meta-analysis of the outcomes of 50,000 planned homebirths (Hutton et al., 2019; Reitsma et al., 2020). The results of this study show that regardless of parity, there is no significant difference in neonatal outcomes between hospital and homebirth.

In addition, women who start their labour planning to give birth at home are:

- 40% less likely to have a caesarean section
- 50% less likely to have an instrumental birth (forceps or ventouse)
- 70% less likely to have epidural anaesthesia
- 40% less likely to have a 3rd or 4th degree tear (tear involving the anal sphincter)
- 60% less likely to receive a hormone drip to speed up labour
- 30% less likely to have a postpartum haemorrhage
- 75% less likely to have an infection postnatally.

These are powerful outcomes and reinforce confidence in the safety for women and their babies of choosing to birth at home, even if they then transfer to hospital in labour.

However, decision-making is a multifaceted process 'involving personal and non-clinical factors' (Stone, 2016), and as clinicians, but also advocates for women, we must ensure we talk about evidence separately from decision-making as evidence is not the only thing that informs decisions (Wickham, 2016). In my experience with the homebirth team, when making a decision about homebirth, women are less likely to be reviewing evidence-based data and more likely to draw on common-sense judgements about what constitutes risk in everyday life, with an acknowledgement that scientific evidence is not straightforward given the unpredictability and social nature of birth.

Some women and men see homebirth as an odd, backward, uninformed choice or simply not for 'people like us'. Our experience at the Birmingham Women's Hospital is that the demographic of the women who choose a home-birth with our team almost exactly reflects the demographic of Birmingham itself. Women need to see images of all kinds of women having homebirths to feel that it is relevant to them. Having a selection of images to show, or a short video, can have a positive effect on changing some deep-seated beliefs about the relevance of homebirth for certain groups of women. Recognising this, we have made video interviews with several of our homebirth women which we have posted online. In addition, we have an Instagram account where we post images of our midwives and maternity support workers when they have assisted at a homebirth.

Ultimately, concerns over safety are often not the reason a woman and/or her partner dismiss the idea of homebirth. In my experience, the real issue is the strong cultural association between birth and hospital. The default position for most women when imagining/planning their birth is for it to be in hospital.

Changing this mind-set requires a seismic shift in thinking. So, how can we promote this shift? Below are some of the key triggers which appear to help women and their partners decide that homebirth may be for them.

## Birth Stories

Hearing accounts of women's births first-hand seems to have the biggest impact on decision-making for women and their partners. Prior to the COVID pandemic, we held regular 'meet the team' events to which anyone considering a homebirth was invited. At these events, we talked about the practicalities of homebirth, and couples met the team of midwives and maternity support workers. In addition, we invited new parents who have birthed with us at home to talk about their experiences. We also invited couples whose birth started at home but who were transferred into hospital in labour. Without exception, such couples were positive about their decision to plan a homebirth. During the pandemic and currently, we have moved to an online Zoom event which allows more couples to participate. We include a recorded interview with a couple who birthed at home. These events provide parents-to-be with an insight into the practical and emotional issues around homebirth and have a dramatic effect on chipping away at the deep-seated cultural belief that birth in hospital is the 'right' thing.

## Home Comforts

As a team, we take every opportunity to talk to women antenatally about the period after having a homebirth. This seems to resonate particularly with women who have had a hospital birth previously. We may talk about a recent birth we have been at where the woman's other children woke up and came downstairs to meet their new sibling, with mum tucked up on the sofa with a mug of tea from her own kitchen. We mention how nice it is to have a bath in your own bathroom and that the partner does not have to leave after the birth. These small, practical details can be enough to change someone's opinion about homebirth or to strengthen their resolve to choose this option, particularly if a previous postnatal experience in hospital was not seen as particularly positive.

## Birth Preparation Talk

As a student midwife, I had an elective placement with a team of community midwives in Torbay in the south-west of England where there was a particularly high homebirth rate. I was keen to see what made a difference there. One thing that particularly stood out for me was the point at which midwives discussed where the baby would be born. This was left until around 34 to 36 weeks as it was felt that a woman would be more focused on such a discussion at this point in her pregnancy. The Head of Midwifery for this Trust, which has a homebirth rate of 12%, explained that place of birth should never be a tick box question at the beginning of pregnancy. She compared this to being asked in March what you would like to eat at the office Christmas dinner. In most parts of England, women are 'booked' at the beginning of pregnancy and encouraged to choose their place of birth then. The issue is generally not raised again. At the Birmingham Women's Hospital, community midwives can confidently encourage low-risk women to consider a homebirth at various points in their pregnancy knowing that our specialist homebirth team is available and ready to support women if they choose this option.

Once a woman and her partner have decided they would like a homebirth, our team takes over their antenatal care. A priority for our team has been to provide continuity of carer wherever possible as we know this offers significant benefits for mothers and babies, and women report high levels of satisfaction when they see the same midwife regularly (Sandall, 2017). Because we get to know our women and have relatively small caseloads, we are able to spend the time needed to prepare families for homebirth. Discussions take place at various points in the pregnancy, very much led by the woman, but with the ultimate objective of being fully prepared by 36 weeks. Some issues that come up in the antenatal period are as follows.

## Arrangements for Other Children

What to do with other children is an issue some women are concerned about. We advise that there should be someone available to care for the children should they wake up or become distressed during labour, or should the woman need to transfer into hospital. This could be a neighbour or relative available at the end of a phone. In reality, this has rarely been a problem – women seem to have a sense of when it is safe to give birth, and for many, this is once they have put their children to bed for the night or sent them off to school for the day!

## Who Can Be at the Birth?

Some women wish to have many people around them for birth; others want a private event. Most of the homebirths we have attended have been quiet and intimate, but a few have involved large numbers of friends and/or family members and take away pizzas!

## Using a Birth Pool

We advise women to think about getting a pool. We are great advocates for the use of water in labour, with 60% of women we care for using water to relieve pain in labour and a home waterbirth rate of 50%. We know that immersion in water can make labour quicker and more straightforward. Women also report high levels of satisfaction with using a pool for labour and/or birth (Cluett & Burns, 2009). When the pool arrives, we advise the couple to practise inflating it and to check that the attachments fit the tap – both things they will not want to struggle with for the first time once in labour! Linked with water for pain relief is the issue of entonox (gas and air). Most multiparous women will have used entonox at some point in their previous labour and are relieved to know that it will be available at home.

If a woman chooses not to get a pool, we have a discussion about where she thinks she would like to give birth. This is a useful opportunity to talk about upright positions for labour and to dispel any myths about the need to give birth on a bed – something the woman may have done at a previous hospital birth. Many women envisage giving birth downstairs, with the sofa proving helpful to kneel on or lean against whilst pushing. The discussion on where in the house to give birth provides an opening to mention our equipment and setting up a resuscitation area. We explain that we do this for every birth and reassure couples that some initial help with the first breath is occasionally needed. Rather than worry couples, this information seems to reassure them that we are fully prepared for every eventuality.

## Transfer in Labour

Couples sometimes ask (and we will always tell them if they do not) about how and why they may need to transfer to hospital in labour. We tell couples that safety is our first priority and that if we feel there is a need to transfer, this will be via the emergency ambulance service. A discussion of the issue of transfer seems to reassure couples rather than induce anxiety.

## What Kit Will I Need and Will There Be a Lot of Mess?

The main 'kit' a woman needs for a homebirth is a large quantity of towels for baby and for mum, particularly if using a pool, and one or two plastic sheets to cover furniture. Couples are relieved to know that even though there is unlikely to be much mess, any waste is disposed of by the midwives. This includes the placenta unless the couple wish to keep it. Several of our families have kept their placentas to add to smoothies, cook with onion and garlic, plant in the garden or even to make into a piece of art!

## Managing the Pain of Labour

Many of the primiparous women we care for have attended antenatal classes provided by the Birmingham Women's Hospital which focus on breathing techniques, movement and upright positions. We do not provide a particular antenatal education session for homebirth women because we take the approach that everyone is likely to need something different and we are able to provide individualised preparation. For some women, we offer a one-to-one hypnobirthing session; for others, our 34- to 36-week talk will include a practical session on relaxation, breathing, positions and movement for birth, including a discussion of strategies based on the women's own coping repertoire. Homebirth women tend to have an innate sense that they will be able to manage in labour and at least want to try to see if they can cope! If labour is straightforward, this determination, coupled with being in a relaxed, supportive environment, usually results in a woman coping well with labour and birth. It can be helpful to point out to women planning their first baby at home that very few women planning a homebirth with us have transferred to hospital in labour for more pain relief.

For women having their second or subsequent baby, birth preparation will vary according to the woman's previous birth(s). Some women will be quite anxious about their ability to cope, based on a previous traumatic experience in hospital. For these women, we focus on issues of relaxation, breathing and movement and also talk about the likelihood that this birth will be quicker and that their coping strategies will not have to be employed for too long! We also aim to unpick some of the issues from the previous birth which caused distress if these have not been discussed earlier in pregnancy.

## Early Labour

An important part of any antenatal birth preparation is discussing coping strategies for early labour. For primiparous women, the ability to remain calm, hydrated and nourished in early labour is vital, whether having a home or hospital birth. Women booked with us know they can call us for advice at any point in their labour and that if they need support, we will come out to them in early labour. Knowing someone is at the end of the phone who will come when needed seems to help women cope for longer before calling us. If we visit a woman in early labour, we have the opportunity to remind her and her partner about coping strategies, and this appears to give them the confidence and strength to cope with what can be a long latent phase.

For multiparous women, our advice is somewhat different. We know that second and subsequent babies can make a quick appearance after the start of labour. We advise all our multiparous women that they should not wait too long to call us and that we would rather come for a false alarm than miss the birth of the baby! This does mean that we may make several visits, but it also means that we have missed very few births.

## Conclusion

In an environment where the vast majority of births are in hospital, it is a challenge to find ways to help women question deeply held beliefs. However, women prioritise their baby's and their own safety (Paranjothy & Thomas, 2001), and we now have the evidence that homebirth is safe. When women and their partners recognise that birth is a deeply social act, they begin to see the advantages and relevance for them of homebirth. Caregivers in the antenatal period have the opportunity to dispel myths and to offer birthing women an alternative discourse outside the cultural norm. Through a combination of information giving, story-telling and continuity of midwifery care, the number of women choosing homebirth has substantially increased in Birmingham.

## Practice Pointers: For Health Professionals Supporting Women's Decision-Making about Place of Birth

* Consider where your own, perhaps unconscious, bias/preferences for place of birth come from.
* Become familiar with the latest evidence on safety for mother and baby of homebirth.
* Encourage women to read real-life stories about homebirth or watch homebirth and waterbirth videos on YouTube. This can help provide a counter-balance to the hospital-centric focus on birth in the media.
* Talk to women postnatally about their experience of homebirth to increase your depth of knowledge about what is important to women.

## References

Birthplace in England Collaborative Group (2011) Perinatal and maternal outcomes by planned place of birth for healthy women with low risk pregnancies: The Birthplace in England national prospective cohort study. British Medical Journal, 343:d7400.

Cluett, E.R., Burns, E. (2009) Immersion in Water in Labour and Birth. Cochrane Database of Systematic Reviews, 2:CD000111.

Hutton, E., Reitsma, A., Simioni, J., Brunton, G., Kaufman, K. (2019) Perinatal or neonatal mortality among women who intend at the onset of labour to give birth at home compared to women of low obstetrical risk who intend to give birth in hospital: A systematic review and meta-analyses. The Lancet, 14:59–70.

National Maternity Review (2016) Better Births – Improving outcomes of maternity services in England. A five year forward view for maternity care. Available at: England.maternityreview@nhs.net <accessed, 14 Nov, 2021>

Office for National Statistics (ONS) Births in England and Wales (2019) Available at: www.ons.gov.uk <accessed 28 Oct, 2021>

Paranjothy, S., Thomas, J. (2001) Royal College of Obstetricians and Gynaecologists Clinical Effectiveness Support Unit - National Sentinel Caesarean Section Audit Report. London: RCOG Press.

Reitsma, A., Simioni, J., Brunton, G., Kaufman, K., Hutton, E. (2020) Maternal outcomes and birth interventions among women who begin labour intending to give birth at home compared to women of low obstetrical risk who intend to give birth in hospital: A systematic review and meta-analyses. The Lancet, 21:1–10.

Sandall, J. (2017) The Contribution of Continuity of Midwifery Care to High Quality Maternity Care. Royal College of Midwives: RCM Press.

Stone, M.H. (2016) The evidence and the decision are two quite distinct things. British Medical Journal, 353:i2452.

Wickham, S. (2016) Evidence and decisions: Two different things. Available at: www.sarawickham.com <accessed 28 Oct, 2021>

# 16

# THE POWER TO TRANSFORM

## Freeing Women's Instinctual Potential for Giving Birth through Body-Centred Preparation in Pregnancy

*Janet Balaskas*

Janet Balaskas has been a birth activist for many years and became well known in the UK in the 1980s for her work around 'Active Birth' – a term that she herself coined. She is the author of many books and is a renowned childbirth educator. She trains birth educators around the world and was the founder of the Active Birth Centre in London and its director for four decades. She now works online to reach a wider global audience.

In this chapter, Janet describes her philosophy of Active Birth. She shares her best practice ideas for educating and supporting women to work with their bodies to realise their potential to give birth to their babies powerfully and joyfully.

★

I trained as a birth educator in the UK after the birth of my first daughter in 1979. My inspiration came from the book, 'Childbirth Without Fear' by Grantly Dick-Read. I read this book three weeks before giving birth and it was just the inspiration I needed to trust my intuitive feeling that I knew how to give birth naturally, like all other mammals. It turned out to be true.

However, first, I had to travel back to my homeland, South Africa, to find a small and peaceful place to give birth. In the UK, most women were having to contend with the trend for birth in large hospital units with very limiting protocols. 'Active Management of Birth' was commonly practised, involving widespread use of induction, epidurals and electronic monitoring, with the mother on a bed in a semi-recumbent position.

Women's education for birth was mainly cerebral, learning about interventions and how to manage or resist them. Breathing 'techniques' were taught and provided some help – but the main problem was that women were lying on their

DOI: 10.4324/9781003223771-19

backs or semi-reclining during labour and birth. This passivity was mirrored in antenatal classes which were largely information-based, with very little active participation.

I realised that this method of birth preparation was neither empowering nor effective. The outcomes were not good, with very few women who attended classes giving birth naturally. So, I set off to research the history and ethnology of childbirth and discovered that women being mobile and upright for birth was a universal, cross-cultural practice going back to prehistory.

## The Pelvis First

A deeper study of the anatomy of the female pelvis revealed how it is essentially shaped and designed for upright birth. I saw clearly how the baby could navigate the diameters of the pelvis more easily with the help of gravity. I noticed how the generous curve of the sacrum was like a slide, shaped to guide the baby down and forward. I learned about the softening of the pelvic ligaments during pregnancy in response to the hormone relaxin, so that the bony pelvis became more mobile and 'expandable' by the time of birth to accommodate the baby's descent.

I began to carry a model pelvis and doll with me to classes and to demonstrate the journey of the baby through the pelvis to parents and professionals alike. I explained the importance of utilising the help of gravity to enable an easier angle of descent for the baby. I also talked about how forward leaning upright positions maximised the space in the pelvis owing to the increase of the diameters of the inlet and outlet, and how they ensured better blood circulation, more effective uterine contractions and more easily managed pain. While explaining, I invited participants to get up and feel on their own body what I was talking about. Around this time, I also wrote the Active Birth Manifesto, which listed the research evidence on which my classes were based, and my book, 'Active Birth', was published in the early 1980s. It is still in print and has a global reach.

Four decades later, I continue to do the pelvis demonstration in my classes – it always comes first – and to teach professionals to do it, offering courses online. It is a powerful visual means of convincing people of the benefits of an Active Birth.

It also does wonders in terms of getting the fathers on board. They can easily relate to this common-sense demonstration of the basic mechanics of birth and the main benefits of an active birth. Women become inspired and confident as they learn how their bodies are designed for birth. Upright positions make total sense to them. In pregnancy, they become less fearful and more relaxed – and more empowered during birth, by the ability to envisage and understand what is happening in their bodies.

## Birth Physiology

My understanding of birth physiology has developed over the years, inspired especially by Dr. Michel Odent and Dr. Sarah Buckley and their work on the hormones that drive the process of birth and help the mother through the experience.

Listening to my body during three spontaneous home births, I came to a new understanding of physiology, in particular the actions of the uterus in co-ordination with the hormones that drive labour forward. My use of language in classes changed, as I realised that the cervix was absorbed upwards into the body of the uterus as baby descends, rather than 'dilating' from 0 to 10 cm as is commonly perceived. Contractions could be much better described in the way women experience them, as waves, rushes, pulsations, or surges.

The uterus, and what I call its pulsating 'pull push' actions, can be described as undulating movements, like a jelly fish in the deep ocean. I explain that the so-called 'three stages of labour and birth' are in fact more of a progressive flow, where what happens in one 'stage' is inherent in what has happened earlier. For example, the baby is pushed down not just during birth, but is nudged down little by little by the uterus every time it pulsates throughout the whole of labour. Then, when the cervix is fully absorbed upwards into the body of the uterus, and the baby's head has already descended into the top of the vagina, the 'surges' become 'urges' and the thickened uterus pushes the baby down. This is most effective in the context of upright birth, where gravity aids the process. The language I use is physiological.

## Start of Labour

Another important topic is the role that the baby plays in initiating labour, softening the internal tissues or the 'birth path', stimulating uterine activity. It comes as a surprise to parents to know that the baby, when ready to breathe and to be born, produces the hormones that help to start the labour and end the pregnancy. They are fascinated to learn how mother, baby, uterus, pelvis and hormones all play their part throughout the birth process.

This is a summary of the theoretical side of my teaching and takes me about two hours to complete; the rest is all practical. At the end, the question I'm most frequently asked is, 'Why doesn't everyone know this?' Why indeed! My aim is to inspire confidence, challenge conditioned mindsets about birth and help women and their partners to realise that they can be active participants in the birth of their babies and can trust their own bodies to give birth.

## Practical Work

Once the theory session is over, we can then embark on the practical, experiential way of learning that is so different from the cerebral approach used in many antenatal classes. Couples or mothers try different positions and movements, doing breath-work and using touch that may help in labour, while the information they need is woven in as they rehearse the 'dance of labour'. Thanks to the earlier theoretical input, partners usually let down their defences, and it always surprises me how the atmosphere in the room becomes intimate – allowing the oxytocin to flow!

While the whole group participate in practice for labour, I select one woman or couple at a time to role play birth in each upright birthing position while the others watch. This enables the participants to envisage what birth in an upright position looks like, how the baby emerges and what the role of the midwife and the partner is. Everyone gets a turn. It's a very lively session involving lots of laughter, especially when I show the dads how to catch a baby with mum on all fours just in case they should need to (it does occasionally happen!).

Finally, to illustrate the first hour after birth, I ask one couple to be the new parents and the rest of the group to form a circle around them to create an atmosphere of warm intimacy – a 'love bubble'. Mum sits with baby (doll) in her arms, then as adrenalin levels fall, she lies back on a beanbag with the baby on top of her 'tummy to mummy' and skin to skin – an easier way for many women to breastfeed and to achieve a good latch from the start. I take about an hour to discuss all the issues about the placental transfusion and blood flow through the cord, options and recommendations for cutting the cord, as well as options for what to do with the placenta. I keep mum warm, dad by her side, and encourage them to take the time they need to birth the placenta (under the discreet observation of the midwife), possibly waiting until the placenta is born before cutting the cord, so they can see the 'whole baby', including placenta and intact cord.

My approach is to start with a clear vision and understanding of the physiological and along the way to include how parents can remain as close to it as possible in other circumstances, while benefiting from medical expertise when necessary.

## Integrating Interventions

Finally, you may wonder how I help women and their partners in the event of their needing medical intervention, when the agenda has to change and the birth they need is very different from the birth they planned.

I offer suggestions which combine active birth wisdom with managing interventions – for example, suggesting alternatives such as lying on the side with the upper body raised, rather than the usual semi-recumbent position for epidurals or inductions, and skin-to-skin contact and delayed cord cutting after a caesarean section.

My aim in addressing the 'What if...?' question is to encourage women to have a strong commitment to work towards the birth they would like, but always to keep an open mind. In a session I call, 'The Wise Woman', I encourage women to communicate their needs to their attendants, ask questions and apply elements of what they have learned in the event of interventions to achieve a positive outcome. An Active Birth is one in which the woman remains not only in charge of her body, but also in charge of her choices and decisions, assisted in both by her attendants.

## Pregnancy Yoga

In addition to Active Birth workshops and weekend courses, I also offer weekly pregnancy yoga classes for women where I teach relaxation, breathing and simple yoga postures that increase comfort in pregnancy and prepare both body and mind for birth and mothering. As a yoga student myself in the late 1970s, I noticed how many of the postures seemed like ideal preparation for active labour and birth. I started a small weekly class, wrote a book and have since watched pregnancy yoga grow from its earliest beginnings into a global phenomenon.

Women really value the opportunity to relax, have a gentle stretch and let go of their daily concerns. Lying down on the yoga mat provides a refuge from the pressures of life and a chance to increase connection with the body, breath and baby that modern women really need. I can get to know the women who come to yoga and help them with their emotional preparation for birth and mothering, identifying when there are unexpected issues that need to be explored.

They learn to follow their breathing, discover gravity and turn their attention inwards as they release tension and experience ease and relaxation in its place. These ongoing classes have the effect of creating 'body memory' that will be there for them during labour.

## Conclusion

In my experience, when a woman's preparation for birth is experiential and body-centred, she is usually far more relaxed and confident in the last trimester than she was earlier and is looking forward to the birth. She is empowered not only to trust her body, but also to trust her wisdom and to feel relaxed and safe, knowing that she has within her all the resources she needs.

Fear is transformed into confidence, pain into pleasure and joy. The Active Birth Movement has, I believe, had a transformative effect on the culture of birth, inspiring midwife-led care, the creation of birth centres which are custom designed for natural active birth and the use of birth pools instead of epidurals. Although there is still a very long way to go, great advances have been made in the course of my career. The women arriving in hospital with a birth ball, a big bag of cushions and asking for an Active Birth have been leading a global revolution. Now, more women can look towards having a wonderful natural birth without intervention. For those who may need medical help, staying as close to the physiological as possible and applying the main principles of what they have learned can make almost every birth a positive experience.

Women have an instinct for giving birth, just as babies have an instinct to be born. Birth is a biological, physical process common to all mammals. We birth with our bodies, and we connect with instinct through the body. We learn most effectively by doing. I believe it is essential that birth preparation should be experiential, body-centred and minimally information-based, with the intention of awakening the innate birthing instinct.

## Practice Pointers

- Encourage freedom of movement and spontaneous breathing.
- 'Teach by doing' with partner participation.
- Use relatable 'physiological' language.
- Use role play to demonstrate upright birth.
- Engage participants in experiential learning – the body remembers, the mind forgets!
- Have confidence in the amazing physiology of the birth process.

# PART IV

# Education and Support for Parents of Twins

## Introduction

Twins have always evoked great interest on the part of researchers and society at large. There is something eternally intriguing about two (or more) babies who have shared their mother's womb at the same time and who are born within minutes of each other. Educators may provide specialist antenatal and postnatal sessions for parents who are expecting or have newborn twins. To be able to offer accurate, practical information in response to the many questions these parents have is important. Questions about sleeping, feeding and relationships are likely to be the most common.

The first chapter in this section looks at safe sleeping advice for parents of twins in relation to prematurity, co-bedding and the risk of sudden infant death syndrome. In the second chapter, the idea that breastfeeding two babies is neither sensible nor even possible, especially if the babies need special or intensive care, is challenged. Provided that parents are offered consistent and well-informed guidance, along with strong support to enable careful planning and persistence, it is perfectly possible to feed twins and most parents of twins will find breastfeeding easier in the mid- to long-term than formula feeding.

People are fascinated by the relationship between twins and by the way in which their parents choose to bring them up – similar names, identical clothes, the same presents, or deliberately different. The third chapter in this section examines the complex relationship between parents and their twins and between the twins themselves, reminding practitioners that each twin is a unique individual – his or her own person – and that the individuality of each child needs to be acknowledged and celebrated by parents in their parenting.

DOI: 10.4324/9781003223771-20

# 17

# SLEEP PATTERNS OF TWINS

*Helen Ball*

There is comparatively little research on the sleep of twins and multiples compared to the large amount of research on singleton babies. Among the few published papers, key topics addressed involve a) issues around co-bedding, both in home and neonatal intensive care unit (NICU) settings; b) sudden infant death syndrome (SIDS) and the implementation of safe sleep recommendations for twins; and c) sleep patterns of twin infants and their parents.

★

Co-bedding refers to siblings sharing the same surface during any sleep period, for example being in the same cot together. Most research into co-bedding has focussed on twins with special health needs (see below); nevertheless, the practice of co-bedding twin infants is common, and parents do it for multiple reasons.

A New Zealand survey study found co-bedding was popular, especially among parents with younger twins – 52% of 109 twin pairs co-bedded at six weeks of age, 31% at four months, and 10% at eight months (Hutchinson et al., 2010). Likewise, in a home interview study of 104 parents of twins in the United States, Damato et al. (2012) found more than 65% of twins were co-bedded at four weeks of age while 42% were co-bedded at 13 weeks of age. Room sharing was reported by 64% of families at four weeks of age and by 40% at 13 weeks.

In the United Kingdom, Ball (2006, 2007) investigated parents' perspectives and concerns about co-bedding and employed video data to assess potential risks and benefits of co-bedding compared to separate sleeping, concluding that:

- Co-bedding facilitates rooming-in and thus can influence the reduction of SIDS risk

DOI: 10.4324/9781003223771-21

- Make-shift barriers separating co-bedded infants are unnecessary and can result in harm
- Hospital practices influence parents' behaviour – co-bedding was more popular among parents whose babies were co-bedded in hospital
- Parents find that co-bedding makes night-time care easier due to sleep synchronisation of twins.

No evidence was found to support parents' concerns that co-bedded twins would disturb, overheat or suffocate each other. Parents' reasons for sleeping infants together were supported by the observation that co-bedded twins had synchronous sleep patterns and were subjectively easier to care for; this in turn might relate to co-bedded infants remaining in the parents' room for longer.

The specialist literature for practitioners addresses the question of co-bedding in the NICU. Prior to birth, twin foetuses are in constant contact in utero, giving rise to a synchrony in movement and co-regulation in biological measures. It is therefore thought that close contact is beneficial to their wellbeing in the extra-uterine environment (Hayward et al., 2015).

While the benefits are still being investigated, studies have found that with co-bedding, preterm twins have fewer adverse health issues and longer durations of quiet sleep than non-co-bedding preterm twins. Co-regulation of infant heartbeats means that co-bedding infants have significantly lower heart rates and lower stress levels overall (Hayward et al., 2015) Co-bedding provides comfort to twins undergoing stressful procedures, comparable to the presence of a mother (Campbell-Yeo et al., 2009), and co-bedding attenuates the stress response of preterm twins undergoing heel lance procedures (Badiee et al., 2014; Campbell-Yeo et al., 2014).

The position statement of the US National Association of Neonatal Nurses (NANN) (2012) on co-bedding of twins and higher-order multiples is non-prescriptive, highlighting the lack of sufficient knowledge and recommending the development of clinical protocols to ensure optimal care of multiple-birth infants. The American Academy of Pediatrics (2016) recommends *against* co-bedding twins, justifying this position with the same argument: lack of evidence.

## SIDS and Safe Sleep for Twin Babies

The high prevalence of prematurity and low birth-weight places twin infants at increased risk for sudden infant death syndrome (SIDS). However, SIDS reduction recommendations are aimed at singleton infants and require tailoring for families with multiples (Damato et al., 2016). Both US and UK families face challenges adhering to recommendations to reduce SIDS risks (Ball, 2006; Haas et al., 2017), such as that babies should be placed to sleep on their backs and should remain in the same room as their parents for at least the first six months. When US parents of triplets and quadruplets were recruited from an online support group to complete a survey of infant care practices, it was found that fewer than 80% of babies slept supine, and only 50% shared their parents' bedroom (Haas et al., 2017). This mirrored the UK findings of Ball (2006) that while co-bedded infants slept in their parents' room, twins sleeping in separate cots were moved into their own room by three months.

While most twins are initially co-bedded in a side-by-side position, parents use a variety of co-bedding configurations. These are not all equally safe: Diagonal positioning is unsafe if used with blankets as these are difficult to secure in this position, but with the use of sleeping bags, it is less hazardous. Parents should avoid co-bedding twins in a Moses basket or small bassinette due to lack of space (Ball, 2006).

## Sleep Patterns of Twin Infant and Parents

The sleep patterns of twin babies generally reflect those of singletons (Bartlett & Witoonchart, 2003), the major difference being gestational age. Because twins are often born early, they follow a sleep trajectory aligned with their gestational age rather than birth age. Care should be taken to avoid comparisons with babies who were born later in their gestational development. If twin babies sleep differently from singletons, any differences generally relate to prematurity and/or the amount of time they have spent in an incubator. If babies have experienced a prolonged stay in a NICU, they are likely to be unsettled at home initially due to the dramatic change in environment. Environmental temperature, for instance, may affect their sleep, and twins may achieve better sleep and thermal stability if placed together. Preterm twins will have smaller stomachs and require more frequent feeding than babies of the same chronological age, which will affect the frequency of night waking. Many parents find that their twins' feeding and sleeping patterns become synchronised if they are fed and slept together.

Two other potential differences between the care of multiples and that of singletons are that multiples are more likely to be cared for according to a schedule and are more likely to have several different carers. Both strategies help parents cope with looking after more than one baby, especially if they have other children to care for as well. However, both strategies might also be difficult for babies to adapt to if they have to 'wait their turn' to be fed or comforted, or if they receive inconsistent care from a variety of carers. There is little evidence to draw on, but one suggestion consistent with infants' needs is for parents to designate helpers to take care of the household, the laundry, and feeding the parents, rather than handing over care-giving responsibilities for the babies to others.

Parents of twin infants are generally keen to know when their babies will start sleeping through the night, and how to cope with the night-time care of two babies. Damato and Burant (2008) used actigraphy and sleep diaries to examine parental sleep and fatigue at 2, 12, and 20 weeks following the birth of twins. Fathers obtained less night sleep (5.4 hours) and less 24-hour sleep (5.8 hours) than mothers (6.2 hours night sleep and 6.9 hours in 24 hours). However, mothers experienced more sleep disruptions (mean 2.3 vs 1.0). Morning and evening fatigue levels did not differ between parents, and sleep efficiency (sleep duration represented as a percentage of total time in bed) increased linearly over time for both parents.

In comparison, mothers of single infants had, on average, four disruptions of sleep per night and were awake for 28% of the time after onset of sleep in the first two to three weeks postpartum. The night-time experiences of mothers were therefore similar, regardless of whether they were caring for one infant or more. Fathers of single infants, however, obtained more sleep than mothers. When it comes to night-time care-giving, fathers are minimally affected by one infant, but have greater involvement when there are two.

The prolonged effects of sleep disruption include increased sleepiness, depression, and decreased cognitive performance, together with a higher risk of illness and decreased ability to cope with demands. These contribute to postpartum depression (PPD) with mothers of twins being at increased risk. Parents of twins, and those caring for them in a personal or professional capacity, should therefore be vigilant for signs of PPD in both mothers and fathers and seek or offer support should PPD be suspected.

Ionio et al.'s (2021) systematic review investigated how parents of twins approach the care of their infants after birth and found a lack of ethnic diversity among the parents who participated in the included studies. Cultural differences could drive differences in parents' decisions regarding caring for their twins, and more research is needed to examine this.

## Routines or Schedules

When coping with new babies (singletons or multiples), developing routines can help parents cope, providing structure and an order to do things in, and encouraging the division of tasks between partners. Routines are not prescriptive and all families develop different ones; they have flexibility and can be varied as necessary. Schedules, on the other hand, can create stress rather than reduce it as they are often rigid, and babies don't stick to the clock. Schedules can become a source of conflict when they constrain family life. Parents of multiples are often tempted to implement sleep training to eliminate night-time disruption. However, sleep training is a controversial practice often undertaken for the benefit of the parents rather than the infant(s). It works under certain conditions, but it breaks the synchrony between parents and baby and causes babies stress. Researchers recommend that sleep training is not appropriate for babies under six months old.

## Conclusion

Caring for twins presents unique challenges that require specific choices to be made. The parents of twins would benefit from additional and specially developed advice from health professionals for considering and implementing adequate sleep and feeding practices that reduce parental fatigue and stress, reduce SIDS risks, and promote parent–twin relationships.

## Practice Pointers

- Parents of twins face various challenges in the first weeks after delivery, highlighting a need for health professionals to provide specific support during the postnatal period and monitor for signs of postnatal depression.
- Assessment tools to help identify barriers and facilitators to implementing safe sleep practices with multiples would be useful to inform support strategies for parents.
- The development of NICU clinical protocols around co-bedding would ensure optimal care of multiple-birth infants.

## References

American Academy of Pediatrics Task Force on Sudden Infant Death Syndrome (2016) SIDS and other sleep-related infant deaths: Updated 2016 recommendations for a safe infant sleeping environment. Pediatrics, 138(5):e20162938.

Badiee, Z., Nassiri, Z., Armanian, A. (2014) Cobedding of twin premature infants: Calming effects on pain responses. Pediatric Neonatology, 55(4):262–268.

Ball, H.L. (2006) Caring for twin infants: Sleeping arrangements and their implications. Evidence-Based Midwifery, 4(1):10–16.

Ball, H.L. (2007) Together or apart? A behavioural and physiological investigation of sleeping arrangements for twin babies. Midwifery, 23(4):404–412.

Bartlett, L., Witoonchart, C. (2003) The sleep patterns of young twins. The Journal of Family Health Care, 13(1):21–23.

Campbell-Yeo, M.L., Johnston, C.C., Joseph, K.S., Feeley, N.L., Chambers, C. et al. (2009) Co-bedding as a comfort measure for twins undergoing painful procedures (CComForT Trial). BMC Pediatrics, 9:76.

Campbell-Yeo, M.L., Johnston, C.C., Joseph, K.S., Feeley, N., Chambers, C.T. et al. (2014) Co-bedding between preterm twins attenuates stress response after heel lance: Results of a randomized trial. The Clinical Journal of Pain, 30(7):598–604.

Damato, E.G., Brubaker, J.A., Burant, C. (2012) Sleeping arrangements in families with twins. Newborn and Infants Nursing Reviews, 12(3):171–178.

Damato, E.G., Burant, C. (2008) Sleep patterns and fatigue in parents of twins. Journal of Obstetric, Gynecologic and Neonatal Nursing, 37(6):738–749.

Damato, E.G., Haas, M.C., Czeck, P., Dowling, D.A., Barsman, S.G. (2016) Safe sleep infant care practices reported by mothers of twins. Advances in Neonatal Care, 16(6):E3–E14.

Haas, M.C., Dowling, D., Damato, E.G. (2017) Adherence to safe sleep recommendations by families with higher-order multiples. Advances in Neonatal Care, 17(5):407–416.

Hayward, K.M., Johnston, C.C., Campbell-Yeo, M.L., Price, S.L., Houk, S.L. et al. (2015) Effect of cobedding twins on coregulation, infant state and twin safety. Journal of Obstetric, Gynecologic and Neonatal Nursing, 44(2):193–202.

Hutchinson, B.L., Stewart, A.W., Mitchell, E.A. (2010) The prevalence of co-bedding and SIDS-related child care practices in twins. European Journal of Pediatrics, 169(12):1477–1485.

Ionio, C., Mascheroni, E., Landoni, M., Gattis, M. (2021) Caring for twins during infancy: A systematic review of the literature on sleeping and feeding practices amongst parents of twins. Journal of Neonatal Nursing, doi.org/10.1016/j.jnn.2021.08.017.

National Association of Neonatal Nurses (2012) Cobedding of twins or higher-order multiples. Advances in Neonatal Care, 12(1):61–67.

# 18

# BREASTFEEDING TWINS

*Kathryn Stagg*

When a parent finds out they are expecting a multiple birth, this can cause a wide variety of emotions – shock, love, excitement, worry and even panic. One of the biggest concerns for many parents is whether they will be able to breastfeed their babies.

The good news is that it is very possible to breastfeed twins or even triplets. There are some difficulties to negotiate, but with expert breastfeeding support, these can be overcome.

★

There is little research into the effectiveness of interventions designed for twin families (Whitford et al., 2017). Twins are more likely to be born prematurely; in almost 60% of twin pregnancies, babies are born before 37 weeks (Macones, 2005). Twin babies are more likely to be born smaller than singletons, often because growth in a twin pregnancy slows in the third trimester due to lack of space.

Many twins are born between 36 and 37 weeks' gestation. This means they are at greater risk of developing jaundice (Ruth et al., 2014) and hypoglycaemia (Loftin & Habli, 2010). They are more likely to be sleepy and difficult to feed, and also to have feeding difficulties in the early weeks (Ayton et al., 2012), and so need supplementation with expressed breastmilk or formula.

However, all of these difficulties can be overcome with time and support. As long as the supply of breastmilk is protected, twin parents can generally move towards exclusive breastfeeding if they wish, as their babies grow and their coordination improves.

DOI: 10.4324/9781003223771-22

## Preparing to Breastfeed

Before their babies are born, parents should have a *positive* conversation with healthcare professionals. Professionals need to be mindful of the language they use. Often parents report that they have been told it will be too difficult or, indeed, not possible to breastfeed their babies. This is not the case, and parents should be encouraged to give breastfeeding a try. There is no harm in being realistic; breastfeeding can be a difficult journey. But having twins is a difficult journey in itself and in the long run – once breastfeeding is established – the mothers I have supported have generally found it far easier than bottle feeding.

## Signposting to Support

Healthcare professionals can signpost parents to the most appropriate local breastfeeding support – if possible, an experienced breastfeeding counsellor or International Board Certified Lactation Consultant (IBCLC). An IBCLC is a health-care professional who specialises in the clinical management of breastfeeding. Consultants have undertaken at least 90 hours of lactation education and must have had considerable experience of providing breastfeeding care before they can take the exam leading to qualification by the International Board of Lactation Consultant Examiners. These breastfeeding specialists have the training and experience to support parents in a breastfeeding journey that may be quite complicated.

Healthcare professionals can also point parents in the direction of their local twins club. This can be a great source of emotional support, especially if there are other breastfeeding parents attending the group. Even if there are none, nobody understands what it is like having multiple babies better than other parents of multiples.

Good quality online support can be found in the UK via Facebook groups such as Breastfeeding Twins and Triplets UK and via the Twins Trust.

Going along to a 'Preparing to Breastfeed' session will inform parents about the practical elements of breastfeeding and normal newborn behaviour. Some hospitals also offer a specialist twins session. Accessing antenatal education at around 30 weeks' gestation is a good idea, in case the twins are born prematurely.

## Harvesting Colostrum Antenatally

Research shows that from 36 weeks of pregnancy, mothers can begin hand expressing and harvesting colostrum (Forster et al., 2017) and that doing this increases maternal confidence in breastfeeding (Brisbane & Giglia, 2013). It is generally best to hand express due to the small quantities of colostrum involved. If birth has been scheduled for before 37 weeks' gestation, parents can discuss with their doctor or midwife whether it is appropriate to begin hand expressing before 36 weeks. Drops of colostrum can be sucked straight into a syringe from the nipple or expressed into a sterilised teaspoon or small pot and then sucked up into a syringe. Colostrum should be frozen in syringes clearly labelled with the date of expression, the mother's name and her hospital number and taken to the hospital at delivery. Parents should inform staff when booking-in that they have colostrum stored, so that it can be used for any supplementary feeds needed, or if the mother is unable to feed after the birth.

All staff on delivery and postnatal wards should be informed that the mother would like to breastfeed. If formula is advised, reasons should be given and risks discussed. Parents should be supported to use expressed breast milk to supplement their babies whenever possible. It may also be possible to access donor milk, which is usually preferable if extra milk is needed. Any top-ups should be offered by syringe, cup or paced bottle feeding. Paced bottle feeding mimics breastfeeding in that it involves 'pacing' feeds to allow the baby to be more in control and to recognise when he or she has reached satiety. The baby is fed more slowly and has to work harder to get the milk as opposed to typical bottle feeding.

## Premature Birth

If the babies are born early and taken to the neonatal unit, the mother should be supported to hand express as soon as possible after the birth (ideally within six hours). Following this, hand expressing should be encouraged every two to three hours to prime the prolactin receptors and ensure a full milk supply (Hill et al., 2005). Once her milk begins to come in, or if large volumes of colostrum are being extracted, the mother should move onto a hospital grade pump. Some hospitals have pumps with a preemie setting and these can be used for expressing colostrum. Some mothers respond better to a pump than to hand expressing, so it is worth trying if hand expressing is not working well.

Colostrum, and later milk, can be put straight into the feeding tube as soon as the babies are ready to take feeds. Every mother wishing to breastfeed should be supported to pump eight to twelve times in 24 hours. Breast massage before and during the expressing session should also be encouraged, as research shows this can increase milk output (Morton et al., 2009). Double pumping also results in higher milk volumes (Fewtrell et al., 2016).

Kangaroo care should be supported as soon as the babies are stable. Preterm babies become more stable more quickly when held skin to skin (Bergman et al., 2004). Frequent and extended skin to skin has also been associated with earlier exclusive breastfeeding and higher volumes of milk when expressing (Nyqvist, 2007).

Rooting has been observed as early as 28 weeks' gestation in very premature babies, and longer sucking bursts at 32 weeks; so, once babies are stable, they can be given the opportunity to try the breast (Nyqvist et al., 1999). To begin with, the babies may just lick or nuzzle and perhaps latch on and have a few sucks. The majority of their feeds will continue to be via a feeding tube and pumping continues to be necessary.

Skilled breastfeeding supporters can assess when the babies are feeding well enough to move towards exclusive breastfeeding. Some will be ready to do this at or before 36–37 weeks' gestation; others will take longer and it may be only at 40 weeks' gestation, or more, when they can stop receiving top-ups.

## Birth at 36 to 37 Weeks

Many twins are born at 36 to 37 weeks' gestation. This is considered a full-term pregnancy for twins; however, it is important to remember that this is still quite early in terms of the babies' development. Due to immature brain development and suck pressure, they are more likely to be sleepy and hard to rouse, to fall asleep easily at the breast, to have short sucking bursts or to be uncoordinated in their suck, swallow, breathe pattern, which is significantly associated with suboptimal breastfeeding (Meier et al., 2013). Some will be able to breastfeed exclusively and transfer enough milk; some will not. A skilled breastfeeding assessment should be offered to ensure the babies are feeding well enough to exclusively breastfeed.

The babies may be too sleepy to cue for feeds. If this is the case, parents should be encouraged to feed no later than three hours from the start of the previous feed, thus ensuring a minimum of eight feeds a day (Nyqvist, 2007).

If the babies are not feeding effectively, a feeding plan incorporating time at the breast, pumping and topping up, or 'triple feeding', may be necessary. It should be stressed that this is a short-term intervention until the babies are feeding more effectively and can move towards exclusive breastfeeding. Support for the mother is essential during this time.

Even if a large proportion of the babies' feeds are formula, it is still possible to move towards exclusive breastfeeding, if that is what the parents wish to do. As the babies begin to breastfeed more effectively, top-ups of formula can be gradually reduced, then stopped. There is little research to say when the window of opportunity closes as far as establishing exclusive breastfeeding is concerned. With good breastfeeding support both online and face to face, many families can move towards exclusive breastfeeding after a difficult start.

## Responsive Breastfeeding

Once the babies are feeding efficiently and waking themselves before or around the three hours' mark, are past their due date and gaining weight as expected, the mother can follow their lead and move to responsive feeding. The average breast-fed baby aged one to six months feeds 11 times in 24 hours, with a range of six to 18 feeds (Kent et al., 2006). Parents should be reassured that frequent feeding is normal. If tandem feeding, parents can follow the feeding cues of the hungrier or more alert baby and wake the other so as to feed both together.

## Tandem Feeding

Tandem feeding, that is feeding the twins together, is a useful skill, but not essential. It enables the mother to settle both her babies at once and can help stimulate her milk supply. Tandem feeding maximises the time off for the mother in between feeds and encourages the babies to nap at the same time.

It is the mother's choice whether she tandem feeds all the time, occasionally or not at all. Some mothers prefer to have some one-to-one time with their babies or find tandem feeding physically overwhelming and prefer to feed each baby separately.

Babies can successfully tandem feed from early on. If one baby is feeding better than the other, tandem feeding can help the poorer feeder as the stronger baby does all the hard work of stimulating the mother's let down reflex and maintaining the flow of milk. Research suggests that when tandem feeding, the milk has a higher fat content and the mother experiences more frequent let downs, which can help a weaker feeder (Prime et al., 2012).

Many mothers wonder whether they should give each baby a different breast from feed to feed, or from day to day, when tandem feeding. Swapping means that each eye and each ear of both babies will be stimulated by being on top during different feeds, and that if one breast has a stronger flow (which is quite normal), both babies will benefit. However, not swapping may mean that each baby gets more 'personally tailored' breastmilk (Al-Shehri et al., 2013).

## Combination Feeding

Parents of twins may decide that combination feeding, i.e. feeding their babies a mix of breastmilk and formula, is necessary. The mother may have insufficient glandular tissue in her breasts, or a poor start to breastfeeding may have compromised her supply. The mother may feel that she needs to have a break from breastfeeding, get some sleep or spend time with older children. Combination feeding is always better than giving up breastfeeding completely. It is surprising how many families do not realise that it is an option, believing that breastfeeding is an all or nothing undertaking. As always, breastfeeding professionals need to listen to parents' feeding goals and try to understand their personal situations. Many families fall into a pattern of giving their twins one or two bottles a day at set times and breastfeeding responsively for the rest of the time. This can work well as it means that breastfeeding can be increased as and when the babies' needs change.

## Breastfeeding and Mental Health

Many parents expecting twins experience a lack of control. Twin pregnancy is higher risk (Cheong-See et al., 2016), so birth choice is reduced; there's a higher chance of interventions during labour and premature birth is more likely. Twin parents are also more likely to experience postnatal depression (Wenze et al., 2015). Looking after more than one baby is very difficult, no matter how they are fed.

However, mothers who meet their personal goals for breastfeeding duration have been shown to be at lower risk of postnatal depression, while mothers who plan to breastfeed but do not go on to do so are at higher risk (Borra et al., 2014). Breastfeeding is about far more than nutrition. It is a wonderful way to bond with twin babies, to soothe, settle, love and give immunity to them, even if some of their nutrition is provided in another way. Therefore, skilled support should always be available for parents of multiples who wish to breastfeed.

## Practice Pointers

- It is possible to breastfeed multiples, and if the parent wishes to do so, it is important that they receive adequate support to achieve their goal.
- Barriers to breastfeeding include preterm, late preterm and early term birth as well as the issues of logistics around feeding more than one baby.
- Frequent and efficient removal of the milk, preferably by the babies with a good latch, or by hospital grade double pump if the babies are not breastfeeding or are struggling, should ensure milk production is established.
- Each baby's breastfeeding skills need to be assessed. One baby in a set of multiples can struggle to feed more than another. Feeding plans should be adjusted accordingly.
- Many parents find breastfeeding to be easier than other methods of feeding once the hurdles of the first few weeks are overcome.

## References

Al-Shehri, S., Henman, M., Charles, B.G., Cowley, D., Shaw, P.N. et al. (2013) Collection and determination of nucleotide metabolites in neonatal and adult saliva by high performance liquid chromatography with tandem mass spectrometry. Journal of Chromatography, 931:140–147.

Ayton, J., Hanson, E., Quinn, S., Nelson, M. (2012) Factors associated with initiation and exclusive breastfeeding at hospital discharge: Late preterm compared to 37 week gestation mother and infant cohort. International Breastfeeding Journal, 7(16). doi:10.1186/1746–4358-7-16

Bergman, N.J., Linley, L.L., Fawcus, S.R. (2004) Randomised controlled trial of skin to skin contact from birth versus conventional incubator for physiological stabilization in 1200–2199 gram newborns. Acta Paediatrica, 93(6):779–785.

Borra, C., Iacovou, M., Sevilla, A. (2014) New evidence on breastfeeding and postpartum depression: The importance of understanding women's intentions. Maternal and Child Health Journal, 19(4):897–907.

Brisbane, J., Giglia, R. (2013) Experiences of expressing and storing colostrum antenatally: A qualititive study of mothers in regional Western Australia. Journal of Child Health Care, 19(2):206–215.

Cheong-See, F., Schuit, E., Arroyo-Manzano, D., Khalil, A., Barrett, J. et al. (2016) Prospective risk of stillbirth and neonatal complications in twin pregnancies: Systematic review and meta-analysis. British Medical Journal, 354:i4353.

Fewtrell, M.S., Kennedy, K., Ahluwalia, S., Nicholl, R., Lucas, A. et al. (2016) Predictors of expressed breast milk volume in mothers expressing milk for their preterm infant. Archives of Disease in Childhood, 101(6):F502-F506.

Forster, D.A., Moorhead, A.M., Jacobs, S.E., Davis, P.G., Walker, S.P. (2017) Advising women with diabetes in pregnancy to express breastmilk in late pregnancy (Diabetes and Antenatal Milk Expressing [DAME]): A multicentre, unblinded, randomised controlled trial. Lancet, 389(10085):2204–2213.

Hill, P.D., Aldag, J.C., Chatterton, R.T., Zinaman, M. (2005) Primary and secondary mediators' influence on milk output in lactating mothers of preterm and term infants. Journal of Human Lactation, 21(2):138–150.

Kent, J.C., Mitoulas, L.R., Cregan, M.D., Ramsay, D.T., Doherty, D.A. (2006) Volume and frequency of breastfeedings and fat content of breast milk throughout the day. Pediatrics, 117(3):e387-e395.

Loftin, R.W., Habli, M. (2010) Late preterm birth. Obstetrics and Gynecology, 3(1):10–19.

Macones, G. (2005) Multiple birth. In: Taeush, W., Ballard, R., Gleason, C. (Eds.) Avery's Diseases of the Newborn (8th Ed.). Philadelphia: Elsevier: 57–62.

Meier, P., Aloka, L., Patel, M.D., Wright, K., Engstrom, J.L. et al. (2013) Management of breastfeeding during and after the maternity hospitalization for late preterm infants. Clinics in Perinatology, 40(4):689–705.

Morton, J., Hall, J.Y., Wong, R.J., Thairu, L., Benitz, W.E. (2009) Combining hand techniques with electric pumping increases milk production of mothers with preterm infants. Journal of Perinatology, 29(11):757–764.

Nyqvist, K.H. (2007) Breastfeeding preterm infants. In: Genna, C.W. (Ed.) Supporting Sucking Skills. Boston, MA: Jones and Bartlett: 153–180.

Nyqvist, K.H., Sjoden, O., Ewald, E. (1999) The development of preterm infants' feeding behaviour. Early Human Development, 55(3):247–264.

Prime, D.K., Garbin, C.P., Hartmann, P.E., Kent, J.C. (2012) Simultaneous breast expression in breastfeeding women is more efficacious than sequential breast expression. Breastfeeding Medicine, 7(6):442–447.

Ruth, C.A., Roos, N.P., Hildes-Ripstein, E., Brownell, M.D. (2014) Early term infants, length of birth stay and neonatal readmission for jaundice. Paediatrics and Child Health, 19(7):353–354.

Wenze, S.J., Battle, C.L., Tezanos, K.M. (2015) Raising multiples: Mental health of mothers and fathers in early parenthood. Archives of Women's Mental Health, 18:163–176.

Whitford, H., Wallis, S.K., Dowswell, T., West, H.M., Renfrew, M.J. (2017) Breastfeeding education and support for women with twins or higher order multiples. Cochrane Database. doi:10.1002/14651858.CD012003.pub2.

# 19

# HELPING PARENTS UNDERSTAND AND NAVIGATE THE TWIN BOND

*Joan A. Friedman*

All too often, children of multiple births are thought of as a singular unit. They're known as 'the twins' rather than two separate people. Encouraging individuality when raising twins requires a discriminating appreciation for each twin's emotional needs. This chapter outlines the essential principles that help cultivate a heathy twinship and a harmonious parent–child relationship while still nurturing the unique sibling bond.

★

The core tenet of my philosophy is that parents and professionals need to treat twins as two distinct children who happen to be born at the same time. This perspective goes far beyond the conventional advice to dress twins differently and choose names that don't begin with the same letter of the alphabet. Authentically perceiving and treating twins as two unique children may involve fundamentally changing your mind about what it means to be a twin and adjusting expectations about how twins should interact.

## The Twin Mystique

In order to consider a new perspective on how to raise emotionally healthy twins, it's important to think about how twins are romanticized in Western cultures. Stereotypically, most people think of twins as soul mates connected to each other through a kind of sibling extra-sensory perception. Many of us assume that one twin not only knows what the other is thinking and feeling but can also fill in the empty spaces in the other's persona. It is assumed that each feels lost without the other and that they seek to preserve their twosome status even as adults. Non-twins fantasize that in a twin relationship, one twin always knows what the other

DOI: 10.4324/9781003223771-23

one wants and needs, and for this reason, it is generally felt that twins are each other's pre-destined partner and confidant.

Each of these assumptions contributes to what I call the 'twin mystique', and it has been around a long time. There is something inherently captivating about the idea of having a double, because it invokes a human longing for an intimate, lifelong companion who thoroughly understands us. With such a companion, we feel we would never be abandoned or alone. People project this longing onto twins and see them as enjoying an idealized, intermingled relationship.

Twins can indeed be lifelong friends and can fulfill many emotional needs for each other. But if they are expected to fulfill the fantasy of telepathic soul mates who inhabit a mysterious world of their own, they will never be free to develop as separate individuals.

## Managing Mixed Emotions

Professionals who work with twins moms-to-be should model a measured response to the news. Not every woman will react well to a flippant remark such as 'double trouble'. Being sensitive to each individual's experience is essential. Finding out about a twins pregnancy can elicit a myriad of emotions on the part of the mother and father, some of which they may feel guilty or ashamed about. Even if the parents had anticipated the possibility of twins owing to in vitro procedures or genetic history, learning for certain that they'll be bringing two babies into the world is an emotional jolt. Parents' responses can include shock, ambivalence, anxiety and distress, as well as pride and fulfillment.

If they are first-time parents-to-be and have struggled to get pregnant or undergone months – even years – of in vitro treatments, their initial reactions are, of course, elation and triumph. Women feel they finally belong; they are at last entitled to join the most primal and meaningful of sororities: birth mothers. Men who have experienced with their partners the possibility of permanent infertility may feel especially validated and proud about having twins. After trying, failing and trying again and again to help create a baby, they are now thrilled to be expecting two. Chances are words such as 'grateful', 'blessing', 'ecstatic' and even 'miracle' describe how both feel about the news. Even expectant parents who have not undergone in vitro treatment are generally delighted to find out that they'll be having twins.

However, there are the less-than-joyful, yet very common emotional responses, many of which parents expecting twins tend to keep under wraps. First, there is the shock – contemplating the reality of two babies instead of one: being pregnant with them, delivering them and somehow managing to care for them. Parents worry that they won't be able to handle the physical work of taking care of two babies at once, that they won't be able to give each baby adequate attention or be able to cope financially. If they already have children, they worry about devoting enough time to them once the twins arrive. Women who work outside the home may fear a loss of identity due to the need to cut back on working hours or put their career on hold. Parents are also concerned about the increased physical risks for the babies and the mother during pregnancy. Common concerns include intrauterine growth restriction (IUGR), pre-eclampsia, gestational diabetes and needing bed rest or hospitalization during the pregnancy. Concerns about labor and birth include placental abruption, pre-term labor/delivery, cesarean birth, low birth weight and fetal demise/loss. For all of these reasons, expectant parents of twins may secretly wish they were having only one baby and feel guilty for harboring such thoughts.

## Core Guidelines for Supporting Parents of Twins

a) Help parents think of the twins as unique individuals

Twins need to be seen and addressed as individual children who will grow up to be individual adults. If parents relate to them as 'twins' rather than as separate beings, the twins will relate to each other and the world as 'twins' because that will be the reality they know. Helping parents to think of their babies as distinct individuals from the moment they are told that they are pregnant with twins will ensure that the babies/children/adults think of themselves as unique. The twins are defined by many more influences than simply their relationship to each other inside or outside the womb. In the first stages of life, the parent–child relationship, not the intrauterine communication between the twins, is the most important aspect of a child's development.

b) Help parents understand that they will have different feelings for each child

Even parents of singletons can feel guilty about having different feelings for each of their children. Parents of twins tend to feel such guilt more strongly. A core emotional dilemma facing many new parents of twins is feeling more attached to one baby than the other.

However, if we accept that our children are unique, it only makes sense that they will elicit different feelings in us. Feeling impatient with one twin baby and delighted by the other, feeling angry at one two-year-old's willfulness and relieved that the other plays happily by herself or even a feeling of having more in common with one pre-teen twin than the other does not mean that parents love one child more than the other. Accepting different feelings in response to each child's behavior and personality acknowledges their uniqueness.

Parents of newborn twins need to understand the challenges of bonding with two babies, and that their relationship to each is fluid and changeable. The healthiest way for parents to negotiate this initial phase of getting to know each of their babies is to be honest and authentic about their feelings. Yet, some parents are so upset by their feelings of favoring one baby over the other that they can't acknowledge or discuss the emotional turmoil they're going through. Many insist that they have no preference, that they love both babies the same. Yet, when parents acknowledge that they prefer one baby over the other for various reasons, they not only unburden themselves of troubling feelings, but they can take whatever steps might be necessary to avert a potential problem. Preferences reveal the distinctions between two babies whose relationship with their parents and whose emerging personalities are unique. Ambivalent feelings about parenting babies are normal and have nothing to do with loving or caring about them.

c) Support parents to have 'alone time' with each child

Every infant requires one-on-one time with his or her parent; it is a basic human need. A child cannot feel known to his parent, and a parent cannot adequately know her child without regular, focused time together which enables the parent to attune to the baby's emotional and physical communications.

As a baby experiences being responded to again and again, a secure attachment develops. He comes to expect that he will be appropriately nurtured when he is hungry or tired, happy or excited. Enabling him to get to know his parent – and feel known by her – lays the foundation for his sense of who he is in relation to the world. The need for alone time with parents does not end at infancy. Parents of twins need to offer each child regular one-on-one time throughout their childhood.

Even when parents of twins believe wholeheartedly in the importance of nurturing their children's individual identities, and even though they may long for exclusive time with their babies beyond basic care-taking duties, there can be a certain resistance to undertaking the alone time strategy. There are several reasons for this. First of all, a parent's need to prove their parental competence may inhibit them from spending time alone with each child. There may be the sense that 'I desperately wanted these babies and I'm determined to show that I can handle caring for both of them at the same time'. Another factor is a parent's concern about bonding equally with each baby. Although parents may acknowledge that it's natural to have different responses to their babies' distinct temperaments and demands, they may nonetheless worry that if they spend time alone with each child, they might bond with one more than the other and thus be guilty of 'unequal' treatment. Finally, the 'twin mystique' feeds the erroneous notion that separating twins is somehow unhealthy. Parents are led to believe that if they separate their babies even for relatively short periods of time, the sibling bond will be diminished or harmed.

Yet, in reality, alone time generally relieves parents of the sense that they're not meeting either child's needs properly or are meeting one baby's needs more than the other's. When parents spend one-on-one time with each baby, they experience a positive emotional reaction rather than a guilty or conflicted one. They receive satisfaction and fulfillment from bonding with their babies, but unless they create alone time with each child, this can't happen. Alone time helps parents celebrate each baby rather than feeling guilty about 'inequality' or 'unfairness'.

d) Help parents not to worry about providing a fair and equal childhood for the twins

Just as it is impossible to create a completely safe environment for children, it is also impossible to create a fair and equal one. Yet, most parents, especially parents of twins, understandably feel the need to try to do just that. In fact, an important part of parents' job is to help their children learn how to adapt to or overcome unfair circumstances. Parents who attempt to create a 'fair and equal' environment for their twins, however well-meaning, give them a false impression about themselves and the world and inhibit their ability to deal with life's inevitable inequalities.

e) Help parents understand that their twins do not need to be each other's constant companion or surrogate parent

It can be a relief for parents to assume that their twins want to be together and take care of each other. As young children, the twins may seem like built-in playmates; as they get older, they may appear to enjoy being each other's best friend and most trusted confidant. One twin may take on the role of surrogate parent, seeing to the other's emotional needs. However, when 'two much togetherness' shuts out parents and others, twins don't learn how to socialize in an age-appropriate manner. And the lack of psychological boundaries between twin children can lead to confused roles and, sometimes, inappropriate behavior.

When twins parent each other, they may develop an intense need to maintain an emotional equilibrium. This means that, in order not to disturb their overly close connection, each child denies her own feelings or prevents herself from branching out on her own for fear of upsetting the other. When twins become each other's parental figure, it can be a sign that their real parents are not adequately fulfilling their parental roles. Every child, even those who have a close relationship with a sibling, needs focused attention, guidance and emotional support from their parents.

Parents of twins are understandably impressed with their children's compassion toward each other and their overall ability to get along. They may seem to have interpersonal skills that singletons of the same age don't have. Parents may boast about how the twins take care of one another, share their possessions and play with each other for long periods of time.

Since twin togetherness is taken for granted as an inherent aspect of the twin relationship, it may not occur to parents that their children might be missing an important part of their social and emotional education by not having the experiences singletons have. When children cling to the safety net of their friendship with their twin, many have difficulty forming relationships and making friends outside the family. A twin relationship involving too much togetherness can push compassion into the unhealthy realm of negating one's own abilities, desires and goals. If twins go through their childhood as a couple, they miss out on the experience of being an individual, of testing their own behavior and personality against new people with whom they interact.

One twin taking care of the other may seem natural and loving. However, it is important for parents to understand that when the caretaker role characterizes one twin's interactions with his sibling, or when the cared-for twin expects his twin's attention and can't seem to function without it, the relationship is seriously interfering with each child's ability to become his own person.

## Fathers and Babies, Fathers and Mothers

Having twins provides an expanded opportunity for a father to be involved with his children when they're babies. A father's participation in early childcare always enriches a child's life, but with twins, it is a necessity. When twin babies are fortunate enough to have the full involvement of both parents, they don't have to struggle as much over sharing their mother, and they enjoy the added benefit of getting to know their father intimately from day one. Not only does a dad's involvement lessen a mother's burden and help lay the foundation for a stronger bond between the father and each child, but it can also create a happier relationship between the parents.

However, men may feel profoundly confused by their partners' emotional swings. On the one hand, new moms may be resentful that their spouses are not helping out more with the babies, and at the same time, criticize themselves for needing help. Many judge their maternal adequacy in terms of how well they can handle their parenting duties without assistance. Needing help may engender feelings of dependency which can lead to anger. Some moms may displace their self-criticism for feeling unable to manage two babies without help by getting angry with their husbands and partners.

The new dad is also going through his own emotional changes. He may feel disconnected from and abandoned by his partner and replaced by two tiny, needy babies whom he's trying his best to adjust to. He may attempt to help with childcare chores, even take on an equal parenting role, but the mother may be so critical of his efforts that he feels ineffectual and unappreciated.

Professionals and others seeking to help families with young twins need to remember the father's or partner's need for support as well as offering suggestions on how he or she can help the mother through the exhausting first months and year of the twins' lives. Partners need to understand the need of the new mother for compliments on what a wonderful job she is doing. The slightest hint of disapproval of her mothering can be construed as intensely critical or disparaging, especially in the initial months after the babies' arrival. Partners who simply ask how they can help or take charge of what needs to be done will be cherished!

## Practice Pointers

### Tips for Professionals to Share with Expectant Parents of Twin Babies

- Arrange enough outside help for the first few months of your babies' lives. If a nanny or babysitter is beyond your budget, compile a list of trusted friends, relatives or neighbors who might be willing to pitch in, even for an hour or two a week.
- Sit down with your partner and devise a workable plan for each of you to spend alone time with each baby. The more prepared you are ahead of time, the less frazzled you'll be when your babies arrive – and the more benefit your children will derive from the alone time spent with each of you.
- When buying or borrowing necessary baby items, don't forget to include a single buggy so that you can take each baby out separately during your alone times.
- As you get ready to bring two new babies into your family, continue to think about each child as a distinct individual whom you will get to know and cherish as his or her own unique person.

### Tips for Professionals to Share with New Parents of Twin Babies

- Make sure that you provide each baby with experiences apart from his or her twin so that each one has the chance to be an individual.
- Try to avoid comparing one baby's milestone moments to the other's. Each child develops at his or her own pace.
- Use your alone times with each baby to discover each one's unique personality.
- Don't feel guilty about preferring one baby's behavior over the other's. Your preferences don't mean that you love that baby more; your preferences reveal that you perceive your babies as distinct beings.
- Find a peer support group where you can openly discuss the parent-of-twins emotional overload that you're likely to be experiencing.

### Tips for Professionals to Share with Parents about Encouraging Individuality

- Take separate photos of each twin with mom and dad as well as photos of each twin by him/herself.
- Sing happy birthday twice with two separate cakes or cupcakes!
- Give different birthday presents in the same genre – for example, a dump truck and a crane.
- Buy or borrow an inexpensive single buggy to have on hand for alone time with each twin.

- Describe personality traits rather than labeling your twins. For example, instead of labeling one child 'shy' and the other 'sociable', you can say one twin loves being the center of attention while the other one needs more time to get accustomed to new situations.

## Tips for Professionals to Share with Fathers/Partners of Twin Babies

- Be as involved as possible from the beginning of your babies' lives. This will help you establish your role as a father, ease the mother's exhaustion, and most importantly, help you to form a unique relationship with each baby. Get to know each child separately, apart from his twin and his mother.
- Help the mother spend alone time with each baby by spending time alone with the other baby. This way you'll both feel uniquely connected to each child.
- Make your own plans for alone time with each baby/toddler, choosing activities you and the child enjoy. This way, you won't feel as if you're being controlled by your partner and lack independence as a parent.
- Let the mother know that you are supportive of her getting the outside help she may need. New moms tend to be hard on themselves and may view the need for help as a measure of inadequacy. Reassure her that this is definitely not the case.
- Make time, if at all possible, to be together with your partner – just the two of you. With all that you're both going through, you need experiences that help you reconnect and enjoy each other's company away from your babies.
- Think about reconnecting primarily with physical affection rather than sexual contact in the initial period after the babies' births. In time, this will lead to greater intimacy.
- When your partner reveals how distraught she is by all that is expected of her as a new mother of twins, don't feel you have to come up with specific solutions. She will appreciate just being listened to.
- The greatest support you can give your partner is time, patience, love and affirmation.

## Bibliography

The following books, papers and resources have informed the writing of Joan Friedman's chapter.

Bacon, K. (2006) 'It's good to be different': Parent and child negotiations of 'twin' identity. Twin Research and Human Genetics, 9(1):141–147.

Beebe, B., Lachmann, F. (2005) Infant Research and Adult Treatment: Co-constructing interactions. Hilldale, NJ: Analytic Press.

Burlingham, D. (1952) Twins: A study of three pairs of identical twins. New York: International Universities Press.

Cherro, M. (1992) Quality of bonding and behavioral differences in twins. Infant Mental Health Journal, 13(3):206–210.

Cohen, M. (2003) Sent Before My Time. London: Karnac Books: 19–49.

Duffy, C. (2018) Twin to Twin: From high risk pregnancy to happy family. Coral Gables, FL: Mango Publishing.

Fraga, J. (2018) Psst: Parenting twins can be depressing. Available at: https://www.npr. org/ sections/health-shots/2018/08/29/642716553/pssst-parenting- <accessed 03 Feb, 2020>

Friedman, J.A. (2008) Emotionally Healthy Twins: A philosophy for parenting two unique children. Cambridge, MA: Da Capo Press.

Friedman, J.A. (2014) The Same but Different: How twins can live, love, and learn to be individuals. Los Angeles, CA: Rocky Pines Press.

Friedman, J.A (2018) Twins in Session: Case histories in treating twinship issues. Los Angeles, CA: Rocky Pines Press.

Gottfried, N.W., Seay, B.M. (1994) Attachment relationships in infant twins: The effect of co-twin presence during separation from mother. Journal of Genetic Psychology, 155(3):273–281.

Klein, B. (2012) Alone in the Mirror: Twins in therapy. New York: Routledge.

Lewin, V. (2016) The Twin Enigma. London: Karnac Books.

Noble, N., Bradley, L., Parr, G., Duemer, L. (2017) Fostering twins' identity development: A family issue. The Family Journal, 25(4):345–350.

Sandbank, S.C. (1999) Twin and Triplet Psychology: A professional guide to working with multiples. London: Routledge.

Simon, R. (2016) There is no such thing as a baby: Early psychic development in twins. Contemporary Psychoanalysis, 52(3):362–374.

Stewart, E. (2003) Exploring Twins: Toward a social analysis of twinship. Basingstoke: Palgrave Macmillan.

Winnicott, D.W. (1964) The Child, the Family, and the Outside World. London: Penguin Publishing: 137–140.

Woodward, J. (1998) The Lone Twin. London: Free Association Books.

# PART V
# What Parents Need to Know about Sleeping, Weaning and the Media

## Introduction

While the need to understand the process of labour and birth, and to prepare for this threshold experience, is paramount, numerous research studies have shown that expectant parents are also eager to prepare for the challenges they will meet in the first weeks, months and year of their baby's life. Their urgent need for information and to talk about the postnatal period is sometimes overlooked in antenatal education, and is insufficiently met by opportunities for ongoing parenting education after the birth.

In this section of the book, authors provide both best evidence and guidelines for practitioners when answering parents' questions relating to their babies' sleep patterns, the introduction of solids and media use.

Our evolutionary legacy as human beings shapes our babies' feeding and sleep patterns and their need for proximity to caregivers. However, parents' expectations, based on cultural assumptions, about when and how long their babies will sleep, may be at odds with the solid evidence around sleep duration and night waking. Practitioners can help parents understand that normal infant sleep is characterised by night-time waking at least into the second year of life and that there is a wide range of typical sleep patterns from birth to three. Parents looking for behavioural interventions to address night-time wakings can be introduced to the importance of developing and maintaining a consistent bedtime routine from around six months of age and reducing their involvement at bedtime so as to promote their infants' ability to self-soothe to sleep.

Many practitioners working in the critical 1,000 days will be asked by parents of babies who are around six months to advise them on introducing solids. Evidence stresses the importance of offering babies a variety of foods and of including lumpy and textured foods from an early age. Practitioners who are

DOI: 10.4324/9781003223771-24

caring for the increasing number of families who wish to wean their babies onto a vegan diet should emphasise that an entirely plants-based diet needs careful planning and appropriate supplementation to meet children's essential nutrient needs.

The challenge posed by the proliferation of media is daunting and practitioners may well find themselves being asked to provide guidance to parents. The literature on the impact of early media use on parent-child interactions and children's social-emotional development has expanded considerably in recent years. There is concerning evidence that higher duration of daily media use correlates with lower toddler and pre-schooler language scores. Discussions with parents can focus on both the positive opportunities that media provide for talking together and sharing information and ideas, as well as its potential threat to the quality of the relationship between parents and children.

# 20

# INFANT SLEEP AND FEEDING IN EVOLUTIONARY PERSPECTIVE

*Alanna E.F. Rudzik*

Infant sleep and infant feeding are essential concerns for new parents who are learning to care for an infant. The expectations of infants with regard to feeding and sleep are fundamentally shaped by our evolutionary legacy as mammals and primates, as well as the more recent evolutionary history of our own human lineage. The first part of this chapter provides a review of how our evolutionary legacy affects infant biological expectations for feeding, sleep and proximity to caregivers. At the same time, humans are fundamentally biocultural: our biology is at all times shaped by and intertwined with culture. The second part of the chapter considers how cultural assumptions can shape parental beliefs about infant feeding and sleep, regardless of infants' biological expectations, and provides solid evidence related to infant sleep duration and night-waking. This information can be used to educate and reassure new parents about normal infant sleep.

*

Humans belong to the taxonomic class, Mammalia. Mammals are distinct from others in the animal kingdom in that they nourish offspring using milk produced by the mother's body. Lactation and breastfeeding provided a selective advantage throughout evolution because they allow the mother to buffer the infant from a lack of resources in the environment by mobilising energy and nutrient stores from her own body (Power & Schulkin, 2016). Milk is synthesised from fat, protein, carbohydrates and micronutrients that the mother is able to accumulate prior to and during pregnancy. As a result, even if the infant is born during a period when food is scarce, the infant's growth and development are protected by this evolutionarily novel food source.

DOI: 10.4324/9781003223771-25

The milk produced by different mammalian species has characteristics which have evolved to serve the very different life histories and care strategies of each species (Power & Schulkin, 2016). In some species, offspring are born immature, without the ability to see, hear or move independently (e.g. mice, rabbits) for weeks or months after birth. Offspring are generally part of a litter and are 'cached' (hidden away) by the mother in a warm, secure nest or burrow in early life. The mother will go off to find food and only return to the nest intermittently to feed her young. In line with this care strategy, the mother's milk must necessarily provide enough nutrients, particularly fat and protein, to support the offspring through the period that she is absent (Lozoff et al., 1977). In other species, offspring are born with well-developed senses and ready to travel with their mother within a few hours of birth (e.g. most primates, deer, giraffes). Generally, a mother in these 'carry/follow' species gives birth to a single infant who remains with her at all times, by means of clinging, following or being carried. Infants have constant access to the mother, whose proximity offers the warmth and security that in cached animals is provided by the nest. The milk produced by these mammalian mothers is high in lactose, which provides immediately usable energy, and low in fat and protein, since the infants feed frequently and long periods of separation between mother and infant are unlikely (Lozoff et al., 1977).

Human milk falls into the 'carry' pattern, due to our membership in the primate order. Like our non-human primate relatives (chimpanzees, gorillas etc.) human infants are born with well-developed senses of sight, hearing and proprioception (understanding of where the body is in space) and our evolutionary pattern aligns with a 'carry' strategy of infant care, rather than a 'cache' strategy (Rudzik & Ball, 2021). However, compared to other primates, human infants are extremely neurologically immature at birth, unable to travel independently or to cling to their mothers. This is the result of a trade-off unique to the human lineage. As adults, our brains are far larger than those of other primates but at birth, human infants have achieved only 25% of their full brain size, whereas the infants of other primates are born with brains roughly 50% of adult full size (Ball, 2007). Anthropologists have argued that at around 40 weeks gestation, human mothers reach a ceiling of energy transfer to the fetus which means that the mother's metabolism simply cannot support further brain growth *in utero* (Dunsworth et al., 2012). As a result, human infants are neurologically disorganized at birth and lack the ability to regulate their body temperature and other physiology effectively. These clues tell us that the evolutionary expectation for human infants in the first weeks and months of life is to be within reach of an adult at all times and to breastfeed frequently on demand.

## Human Evolutionary Legacy: Infant Sleep and Infant Feeding

For most of human evolutionary history, infants were fed breastmilk and slept in close proximity to an adult, usually their mother. This would have been a matter of survival, since being left alone would have increased the probability of death or injury from predators or exposure. Infants therefore are hard-wired to 'signal' (cry) when they are apart from their caregivers whether during the day or at night (Ball & Klingaman, 2008). This behaviour is not manipulative; it is simply a way to alert the caregiver that the infant has become separated. The evolutionary pattern of close proximity through the day and night persists in many populations around the world (Alexeyeff, 2013; Morelli et al., 1992; Tahhan, 2008) and indeed was the norm in Western societies until fairly recently (Ball, 2007). However, in modern societies that are Western, educated, industrialised, rich and democratic (WEIRD societies), infant care no longer resembles that provided during most of our evolutionary history (Lozoff & Brittenham, 1979). In the dominant parenting culture of these societies, infants have limited physical contact with caregivers and are often placed in high chairs, playpens, or strollers rather than carried by a caregiver. In particular, sleep most often takes place out of proximity of parents. An entire industry of audio visual monitors, heart rate and temperature sensors and 'smart' cribs/cots has developed in order to reassure parents of the well-being of infants who they have placed in a separate room to sleep. Parents who grew up in WEIRD societies view parent/infant separation for sleep as natural; however, in essence these practices mimic the behaviours shown by caching mammals, as described above. Since human infant physiology and human milk composition have evolved in context of a 'carry' strategy, separation or caching of the human infant can lead to negative consequences for infant health and survival.

Proximity between mother and infant is vital for the establishment and maintenance of lactation and the breastfeeding relationship, an important predictor of infant health outcomes. Separation in the newborn period can delay the onset of full milk production after birth, whereas closer proximity in the early days of life increases the duration of breastfeeding (Ball & Klingaman, 2008; Ball et al., 2006). Breastfeeding through the day and night may also encourage the establishment of day/night rhythms in infants. During pregnancy, the mother's physiology drives fetal circadian rhythms, but after birth, the maternal cues are lost and it takes weeks for the infant to establish rhythms of temperature, stress and sleep hormones (Rudzik et al., 2021). In breastfed infants, the sleep hormone, melatonin, which passes to the infant through the breastmilk, may play a role in advancing the development of day/night compatible sleep patterns, compared to formula fed infants, since formula does not contain melatonin (Arslanoglu et al., 2012). Infants at risk of Sudden Infant Death Syndrome (SIDS) and those who have suffered a life-threatening event show low levels of melatonin when compared with matched controls (Sivan et al., 2000; Cornwell & Feigenbaum, 2006). Lack of proximity between parents and child during sleep has also been identified as a risk factor for SIDS; public health guidelines recommend that infants should be placed to sleep in the same room as their parents for at least the first six months of life (Moon & Task Force on Sudden Infant Death Syndrome, 2016). While Western parents may view bedsharing as unsafe and separation during sleep as normal, Pacific Islanders, Mayans and others view solitary infant sleep as neglectful, abusive and/or risky (Alexeyeff, 2013; Ball, 2007; Morelli et al., 1992).

## Cultural Beliefs about Infant Feeding and Sleep

As mammals, human infants have evolved to be breastfed. Their biological 'expectation' is to be in proximity to a caregiver at all times, and to breastfeed frequently throughout the day and night. However, culture shapes and determines what a parent believes is normal in terms of feeding and sleep. There is a widespread perception in the US and the UK that infants who are breastfed do not sleep as well as those who are formula fed and that their mothers consequently experience worse sleep; family and friends often pressure new mothers to introduce formula to the diet of exclusively breastfed infants in order to improve their sleep (Brown & Harries, 2015; Douglas & Hill, 2013; Rosen, 2008; Rudzik & Ball, 2016). However, studies comparing the sleep of breastfed and formula fed infants have found no significant difference in objective sleep measures between the two groups (Rudzik et al., 2018). Likewise, maternal sleep and functioning are not negatively affected among breastfeeding mothers, as compared to those who formula feed (Doan et al., 2014; Montgomery-Downs et al., 2010). Inaccurate perceptions or assumptions related to infant and maternal sleep can shape parental decisions about whether to breastfeed their infant.

Beliefs about infant sleep that have become part of the broader cultural model can strongly influence parental expectations. In an early study of infant sleep (Moore & Ucko, 1957), researchers followed 104 infants from two weeks of age through to one year to determine at what age they began to sleep from midnight to 5am, a period that was described as 'sleeping through the night'. Using this definition, 70% of the infants in the study began sleeping through the night by the age of three months, a statistic that is widely used by clinicians to provide parents with guidance on infant sleep (Jones & Ball, 2012). However, the results of the study were more complicated than they first appear. Half of the infants who started to sleep through the night by three months of age, approximately 35% of the total sample, began once again to wake at night between six months and one year. Another 10% of the infants in the sample never slept through the night prior to one year of age. Thus, in reality nearly half the studied infants (45%) did *not* sleep through the night consistently starting at three months. Those who *did* sleep through the night, given the definition used in the research, may have been sleeping only for five hours—a period that most parents do not recognise as a full night's sleep (Henderson et al., 2013). When coupled with the lack of information about the feeding method of the infants, the clinical usefulness of the study is doubtful, yet the three-month guideline has become a widely accepted milestone among clinicians and laypeople alike.

Fortunately, high quality data regarding the duration and nature of infant sleep is now available. Galland and colleagues (2012) conducted a systematic review of 34 childhood sleep studies in industrialized countries around the world. This review found that infant sleep in the early months of life is highly variable; between birth and two months of age, the average number of hours of sleep is 14.6, spread throughout the 24-hour day, with an extremely wide range, extending from a lower limit of 9.3 hours to an upper limit of 20 hours. In this early period, infants wake on average 1.7 times per night (range 0–3.4 times). Around three months, as infants begin to consolidate their sleep into a longer period of overnight sleep with supplementary day time naps, the average number of hours of sleep drops by an hour to 13.6, with a somewhat narrower range (9.4–17.8 hours). Between three and six months, infants continue to wake 0.8 times per night (range: 0–3 times). By six months, the average number of hours of sleep drops to 12.9 (range: 8.8–17.0), an average that remains roughly constant through 12 months (12.9 hours) to two years of age (12.6 hours). The variability in hours of sleep declines from six months to two years, from a range of 8.8–17.0 hours at six months to a range of approximately 10–15 hours from 12 months to 2 years. Through 7–11 months, infants wake at night an average of 1.1 times (range: 0–3.1 times) and night-waking continues into the second year of life (0.7 times, range: 0–2.5). Galland and colleagues' work (2012) presents a picture of normal infant sleep that differs substantially from the three-month milestone for 'sleeping through the night' that arose from the Moore and Ucko (1957) study. Infants show great variability in terms of the duration of their sleep, especially in the early months, and night-waking is commonplace through the first and second year of life. Sharing these well-evidenced findings with parents may help to reassure them that their infant's sleep pattern falls within global norms for infant sleep.

## Practice Pointers

- Human infants have evolved to breastfeed frequently both day and night and to sleep in proximity to a caregiver.
- Cultural assumptions that shape parental perceptions of infant sleep and infant feeding often influence whether or not a parent is willing to breastfeed.
- Normal infant sleep is highly variable and is characterised by night-time waking through the second year of life.

## References

Alexeyeff, K. (2013) Sleeping safe: Perceptions of risk and value in Western and Pacific infant co-sleeping. In: K. Glaskin and R. Chenhall (Eds.) Sleep Around the World: Anthropological perspectives. New York: Palgrave Macmillan: 113–131.

Arslanoglu, S., Bertino, E., Nicocia, M., Moro, G.E. (2012) WAPM Working Group on nutrition potential: Chronobiotic role of human milk in sleep regulation. Journal of Perinatal Medicine, 40(1):1–8.

Ball, H.L. (2007) Night-time infant care: Cultural practice, evolution, and infant development. In: Liamputton, P. (Ed.) Childrearing and Infant Care Issues: A cross-cultural perspective. New York: Nova Science Publishers: 47–61.

Ball, H.L., Klingaman, K. (2008) Breastfeeding and mother-infant sleep proximity: Implications for infant care. In: Trevathan, W., Smith, E.O., McKenna, J.J. (Eds.) Evolutionary Medicine and Health: New perspectives. New York: Oxford University Press: 226–241.

Ball, H.L., Ward-Platt, M.P., Heslop, E., Leech, S.J., Brown, K.A. (2006) Randomised trial of infant sleep location on the postnatal ward: Implications for breastfeeding initiation and infant safety. Archives of Disease in Childhood, 91(12):1005–1010.

Brown, A., Harries, V. (2015) Infant sleep and night feeding patterns during later infancy: Association with breastfeeding frequency, daytime complementary food intake, and infant weight. Breastfeeding Medicine, 10(5):246–252.

Cornwell, A.C., Feigenbaum, P. (2006) Sleep biological rhythms in normal infants and those at high risk for SIDS. Chronobiology International, 23(5):935–961.

Doan, T., Gay, C.L., Kennedy, H.P., Newman, J., Lee, K.A. (2014) Nighttime breast-feeding behavior is associated with more nocturnal sleep among first-time mothers at one month postpartum. Journal of Clinical Sleep Medicine, 10(3):313–319.

Douglas, P.S., Hill, P.S. (2013) Behavioral sleep interventions in the first six months of life do not improve outcomes for mothers or infants: A systematic review. Journal of Developmental and Behavioral Pediatrics, 34(7):497–507.

Dunsworth, H.M., Warrener, A.G., Deacon, T., Ellison, P.T., Pontzer, H. (2012) Metabolic hypothesis for human altriciality. Proceedings of the National Academy of Sciences of the United States of America (PNAS), 109(38):15212–15216.

Galland, B.C., Taylor, B.J., Elder, D.E., Herbison, P. (2012) Normal sleep patterns in infants and children: A systematic review of observational studies. Sleep Medicine Reviews, 16(3):213–222.

Henderson, J.M.T., Motoi, G., Blampied, N.M. (2013) Sleeping through the night: A community survey of parents' opinions about and expectations of infant sleep consolidation. Journal of Paediatrics and Child Health, 49(7):535–540.

Jones, C.H.D., Ball, H.L. (2012) Medical anthropology and children's sleep: The mismatch between Western lifestyles and sleep physiology. In: Green, A., Westcombe, A.M. (Eds.) Sleep: Multidisciplinary perspectives. London: Jessica Kingsley Publishers:86–103.

Lozoff, B., Brittenham, G. (1979) Infant care: Cache or carry. Journal of Pediatrics, 95(3):478–483.

Lozoff, B., Brittenham, G., Trause, M., Kennell, J., Klaus, M. (1977) Mother-newborn relationship – Limits of adaptability. Journal of Pediatrics, 91(1):1–12.

Montgomery-Downs, H.E., Clawges, H.M., Santy, E.E. (2010) Infant feeding methods and maternal sleep and daytime functioning. Pediatrics, 126(6):e1562–e1568.

Moon, R.Y. & Task Force on Sudden Infant Death Syndrome (2016) SIDS and other sleep-related infant deaths: Evidence base for 2016 updated recommendations for a safe infant sleeping environment. Pediatrics, 138(5):e20162940.

Moore, T., Ucko, L.E. (1957) Night waking in early infancy: Part I. Archives of Disease in Childhood, 32(164):333–342.

Morelli, G., Oppenheim, D., Rogoff, B., Goldsmith, D. (1992) Cultural variation in infants' sleeping arrangements: Questions of independence. Developmental Psychology, 28(4):604–613.

Power, M.L., Schulkin, J. (2016) Milk: The biology of lactation. USA: Johns Hopkins University Press.

Rosen, L.A. (2008) Infant sleep and feeding. Journal of Obstetric, Gynecologic and Neonatal Nursing, 37(6):706–714.

Rudzik, A.E.F., Tomori, C., McKenna, J.J., Ball, H.L. (2021) Biocultural perspectives on infant sleep. In: Han, S., Tomori, C. (Eds.) The Routledge Handbook of Anthropology and Reproduction. London: Routledge Press:559–572.

Rudzik, A.E.F., Ball, H.L. (2021) Biologically normal sleep in the mother-infant dyad. American Journal of Human Biology. doi.org/10.1002/ajhb.23589.

Rudzik, A.E.F., Ball, H.L. (2016) Exploring maternal perceptions of infant sleep and feeding method among mothers in the United Kingdom: A qualitative focus group study. Maternal and Child Health Journal, 20(1):33–40.

Rudzik, A.E.F., Robinson-Smith, L., Ball, H.L. (2018) Discrepancies in maternal reports of infant sleep vs. actigraphy by mode of feeding. Sleep Medicine, 49:90–98.

Sivan, Y., Laudon, M., Kuint, J., Zisapel, N. (2000) Low melatonin production in infants with a life-threatening event. Developmental Medicine and Child Neurology, 42(7):487–491.

Tahhan, D.A. (2008) Depth and space in sleep: Intimacy, touch and the body in Japanese co-sleeping rituals. Body & Society, 14(4):37–56.

# 21

# SLEEP IN EARLY CHILDHOOD

## The Role of Bedtime Routines

*Angela D. Staples and Leah LaLonde*

Sleep changes rapidly from several shorter periods over 24 hours in the first weeks of life to one nap and one long period of sleep at night by age three. This review covers typical sleep patterns from birth through age three and discusses how parents' attitudes and behaviors change during this period. In addition to parent education about child sleep, we review two behavioral interventions that have been shown to be effective for addressing parent concerns about bedtime resistance and reducing night-time awakenings. These interventions – beginning about six months of age – aim to help parents reduce over-involvement prior to bedtime and in response to night awakenings, to promote their child's ability to self-soothe to sleep. Importantly, establishment of a consistent bedtime routine of 15 to 30 minutes may reduce or prevent both resistance at bedtime and frequent night-time awakenings.

★

The first three years of a child's life is a period of rapid growth in all areas from physical movement to changes in emotional expression to increasingly child-initiated and child-directed social interaction. During this time, sleep also changes dramatically from short periods of sleep throughout the day and night in the first weeks of life to a single period of sleep during the night and, for about half of children, one nap during the day by the second year of life. In addition to consolidating sleep so that most of it occurs at night, children also develop the ability to self-soothe back to sleep after waking during the night. Difficulty self-soothing back to sleep without parental assistance is a common sleep-related concern that parents of young children raise with their pediatrician (Honaker & Meltzer, 2016). Unfortunately, the number of physicians specially trained in childhood sleep problems and sleep disorders is far fewer than what is needed.

DOI: 10.4324/9781003223771-26

For example, in the US, pediatric sleep specialists represent fewer than one-tenth of medical providers (Honaker & Meltzer, 2016). Thus, parents and physicians alike are challenged to find workable solutions for both sleep problems (e.g., bedtime resistance) and sleep disorders (e.g., obstructive sleep apnea). An important caveat is that not all parents view the same sleep behavior as problematic (e.g., Owens, 2008). Thus, we define a sleep problem as those behaviors that parents identify as problematic while keeping in mind this definition likely differs across individuals, families, and cultures. This contrasts with sleep disorders, which have clearly defined medical criteria.

This review does not address sleep disorders such as sleep apnea, in part because treatment is primarily the domain of physicians. Additionally, this review does not address specific socio-cultural factors such as co-sleeping, feeding practices, or environmental factors (e.g., tobacco use, neighborhood noise, type of bedding) – all of which impact both parent and child sleep. Instead, we provide a selective overview of four interrelated topics regarding sleep in early childhood with a specific emphasis on behavioral interventions for sleep problems. First, we briefly review the typical changes in sleep from birth through age three. Second, we highlight parenting practices in relation to child development and cultural context. Third, we summarize effective sleep interventions for young children. Finally, we emphasize the role of the bedtime routine as a relatively straightforward practice that, when implemented early, may prevent the development of sleep problems.

## Typical Development of Sleep

Newborn infants sleep an average of 14–15 hours per 24-hour period, which drops to an average of 12 hours around two to three years of age (Galland et al., 2012). In the first two months, infants sleep approximately nine hours at night and six hours during the day (Sadeh et al., 2009). However, there is considerable variability in night-time sleep such that sleeping as few as six hours at night (with more daytime hours) or as many as 11 hours could both be viewed as typical or not problematic. From birth to age three, the number of hours children sleep at night increases, while the number of hours spent sleeping during the day declines (Sadeh et al., 2009).

While the timing, number, and duration of sleep episodes during daytime varies greatly in early infancy, between 8 and 12 months, daytime sleep consolidates into two nap periods, one in the morning and one in the afternoon (Mindell et al., 2016). Around 18 months, children sleep once per day for one to two hours in the afternoon. By age three, children decrease both the number of naps per week as well as their average duration (Staples et al., 2015), with roughly half of children no longer napping (Iglowstein et al., 2003). There are several factors that contribute to the age at which children stop napping, including both internal (e.g., brain development) and external factors (e.g., childcare) (Kurdziel et al., 2013). While we know that most two-year-old children nap and five-year-old children do not nap, there remain questions about whether there is an optimal or recommended age at which children could or should be encouraged to stop napping (Spencer et al., 2016; Thorpe et al., 2015). One consistent difference between three-year-old children who nap versus those who do not nap is that children who nap sleep less at night (Spencer et al., 2016; Thorpe et al., 2015). However, the total amount of sleep per 24-hour period is similar for children who are and those who are not napping (Thorpe et al., 2015). One implication is that by age three, some children sleep less at night because they are getting the recommended number of hours of sleep when considered over a 24-hour period. Thus, when determining if a child is getting sufficient sleep, parents and physicians should consider sleep over 24 hours and not just the amount of nightly sleep.

In addition to changes in the amount of daytime and night-time sleep, children also develop the ability to self-soothe back to sleep beginning around three months of age, with roughly 80% of children sleeping through the night by nine months (Owens, 2008). Yet, waking once each night every night of the week is common for children ages 6 to 11 months (Sadeh et al., 2009). By age three, waking once during the night declines to approximately three nights each week. The length of time children are awake at night also declines from more than one hour in newborns, to less than 20 minutes by age three (Sadeh et al., 2009), though it should be noted that, like hours of night-time sleep, there is wide variability in both the number and duration of night wakings. It should also be noted that brief periods of arousal happen several times per night, but children do not always signal (e.g., cry) that they are awake (Tikotzky & Sadeh, 2009). Thus, the majority of sleep research on awakenings, which use parent report, provide information about signaled awakenings as opposed to the total number of night-time arousals (Goodlin-Jones et al., 2001).

## Parenting Practices and Sleep

With changes in when and how long children sleep in early childhood, it probably appears self-evident that parenting behaviors surrounding sleep also change. For example, the majority of parents either nurse or bottle feed their infant before putting to bed for the first nine months of life (Sadeh et al., 2009). In contrast, the percentage of children who are nursed or bottle fed after waking during the night declines rapidly from birth to four months and then continues to decline through age three (Sadeh et al., 2009). As infants develop, need for nourishment during the night decreases rapidly, which is typically matched by a decline in parents offering nourishment. In addition to changes in nourishment, attitudes or beliefs about why their infant is waking during the night are another reason for changes in parental response.

Two longitudinal studies, one of first-time mothers (Tikotzky & Sadeh, 2009) and one of mothers and fathers (Reader et al., 2017), found changes in why parents thought their infants were waking and how they viewed their own role in responding to the awakening. Across both studies, parents who reported greater concern about their infants' distress upon awakening also reported intervening more during the night. These concerns and thus the need for immediate intervention, declined over the first year of life for both mothers and fathers. Thus, parental perceptions about the reason for night-time awakenings relate to how and if parents respond to their infant.

Furthermore, mothers and fathers who continue to attribute infant distress as the reason for waking, irrespective of the child's age, tend to increase their involvement (e.g., holding, rocking) to help their child fall asleep. It is precisely this over-involvement beyond when it is needed that has been shown to contribute to the persistence of sleep problems for young children. One implication is that educating parents on the difference between times when their child needs their presence at night (true distress) from times when they do not (brief arousals) may help reduce over-involvement at night.

Along with developmental stage, cultural norms and values also impact parent perceptions of and response to sleep problems. Frequent night wakings, for example, were more likely to be regarded as problematic among parents from primarily Caucasian (PC) countries compared to parents from primarily Asian (PA) countries, whereas the number of naps was more likely to be perceived as problematic by parents in PA countries (Sadeh et al., 2011). There are also differences in parental practices across cultures. For example, fewer than 5% of children from PA countries fall asleep independently compared to about 50% of children from PC countries. Children from PA countries are also more likely to go to bed later and share a room with parents than children from PC countries (Mindell et al., 2010). While these findings demonstrate large-scale cultural differences, there are also likely to be more nuanced differences between parenting practices surrounding children's sleep. One implication is that cultural norms and beliefs may not only play a role in when and why parents seek advice about their child's sleep, but they may also impact whether parents are willing to change their parenting practices, particularly if these changes run counter to their cultural beliefs.

## Interventions for Sleep Problems

Sleep problems for children are classified into two categories: night waking and bedtime resistance (Mindell et al., 2006). At this time, there are no standards for determining when a sleep problem has reached a clinical level as opposed to a behavior that, while problematic, is likely to be temporary (Morgenthaler et al., 2006). For example, awakenings increase around the time infants learn to crawl and then return to pre-crawling levels within two weeks (Scher & Cohen, 2015). Bedtime resistance, such as stalling or refusing to stay in bed, also tends to increase from 12 to 36 months (Jenni et al., 2005), which parallels increasing independence during the day. Thus, parents and practitioners alike are challenged to separate typical age-related changes in children's sleep from those that are frequent, persistent sleep problems. A key factor in determining whether a sleep behavior is temporary, or a sign of a more serious problem, is the extent to which parents view the behavior as problematic.

Behavioral treatments are effective in reducing the two most common types of sleep problems in early childhood – bedtime resistance and frequent night waking (Meltzer & Mindell, 2014; Mindell et al., 2006). In general, these interventions aim to reduce excessive involvement by parents at sleep onset and in response to a night waking. Broadly speaking, treatments fall into three categories: extinction, routines, and preventative education (Morgenthaler et al., 2006). At its core, extinction involves a consistent bedtime routine and requires that parents ignore problematic bedtime behaviors (e.g., whining, fussing, and crying). Graduated extinction, a modified version of the treatment that parents tend to be more comfortable enforcing, involves gradually lengthening the time to respond to a child's stalling at bedtime or in response to night-time awakening. Notably, it is suggested that gradual non-responding should begin around six months of age as a method of preventing the development of sleep problems, though more research is needed to determine whether this approach plays a causal role in preventing sleep problems (Morgenthaler et al., 2006). Routines involve setting a consistent time for getting ready for bed, time to be in bed, and a consistent set of activities prior to bedtime (Meltzer et al., 2010). Parent over-involvement during the bedtime routine (e.g., putting the child to bed after they fall asleep) tends to result in frequent awakenings where the child is unable to soothe themselves back to sleep without parental intervention (Ribeiro et al., 2015). Therefore, the bedtime routine should end with the child being drowsy, but not asleep, so that they learn to fall asleep without the presence of a parent. The same principle applies to night-time awakenings. For children who are already exhibiting sleep problems – bedtime resistance or frequent awakenings – establishment of a nightly routine is recommended along with gradual (or abrupt) non-responding (Meltzer et al., 2010). Finally, preventative education covers a variety of topics and methods that include information about typical sleep development as well as methods for responding to problematic behaviors without inadvertently reinforcing them.

## Benefits of a Bedtime Routine

Of the recommended treatments for sleep problems, two are also recommended practices that are likely to reduce the possibility of the development of future sleep problems: Education and bedtime routines. Notably, education includes information about bedtime routines; specifically, how to set a night-time schedule that supports the development of a child's independence from their parent in falling asleep as well as returning to sleep upon waking at night. There are several aspects of a bedtime routine, including parental warmth and consistency of schedule and activities. Parental warmth includes expressing positive emotions, setting appropriate limits, responsiveness to child cues, and not expressing frustration or anger. Greater observed warmth prior to bedtime was associated with fewer awakenings (Teti et al., 2010), longer duration, and less variability (Hoyniak et al., 2021). There is also preliminary evidence that increasing parental warmth prior to bedtime for children who had a sleep problem was effective in reducing both bedtime resistance and the number of awakenings (Burke et al., 2004).

Greater consistency in the timing and steps of a bedtime routine in a community sample was associated with fewer signaled awakenings and a greater percentage of sleep while in bed (Staples et al., 2015). Importantly, studies have found that it was not the number of steps involved in the bedtime routine, rather it was the consistency of the bedtime routine that was predictive of better sleep (Mindell et al., 2015; Staples et al., 2015). Furthermore, there was a dose-dependent response such that as consistency in routine increased, so did the improvement in the child's sleep (Mindell et al., 2015). Establishing a bedtime routine for children who have already developed sleep problems has also been effective in correcting the problematic behavior within just three nights (Mindell et al., 2017). A separate study found that the benefits of improved sleep following the establishment of a bedtime routine persisted a year following the intervention (Mindell et al., 2011). Of particular interest for parents and practitioners was that the bedtime routine intervention consisted of three steps – bath, massage, quiet activity – that lasted between 15 and 30 minutes. This suggests that to be effective, the bedtime routine need not be elaborate in activities, steps, or time to complete. Finally, a consistent bedtime routine not only reduces frequent night-time awakenings, but it also has been linked to improvement in daytime behavior, regulation of negative emotions and improved parent–child interaction (for a complete review, see Mindell & Williamson, 2018).

## Conclusion

For parents of children with sleep problems, particularly when children are resisting going to bed and/or need their parent to return to sleep after a night-time awakening, establishment of a bedtime routine is strongly recommended. The specific steps in the routine are not as important as the overall tone (calming and positive) and consistency. Specifically, the entirety of the routine should be consistent, including the type of activities, the ordering of activities, and the time at which the routine begins and ends. Finally, the bedtime routine should be repeated as many nights as possible, with every night being best practice. For those working with parents of young children, educating parents early on appears to be the most effective and economical method of reducing or preventing sleep problems. Specific recommendations for parents should also take into consideration individual preferences (e.g., sleep location), family dynamics (e.g., number of children, parent work schedule), and cultural values (e.g., co-sleeping, room sharing) surrounding sleep practices.

## Practice Pointers

- Determining whether sleep behavior is problematic depends on factors such as developmental age and cultural values and norms.
- Extinction, routines, and education about sleep development are effective interventions for families looking to address sleep concerns.
- Establishment of a consistent bedtime routine is recommended for the two most common sleep problems in early childhood: Bedtime resistance and frequent night-time awakenings.
- When the child is six months old, begin establishing a consistent 15- to 30-minute night-time routine, that happens at the same time each night (+/−30 minutes).
- The child should be drowsy at the end of the bedtime routine, but not asleep.
- Suggested bedtime activities are those that convey a sense of calm, warmth, security, and safety such as snuggling, reading, singing a lullaby, or a brief (three- to five-minute) massage.
- Bedtime activities to avoid include watching TV or using portable electronic devices with screens.

## References

Burke, R.V., Kuhn, B.R., Peterson, J.L. (2004) Brief report: A 'storybook' ending to children's bedtime problems: The use of a rewarding social story to reduce bedtime resistance and frequent night waking. Journal of Pediatric Psychology, 29(5):389–396.

Galland, B.C., Taylor, B.J., Elder, D.E., Herbison, P. (2012) Normal sleep patterns in infants and children: A systematic review of observational studies. Sleep Medicine Reviews, 16(3):213–222.

Goodlin-Jones, B.L., Burnham, M.M., Gaylor, E.E., Anders, T.F. (2001) Night waking, sleep-wake organization, and self-soothing in the first year of life. Journal of Developmental and Behavioral Pediatrics, 22(4):226–233.

Honaker, S.M., Meltzer, L.J. (2016) Sleep in pediatric primary care: A review of the literature. Sleep Medicine Reviews, 25:31–39.

Hoyniak, C.P., Bates, J.E., McQuillan, M.E., Albert, L.E., Staples, A.D. et al. (2021) The family context of toddler sleep: Routines, sleep environment, and emotional security induction in the hour before bedtime. Behavioral Sleep Medicine, 19(6):795–813.

Iglowstein, I., Jenni, O.G., Molinari, L., Largo, R.H. (2003) Sleep duration from infancy to adolescence: Reference values and generational trends. Pediatrics, 111(2):302–307.

Jenni, O.G., Zinggeler, H.F., Iglowstein, I., Molinari, L., Largo, R.H. (2005) A longitudinal study of bed sharing and sleep problems among Swiss children in the first 10 years of life. Pediatrics, 115(1):233–240.

Kurdziel, L., Duclos, K., Spencer, R.M.C. (2013) Sleep spindles in midday naps enhance learning in preschool children. Proceedings of the National Academy of Sciences, 110(43):17267–17272.

Meltzer, L.J., Johnson, C., Crosette, J., Ramos, M., Mindell, J.A. (2010) Prevalence of diagnosed sleep disorders in pediatric primary care practices. Pediatrics, 125(6):e1410–e1418.

Meltzer, L.J., Mindell, J.A. (2014) Systematic review and meta-analysis of behavioral interventions for pediatric insomnia. Journal of Pediatric Psychology, 39(8):932–948.

Mindell, J.A., Du Mond, C.E., Sadeh, A., Telofski, L.S., Kulkarni, N. et al. (2011) Long-term efficacy of an internet-based intervention for infant and toddler sleep disturbances: One year follow-up. Journal of Clinical Sleep Medicine, 7(5):507–511.

Mindell, J.A., Kuhn, B., Lewin, D.S., Meltzer, L.J., Sadeh, A. (2006) Behavioral treatment of bedtime problems and night wakings in infants and young children. Sleep, 29(10):1263–1276.

Mindell, J.A., Leichman, E.S., Composto, J., Lee, C., Bhullar, B., et al. (2016) Development of infant and toddler sleep patterns: Real-world data from a mobile application. Journal of Sleep Research, 25(5):508–516.

Mindell, J.A., Leichman, E.S., Lee, C., Williamson, A.A., Walters, R.M. (2017) Implementation of a nightly bedtime routine: How quickly do things improve? Infant Behavior and Development, 49:220–227.

Mindell, J.A., Li, A.M., Sadeh, A., Kwon, R., Goh, D.Y.T. (2015) Bedtime routines for young children: A dose-dependent association with sleep outcomes. Sleep, 38(5):717–722.

Mindell, J.A., Sadeh, A., Kohyama, J., How, T.H. (2010) Parental behaviors and sleep outcomes in infants and toddlers: A cross-cultural comparison. Sleep Medicine, 11(4):393–399.

Mindell, J.A., Williamson, A.A. (2018) Benefits of a bedtime routine in young children: Sleep, development, and beyond. Sleep Medicine Reviews, 40:93–108.

Morgenthaler, T.I., Owens, J.A., Alessi, C., Boehlecke, B., Brown, T.M., et al. (2006) Practice parameters for behavioral treatment of bedtime problems and night wakings in infants and young children. Sleep, 29(10):1277–1281.

Owens, J.A. (2008) Socio-cultural considerations and sleep practices in the pediatric population. Sleep Medicine Clinics, 3(1):97–107.

Reader, J.M., Teti, D.M., Cleveland, M.J. (2017) Cognitions about infant sleep: Interparental differences, trajectories across the first year, and coparenting quality. Journal of Family Psychology, 31(4):453–463.

Ribeiro, A., Liddon, C.J., Gadaire, D.M., Kelley, M.E. (2015) Sleep, elimination, and noncompliance in children. In: Roane, H.S., Ringdal, J.E., Falcomata, T.S. (Eds.) Clinical and Organizational Applications of Applied Behavior Analysis. London: Elsevier: 247–272.

Sadeh, A., Mindell, J.A., Luedtke, K., Wiegand, B. (2009) Sleep and sleep ecology in the first 3 years: A web-based study. Journal of Sleep Research, 18(1):60–73.

Sadeh, A., Mindell, J.A., Rivera, L. (2011) 'My child has a sleep problem': A cross-cultural comparison of parental definitions. Sleep Medicine, 12(5):478–482.

Scher, A., Cohen, D. (2015) Sleep as a mirror of developmental transitions in infancy: The case of crawling. Monographs of the Society for Research in Child Development, 80(1):70–88.

Spencer, R.M.C., Campanella, C., de Jong, D.M., Desrochers, P., Root, H. et al. (2016) Sleep and behavior of preschool children under typical and nap-promoted conditions. Sleep Health, 2(1):35–41.

Staples, A.D., Bates, J.E., Petersen, I.T. (2015) Bedtime routines in early childhood: Prevalence, consistency, and associations with night-time sleep. Monographs of the Society for Research in Child Development, 80(1):141–159.

Thorpe, K., Staton, S., Sawyer, E., Pattinson, C., Haden, C., & Smith, S. (2015). Napping, development and health from 0 to 5 years: A systematic review. Archives of Disease in Childhood, 100(7):615–622.

Teti, D.M., Kim, B-R., Mayer, G., Countermine, M. (2010) Maternal emotional availability at bedtime predicts infant sleep quality. Journal of Family Psychology, 24(3):307–315.

Tikotzky, L., Sadeh, A. (2009) Maternal sleep-related cognitions and infant sleep: A longitudinal study from pregnancy through the 1st year. Child Development, 80(3):860–874.

# 22

# FOOD FUSSINESS IN EARLY CHILDHOOD

## Assessment and Management

*Gillian Harris*

Infants and toddlers are frequently described by their parents as fussy eaters. There is, however, no standard definition of fussiness, and interpretation of a child's behaviour is usually subjective, comparative and age related. So, when we use the term 'fussy', what exactly do we mean? A refusal to accept first complementary foods according to their taste or texture? The toddler who refuses new foods or rejects foods that they used to eat? A child with a small appetite who never seems to finish the foods on offer, or who accepts a food one day but rejects it the next? Each of these 'fussy' behaviours has different contributing factors and so needs to be considered and managed accordingly.

★

Infants readily accept the tastes of the first foods given to them if these are predominately sweet; there is an innate preference for the sweet taste. A preference for all other tastes and taste combinations (sour, salt, umami, bitter), however, has to be learned through exposure (Hetherington et al., 2015). The learned preference for salt is quite quick, sour and umami less so and bitter is difficult, taking longer with more exposure experiences needed. A bitter taste is associated by all mammals with toxicity, so the first time an infant is given broccoli (bitter), they are likely to spit it out and make a face. Parents might then assume that their infant is fussy, rather than just unused to the taste. Unfortunately, this also means that some parents will then stop offering those very tastes that need repeated exposure in the early months to enable acceptance (Harris & Mason, 2017).

Some infants, however, have more difficulty with taste acceptance. Differences in response are genetically determined. One of the most notable responses is to the bitter taste; we find bitter 'supertasters' from infancy to adulthood (Bell & Tepper, 2006). A bitter supertaster will always be so and will never learn to like

DOI: 10.4324/9781003223771-27

the taste of bitter vegetables. There are other differences in taste sensitivity, for example to coriander and to beetroot; for some, these will always taste disgusting. This means that, from the beginning, there will always be some infants reluctant to accept a range of tastes.

There is good evidence (Harris & Mason, 2017) that breastfeeding is beneficial in extending the range of food tastes accepted. This exposes the infant to a variety of tastes within the milk, and this exposure generalizes to a willingness to try new foods. Infant formula, however, has a standard taste. It is therefore important to help those who formula feed to offer a wide taste range in early infancy. It is also important to promote food preparation at home wherever possible. The taste differences between home-cooked foods are more distinct than between commercially produced foods. Research (Harris & Coulthard, 2016) suggests that parents who offer their child home-prepared first foods, as opposed to commercial baby foods, are more likely to report that their child eats a wider range of fruit and vegetables in later childhood.

It has also been observed (Maier et al., 2008) that infants given many foods in rotation during the introductory period of solids are more likely to accept new foods than those introduced to new tastes one at a time. This is because these infants experience a wider range of tastes in the early sensitive period of introduction. The difficulty is in telling the difference between an infant who might accept a taste if you persevere and those who will never accept that taste. If after ten or so small exposures, the infant still shows a real disgust response (gag and grimace), then it is likely that this is an innate dislike rather than a lack of exposure.

## Textured Foods

The introduction of lumpy textured solids, or soft finger foods, has to be done in a timely fashion by at least seven months. Infants who are introduced to textured foods later than ten months may have problems both with the mouth-feel of the food and the ability to process such foods (Northstone et al., 2001). Infants without early experience of lumpy solids, either given by spoon or as finger food, will attempt a 'liquid' swallow (over the back of the tongue) which may well trigger a gag response (Mason et al., 2005). Some parents may then respond to this by further delaying the introduction of solid textured foods (Coulthard & Harris, 2003). These children may then become 'orally defensive'; they dislike the feel of food in the sides of their mouths. They then remain on soft bite-and-dissolve or pureed foods as they progress into their second year.

## Practice Pointers

- Parents with an infant who shows a frequent gag response should be supported in the gradual but timely introduction of textured foods.

- Start with a smooth mash and then progress through easy bite-and-dissolve, and bite-and-melt foods, before more solid textures are introduced. (Easy textures will 'dissolve' on the tongue or can be 'mushed' against the palate.)

## Sensory Hypersensitivity

There are other, more general differences, which impact on an infant's food acceptance and may well lead to the description of 'fussy'. Sensory hypersensitivity, and consequent hyper-reactivity, may well be an innate trait or due to pre- or perinatal distress (Longfier et al., 2016). Children can be hypersensitive to taste, smell, touch and sound; all of these can affect food acceptance and mealtime experiences (Rendall et al., 2022). This difference in reactivity is seen more often in children on the autism spectrum, but not necessarily so.

Infants from the age of four to five months can show differences in sensory sensitivity which determine both how willing they are to taste a new food (Coulthard et al., 2016) and accept lumpy textures in the mouth when these are first introduced. Children later diagnosed with extreme food fussiness are usually reported by the parents as having first refused foods when lumpy textured solids were introduced. These children show sensory reactivity in the texture/tactile domain and often don't like to handle 'sticky' finger foods or to get food around their mouth. They are more reluctant both to allow food to go into the sides of their mouth and to process the more difficult textures (Smith et al., 2005). Children who show sensory reactivity to food properties are those more likely to be anxious about the whole eating process (Farrow & Coulthard, 2012) and who show more extreme food refusal.

## Practice Pointers

- Sensory hyper-reactivity is often reliably reported by parents and can be observed across all domains.
- Parents report not only difficulties with feeding, but also with sleep, crying, reaction to noise and to touch.
- In infancy, tactile hypersensitivity contributing to poor food acceptance can be helped by the use of massage around the face, mouth, hands and arms and by sensory play. (See resources.)

## Neophobia

In most infants, the first year is one of a ready acceptance of new foods, if a range of tastes and textures has been introduced in a timely way. Infants first learn to accept the taste, the smell and then the texture of foods that they eat. A change comes about, however, in the second year. Toddlers begin to attend more to the way their food looks and the way in which it is packaged; this tells them if it is safe to eat. This attention to visual detail leads them into a period of food rejection: The neophobic stage (Pliner, 1994). Food is refused on sight, and toddlers are less likely to try new foods. A food might be rejected because it is the wrong colour (when cooked) or comes in the wrong yoghurt pot. Toddlers at this stage are attending to the 'local' (fine) detail of what they are being asked to eat; a broken biscuit is no longer a biscuit. In addition, foods that have been accepted before might now be refused if their appearance changes on subsequent presentations (Brown & Harris, 2012). This is especially true of all fruit and vegetables, but less likely to be a problem with processed carbohydrates (cookies, McDonald's chips).

The neophobic stage starts at around 20 months and then gradually diminishes over the next three years (Nicklaus, 2009); eventually, most children will increase their range of accepted foods. Neophobia occurs in nearly all children, although some will be more neophobic than others. It is, to some extent, genetically determined – related both to parental neophobia and the child's degree of sensory hypersensitivity (Cooke et al., 2007).

It should be remembered, however, that a child will only learn to accept those foods that have been offered in the early years. If they have only been exposed to a restricted diet, that will be the diet they prefer. A child who has been offered only highly processed fast food will only eat these foods as they progress through the toddler years.

## Practice Pointers

- Most children move out of the neophobia stage without problem. Parents need to be reassured that this stage will pass and advised to use gentle methods to move their child along.
- Forcible feeding techniques (coaxing, bribing, mixing and hiding foods and withholding accepted foods) are all known to be maladaptive, and in some cases, lead to weight loss and long-term food refusal.
- Children at this stage respond best to exposure to new foods through parental and peer group modelling at mealtimes, during food preparation and 'tiny tastes' programmes (Holley et al., 2015; Remington et al., 2012).
- In early childhood, sensory play helps children move on with their willingness to try new foods (Coulthard & Sealy, 2017). (See resources.)

## Avoidant and Restrictive Food Intake Disorder (ARFID)

There are some children, however, who do not move on from the neophobic stage. These children are most likely to be those who are sensory sensitive in at least one domain and often in all domains. This hypersensitivity, often associated with co-morbid anxiety (Farrow & Coulthard, 2012) and contamination fears, leads to hyper-vigilance to detail. Every new food is inspected and any food that doesn't look right will be rejected as 'unsafe' to eat. As the neophobic stage progresses, these children form a strong disgust response to all new foods or variations of known foods. Parents will reliably report that their child had problems with the acceptance of foods from early infancy or at least from 18 months. This reluctance to accept food with difficult, or multiple, textures usually means that the child's diet is confined to easy textures such as purees (yoghurt, commercial baby food), bite and melt (chocolate), bite and dissolve (soft crisps). Some will move onto the more difficult textures (toast, fries), but none will move on to complex texture and taste combinations, for example broccoli, tomato, unprocessed meat or fish and mixed dishes (Bryant-Waugh, 2013).

Unlike their peers, these children are not motivated to increase their range of foods because they want to imitate or be like others. Their fear of food, and the disgust response which develops, can be maintained into adulthood. They might eventually be diagnosed with a genetically determined eating disorder, avoidant and restrictive food intake disorder (ARFID) (American Psychiatric Association, 2013). This is more likely to be observed in those on the autism spectrum, but not exclusively so (Schreck & Williams, 2006). (See resources.)

## Small Appetite or Too Much Food?

The last group of potentially fussy eaters comprises children who are reported as eating too little at mealtimes; they will eat a reasonable range of foods but not 'enough'.

Many parents are not really aware of the portion size appropriate to a toddler and will offer too much food at a mealtime or too many calorie-dense meals and snacks throughout the day. In a small survey (Infant and Toddler Forum, 2016), some parents consistently misidentified an adult portion size as appropriate for a toddler (More & Emmett, 2014). Parents may not understand how little food a toddler needs after the early infancy growth spurt. Parents are also often not aware that toddlers can regulate their energy intake quite well to match their growth needs (Fomon et al., 1975). Not eating 'enough' at mealtimes might be because the child is given high-calorie snacks between meals or is too reliant on milk-based drinks. Parents sometimes forget that milk has calories in it even if the bottle is given at night!

In addition, some parents do not realize that a short child will eat less than a taller child. In some cases, a genetically determined short child will be over-persuaded to 'eat up' to encourage them to grow. Comparisons are made between the 'fussy' child and other children who have good appetites but who may well be 'responsive' over-eaters who are eating more than they need (Syrad et al., 2015).

The final reason for a small appetite at mealtimes is that the parents have become so anxious about feeding that they have resorted to force feeding. This is the most common reason for growth faltering (where there is no underlying medical condition); anxiety reduces appetite (Harris, 2009). Often a child who is made anxious at mealtimes might eat well at snack time when away from the meal table. It should also be remembered that idiosyncratic refusal of foods (which are sometimes accepted) may well be due to mealtime anxiety, tiredness, low appetite or constipation.

## Practice Pointers

- Parents need help to assess whether or not they are offering their child too much food, especially too many calorie-dense snacks.
- If the child is dependent on milk-based drinks, these should be gradually reduced as solid food intake increases.
- Parents might need help to move on from maladaptive feeding strategies and to set up a regime with small frequent meals and snacks throughout the day.

## In Conclusion

The term 'fussy' eater will have different connotations at different ages and stages of infancy and early childhood; management strategies need therefore to be tailored accordingly. If parents are encouraged to introduce complementary foods in the critical early period by offering a wide range of tastes and textures, most infants will eventually accept a good range of foods. There will be some regression during the neophobic stage; however, with gentle family and peer group modelling, this stage too will gradually resolve.

Some children's food refusal will, however, not resolve and this is not the parents' fault. These children are those with sensory hyper-reactivity, ARFID and often (but not always) co-morbid conditions such as autism spectrum disorder. Whatever the parents do, or have done, it has not been causal, although in some cases, strategies such as coercive feeding, mixing, hiding and withholding foods might not have helped.

It is useful to remind parents that, just as most adults are a bit 'fussy', many children will also be a bit 'fussy' about certain food tastes and, more often, food textures. This dislike should be respected.

## Online Resources

- ARFID Awareness: Registered UK charity for the support of children and adults with Avoidant and Restrictive Food Intake Disorder: www.arfidawarenessuk.org
- Sensory Play Toolkit: https://sensoryplaytoolkit.weebly.com/

## References

American Psychiatric Association (2013) Diagnostic and Statistical Manual of Mental Disorders (5th ed.) Arlington, VA: American Psychiatric Publishing.

Bell, K.I., Tepper, B.J. (2006) Short-term vegetable intake by young children classified by 6-n-propylthoiuracil bitter-taste phenotype. American Journal of Clinical Nutrition, 84:245–251.

Brown, S., Harris, G. (2012) Rejection of known and previously accepted foods during early childhood: An extension of the neophobic response? International Journal of Child Health and Nutrition, 1:72–81.

Bryant-Waugh, R. (2013) Avoidant and restrictive food intake disorder: An illustrative case example. International Journal of Eating Disorders, 46(5):420–423.

Cooke, L.J., Haworth, C.M.A., Wardle, J. (2007) Genetic and environmental influences on children's food neophobia. American Journal of Clinical Nutrition, 86(2):428–33.

Coulthard, H., Harris, G. (2003) Early food refusal: The role of maternal mood. Journal of Reproductive & Infant Psychology, 21:335–345.

Coulthard, H., Harris, G., Fogel, A. (2016) Association between tactile over-responsivity and vegetable consumption early in the introduction of solid foods and its variation with age. Maternal and Child Nutrition, 12(4):848–859.

Coulthard, H., Sealy, A. (2017) Play with your food! Sensory play is associated with tasting of fruits and vegetables in preschool children. Appetite, 113:84–90.

Farrow, C.V., Coulthard, H. (2012) Relationships between sensory sensitivity, anxiety and selective eating in children. Appetite; 58:842–846.

Fomon, S.J., Filer, L.J., Thomas, L., Anderson, T.A., Nelson, S.E. (1975) Influence of formula concentration on caloric intake and growth of normal infants. Acta Paediatric Scandinavica, 64:172–81.

Harris, G. (2009) Food refusal in the sensory sensitive child. Journal of Paediatrics & Child Health, 19(9):435–436.

Harris, G., Coulthard, H. (2016) Early eating behaviours and food acceptance revisited: Breast feeding and introduction of complementary foods as predictive of food acceptance. Current Obesity Reports, 5:113–120.

Harris, G., Mason, S. (2017) Are there sensitive periods for food acceptance in infancy? Current Nutrition Reports, 6(2):190–196.

Hetherington, M., Schwartz, C., Madrelle, J., Croden, F., Nekitsing, C. et al. (2015) A step-by-step introduction to vegetables at the beginning of complementary feeding: The effects of early and repeated exposure. Appetite, 84:280–290.

Holley, C.E., Haycraft, E., Farrow, C. (2015) 'Why don't you try it again?' A comparison of parent led, home based interventions aimed at increasing children's consumption of a disliked vegetable. Appetite, 87:215–222.

Infant and Toddler Forum (2016) The supersized issue: Why UK parents are overfeeding. Available at: https://infantandtoddlerforum.org/articles/rethink-toddler-portion-sizes/ <accessed 6 September, 2020>

Longfier, L., Soussignan, R., Reissland, N., Leconte, M., Marret, S. et al. (2016) Emotional expressiveness of 5–6 month-old infants born very premature versus full-term at initial exposure to weaning foods. Appetite, 107:494–500.

Maier, A.S., Chabanet, C., Schaal, B., Leathwood, P.D., Issanchou, S.N. (2008) Breastfeeding and experience with variety early in weaning increase infants' acceptance of new foods for up to two months. Clinical Nutrition, 27:849–857.

Mason, S.J., Harris, G., Blissett, J. (2005) Tube feeding in infancy: Implications for the development of normal eating and drinking skills. Dysphagia, 20:46–61.

More, J.A., Emmett, P.M. (2014) Evidenced based, practical food portion sizes for pre-school children and how they fit into a well-balanced, nutritionally adequate diet. Journal of Human Nutrition and Dietetics, 28(2):135–154.

Nicklaus, S. (2009) Development of food variety in children. Appetite, 52(1):253–255.

Northstone, K., Emmett, P., Nethersole, F. (2001) The effect of age of introduction to lumpy solids on foods eaten and reported feeding difficulties at 6 and 15 months. Journal of Human Nutrition and Dietetics, 14:43–54.

Pliner, P. (1994) Development of measures of food neophobia in children. Appetite, 23:147–163.

Remington, A., Anez, E., Croker, H., Wardle, J., Cooke, L. (2012) Increasing food acceptance in the home setting: A randomized controlled trial of parent-administered taste exposure with incentives. American Journal of Clinical Nutrition, 95(1):72–77.

Rendall, S., Harvey, K., Tavassoli, T., Dodd, H. (2022) Associations between emotionality, sensory reactivity and food fussiness in young children. Food Quality and Preference, 96:104420.

Schreck, K.A., Williams, K. (2006) Food preferences and factors influencing food selectivity for children with autism spectrum disorders. Research in Developmental Disabilities, 27(4):353–363.

Smith, A.M., Roux, S., Naidoo, N.T., Venter, D.J.L. (2005) Food choices of tactile defensive children. Nutrition, 21(1):14–19.

Syrad, H., Johnson, L., Wardle, J., Llewellyn, C.H. (2015) Appetitive traits and food intake patterns in early life. American Journal of Clinical Nutrition, 103(1): 231–235.

# 23

# WEANING A BABY ONTO A VEGAN DIET

*Amanda Benham*

Recently there has been an increase in the number of people adopting plant-based diets in many countries, mainly out of concern for animals but also for health and environmental reasons. The widespread adoption of a vegan diet could result in a substantial reduction in chronic disease and economic and climate-change benefits (Springmann et al., 2016). However, there is a lack of international consensus on the safety and desirability of such diets for infants and children. While some authorities, including the Academy of Nutrition and Dietetics (Melina et al., 2016), the Canadian Paediatric Society (Amit, 2010), the British Dietetic Association (BDA, 2017) and Australia's National Health & Medical Research Council (NHMRC, 2013) hold the position that well-planned vegan diets can be suitable for all age groups, several European authorities have discouraged the use of vegan diets for children (Federal Commission for Nutrition (FCN), 2018; Fewtrell et al., 2017; Richter et al., 2016; Redecillas-Ferreiro et al., 2020). However, experts agree that if an infant is to be weaned onto a vegan diet, the diet needs to be well-planned and supplemented appropriately to meet nutrient needs.

★

While there is a lack of studies specifically on weaning infants onto a vegan diet, there have been several studies of children who are on a vegan diet, including since weaning. A recent review (Sutter & Bender, 2021) on nutrient status and growth in vegan children concluded that from the limited data available, a well-planned and supplemented vegan diet is able to provide the recommended amounts of nutrients for normal growth and can have some benefits, such as prevention of obesity and atherosclerosis. The VeChi Youth Study (Alexy et al., 2021) in Germany has compared the nutrient intake and status of children on

DOI: 10.4324/9781003223771-28

vegetarian, vegan and omnivore diets (aged 6–18 years), finding that a vegan diet can meet nutrient requirements in childhood and adolescence. In a similar study (Desmond et al., 2021) of five to ten years-old children, it was found that the children on vegan diets had healthier cardiovascular risk profiles and had lower adiposity but were shorter and had lower bone mineral content than omnivores.

While there is consensus that a vegan diet *can* be planned to meet nutrient requirements, failure to plan can and has resulted in serious adverse health consequences in infants, such as developmental issues due to vitamin B12 deficiency (Honzik et al., 2010) and rickets due to vitamin D deficiency (Lemoine et al., 2020). Clearly, as with any type of diet, adverse consequences can result if care is not taken to meet nutrient needs.

## Infant Feeding Guidelines for Vegan Parents

Most of the guidelines for the general population relating to complementary feeding also apply to infants being weaned onto a vegan diet. These include:

- Considering age and readiness for introducing 'solids'
- Offering food in a form and texture appropriate for the infant's feeding skills
- Continuation of breastfeeding or the use of a commercial infant formula until 12 months of age (and beyond for breastfeeding)
- Early introduction of iron-rich foods
- Repeated offering of foods that have been refused in the past
- Avoiding adding salt or sugar to foods
- Not delaying the introduction of potential allergens
- Monitoring growth and development.

## Points of Difference

For vegans, a commercial non-dairy infant formula is the only safe alternative to breast milk or dairy-based formula. While some health authorities have advised against the use of soy formula for infants under six months of age, a 2014 review in the British Journal of Nutrition did not find evidence of adverse effects of soy formula (Vandenplas et al., 2014).

While it is currently recommended for the general population that potential allergens (including cows' milk and eggs) be introduced to infants early, this advice may not be appropriate for vegans. There is a risk of increased sensitization to subsequent allergy if foods such as fish, shellfish, eggs and dairy are not consumed regularly after introduction (West, 2017), and so their introduction to infants being raised on a vegan diet to 'test' if they are allergic may be counterproductive. However, as wheat, soy products, peanuts, tree nuts and seeds are good sources of nutrients for children on plant-based diets, these should be introduced at an early stage of complementary feeding and given repeatedly after introduction if there are no adverse reactions (Ierodiakonou et al., 2016). Food allergies in infants weaned onto a vegan diet can make meeting nutrient needs more challenging, and specialised dietary advice is strongly recommended in these cases.

## Meeting Key Nutrient Needs

The essential nutrients requiring specific attention on a vegan diet can be categorised as:

1  Nutrients that are rarely if ever found naturally in plants: vitamins B12 and D
2  Nutrients that may have lower availability in or absorption from plant-based foods: iron, zinc, protein, vitamin A
3  Nutrients typically supplied substantially by animal products on a western omnivorous diet: calcium, protein, omega-3 fatty acids, energy
4  Minerals from plants grown in soil low in these nutrients: iodine and potentially selenium.

Each of these nutrients will be considered in turn.

## Vitamin B12

Vitamin B12 is not naturally found in commonly consumed plant foods, and reports of it being found in useful amounts in mushrooms, tempeh or other fermented foods have been found to be erroneous, as most if not all of the vitamin present is in a biologically inactive analogue form (Dagnelie et al., 1991).

Consequences of B12 deficiency in infants can include growth failure, seizures, hypotonia, microcephaly and developmental delay, and delays in treatment have resulted in permanent developmental abnormalities (Honzik et al., 2010). Although breastmilk concentration of B12 is generally higher in women who are supplementing adequately (e.g. 50 mcg per day), deficiency is still possible in breastfed infants in the absence of maternal deficiency, and breastmilk of vegan mothers may not be adequate to meet the needs of infants, especially from about four to six months of age (Pawlak et al., 2018). Supplementing vitamin B12 daily to breastfed infants of vegan mothers by no later than six months of age is recommended (Baroni et al., 2019), and supplementing from birth is indicated if maternal intake during pregnancy was inconsistent or inadequate.

Vitamin B12 is best supplemented as a stand-alone supplement as some other nutrients in multi-nutrient supplements can convert up to 90% of the vitamin B12 into inactive analogues (Kondo et al., 1982). This can result in falsely raised levels of serum vitamin B12. The amount of vitamin B12 that can be absorbed from a single dose of supplement is limited, so the amount that needs to be supplemented is much higher than the recommended intake from food.

## Vitamin D

Normally, plant-based foods do not contain vitamin D, although some foods may be fortified with it and UV-irradiated mushrooms can provide vitamin D (Cardwell et al., 2018). As vitamin D enhances the absorption of dietary calcium, deficiency can result in compromised bone growth and development. This can result in stunting and rickets, which is characterised by soft, weakened bones and can result in permanent skeletal deformities.

Traditionally, vitamin D was provided largely by the action of sunlight on bare skin, but modern lifestyles and concerns over skin damage and melanoma have resulted in reduced sun exposure and a high prevalence of vitamin D deficiency globally, with 75% of new-borns found to be deficient (Saraf et al., 2016). Darker skin, further distance from the equator and greater degree of skin coverage are known to be risk factors for vitamin D deficiency, but given the high prevalence of deficiency, supplementation of all infants and young children with vitamin D is prudent.

There is, however, a lack of international consensus on vitamin D supplementation for infants and children. While both the American and the European Academies of Paediatrics recommend 400 IU for all infants from birth, other health authorities recommend it only for breastfed infants or only those considered at risk of deficiency, such as infants of dark-skinned or veiled women (Munns et al., 2006).

Not all vitamin D supplements are acceptable to vegans, as vitamin D3 is typically derived from sheep's wool. However, vitamin D3 derived from vegan sources is available and vitamin D2 is normally vegan-suitable.

## Iron

Deficiency of iron in infants and young children is relatively common worldwide and can result in anaemia, increased susceptibility to infections and impaired development (Shubham et al., 2020). While iron is widespread in plant foods, non-haem iron is not always as well absorbed as haem iron, largely due to the presence of naturally-occurring compounds known as phytates. This effect of phytates can be reduced by soaking, fermenting, leavening and sprouting grains and legumes, and serving iron-rich plant foods with foods containing vitamin C and carotenes to further enhance the absorption of non-haem iron (Shubham et al., 2020). For example, fortified cereal can be served with vitamin C-rich fruit at breakfast and at other meals, tofu or legumes and green vegetables can be included, with a squeeze of lemon juice for vitamin C added on serving (vitamin C is heat sensitive and is degraded during cooking).

## Zinc

As with iron, the presence of phytates in plant foods can decrease zinc absorption, while the presence of organic acids and protein can enhance it (Lönnerdal, 2000). Zinc deficiency can result in impaired immunity, poor wound healing, growth failure and neuro-cognitive disorders (Krebs, 2013). It is important that zinc-rich foods be provided at weaning and throughout childhood.

Zinc-fortified baby cereals (where available), tofu and other soy products, legumes and nut and seed butters should be introduced as early complementary foods and remain in the diets of vegan children. As with iron, including a source of vitamin C with each meal and limiting fibre intake will enhance absorption.

## Protein

While ample protein can be obtained from a varied plant-based diet, the somewhat lower digestibility and variable amino acid balance of plant proteins has led to suggestions that protein intake recommendations be increased by up to 30% for children relying on plant proteins (Mangels & Messina, 2001). Overall protein quality can be improved by ensuring different plant sources of protein (e.g. grains and legumes) are included at each meal or no more than six hours apart (Young & Pellett, 1994). This is because amino acids consumed up to six hours apart are able to be used to form 'complete' protein; so, for example, if rice is eaten at lunch at 1pm and beans at dinner at 6pm, the amino acids from each will complement each other. However, if the rice is eaten at 7am and the beans at 6pm, they will not do so.

## Vitamin A

Vitamin A deficiency can result in impaired growth and development, increased susceptibility to infections, night blindness and ultimately blindness (Wiseman et al., 2017). Whereas animal products contain pre-formed vitamin A, plants provide what is known as pro-vitamin A from carotenes, which needs to be converted into vitamin A. This conversion varies between individuals, with around 45% of people having a genetic make-up that can result in a substantial reduction in their ability to convert pro-vitamin A to vitamin A (Leung et al., 2009). Therefore, those affected who are eating a vegan diet may need a higher intake of beta-carotene equivalents than typically recommended. The foods richest in carotenes suitable for infants are cooked and pureed/mashed carrots, sweet potato, kale and spinach.

## Calcium

Consumers of western-style diets have traditionally obtained a substantial proportion of their total calcium intake from dairy products. However, adequate calcium can be obtained on dairy-free diets, with recommended intakes being more easily met if some calcium-fortified foods are included. For infants under 12 months, adequate calcium can be obtained from breast-milk or formula (Bae & Kratzsch, 2018). A full fat fortified soy milk can be given as a drink from 12 months of age. Other plant milks are not as rich in protein, iron and other key nutrients and are not normally recommended for infants and small children. Additional sources of calcium include calcium-set tofu, tahini, almond butter, kale, Asian greens, figs and in some areas, 'hard' calcium-rich water.

## Iodine and Other Trace Minerals

The amount of trace minerals in plant foods depends on where they were grown. In many parts of the world, the soil is depleted of iodine, resulting in a high prevalence of iodine deficiency. Deficiency in infants and young children can result in growth failure, intellectual impairment and thyroid inadequacy (Pearce et al., 2013). Seafood (including seaweeds) tends to be rich in iodine, but some seaweeds (particularly kelp/kombu) can contain dangerously high amounts of iodine and are not recommended, while others may contain excessive amounts of arsenic and other heavy metals (Cherry et al., 2019).

It is recommended that all lactating women should supplement with iodine, with 150 mcg per day recommended in the USA, Europe and Australia (Lazarus, 2014; Leung et al., 2014; NHMRC, 2010). However, based on lower iodine intakes in vegans (Eveleigh et al., 2020) and on intakes required to ensure adequate breastmilk concentration (Dror & Allen, 2018), women on a vegan diet may need to supplement at the WHO recommended level of 250 mcg per day (Untoro et al., 2007). From 12 months of age, iodised salt can be used as a source of iodine for children on vegan diets. In some cases, an iodine supplement will be required to meet the recommended intake.

Selenium is an essential trace element that the diets of some adult vegans have been found to be low in, although evidence of frank deficiency is lacking (Kristensen et al., 2015; Lightowler & Davies, 2000). In areas where selenium levels are low in plant foods, the inclusion of Brazil nut paste will boost intake considerably.

## Essential Fatty Acids

Vegan diets tend to be rich in omega-6 fatty acids, but most plant-based foods are not rich in the omega-3 fatty acids. While adequate amounts of omega-3 alpha-linolenic acid (ALA) can be obtained from a well-planned vegan diet, plants lack omega-3 docosahexaenoic acid (DHA). DHA is important for development of the brain and retina, and it appears that DHA supplementation of infants can result in long-term improvements in mental and psychomotor developmental indices and visual acuity (Shulkin et al., 2018). Most DHA supplements are derived from fish oil, but fish obtain their DHA from algae, and algal-derived DHA supplements suitable for vegans are available.

## Energy

Meeting energy needs on a vegan diet need not be difficult but can be hampered by (i) an excessively high fibre intake and (ii) an inadequate fat intake. Legumes and whole grains are rich in fibre and low in fat, and for this reason it has been recommended that infants should be initially introduced to refined rather than whole grains, that the skin of beans be removed and high fat foods be included daily (Baroni et al., 2019).

## Food and Supplement Intake Recommendations

Various food planning guides specific to children on plant-based diets have been developed (Baroni et al., 2019a; Menal-Puey et al., 2019). The details vary, but it is typically recommended that vegan diets are composed predominately of foods from each of these groups:

- legumes and soy products
- grains and cereals (including iron-fortified) and potato
- vegetables
- fruit
- nut and seed pastes
- fortified plant milk (for older infants and for children).

Supplemental vitamin D is generally recommended from birth, and vitamin B12 supplementation is also recommended from birth for breastfed babies of vegan mothers who did not supplement adequately during pregnancy.

The guidelines and meal plans below are designed to meet infants' needs for essential nutrients and establish a healthy vegan eating pattern.

## About Six Months of Age

When the infant is ready, at around six months of age (and never less than four months) it is recommended that complementary feeding is initiated. Iron-rich foods such as iron-fortified baby cereal, silken tofu or well-cooked red lentils are recommended as first foods. Well-cooked pureed green and other colourful vegetables and cooked/soft fruits can also be offered. It is generally recommended that foods are offered about an hour after breastfeeding, when the baby is relaxed and not too hungry, and ideally at family meal times. Peanut and other nut pastes, tahini, wheat and soy should be introduced one at a time to enable identification of allergens if a reaction occurs. Breastmilk or formula will continue on demand/several times during the day and generally at night also. Supplements of vitamins B12 and D, flaxseed oil and DHA should be introduced, as per Table 23.2.

## About Seven Months of Age

At seven months of age, foods from each of the plant food groups can be offered every day. The recommendations and suggested meal plans below are based on current recommendations, adapted for infants on plant-based diets.

---

### BOX 23.1: SAMPLE MEAL PATTERN BY ABOUT SEVEN MONTHS OF AGE

Meal 1: Iron-fortified baby cereal (made with water, breastmilk or formula) + fruit + 0.5 tsp flaxseed oil
Meal 2: Iron-fortified cereal + vegetable/s + tofu/red lentils + nut butter or tahini

---

## Eight to Twelve Months of Age

---

### SAMPLE MEAL PATTERN BY ABOUT NINE MONTHS OF AGE

Breakfast: Iron-fortified baby cereal (made with fortified soy milk) + vitamin C-rich fruit + 0.5 tsp flaxseed oil + 1 tsp nut butter
Lunch: Iron-fortified cereal or other grain or potato + soy product/legume + colourful vegetables + a squeeze of lemon/lime juice (for vitamin C)
Dinner: Iron-fortified cereal or other grain or potato + soy product/legume + colourful vegetables + 1 tsp tahini + a squeeze of lemon/lime juice (for vitamin C)
Supplements: See Table 23.2.

---

From eight months of age, it is recommended that food starts being offered before breastmilk or formula. An increasing variety of foods from each of the plant food groups should be offered every day. The amount of food consumed will increase according to appetite. Full fat fortified soy milk can be used on cereal and in cooking but should not replace breastmilk or formula or be used as a drink until 12 months of age.

## From 12 Months of Age

Children should be able to eat most family meals with minimal modifications. Fortified soy milk can be given as a drink, as well as used on cereal and in cooking. It is normally recommended that formula and bottle-feeding cease at 12 months of age.

---

### SAMPLE MEAL PATTERN FROM ABOUT AGE 12 MONTHS

Breakfast: Iron-fortified cereal with fortified soy milk + vitamin C-rich fruit + nut butter + 1/2 tsp flaxseed oil (or a tsp of ground flaxseeds or chia seeds)
Snack: Drink of fortified soy milk + crackers or bread with nut butter or hummus
Lunch: Grain product + soy product/legume* + green vegetable + red/orange/yellow vegetable + source of vitamin C (e.g. raw tomato)
Snack: Drink of fortified soy milk plus fresh fruit
Dinner: Grain/potato + soy product/legume* + green vegetable + red/orange/yellow vegetable + high fat food (e.g. nut butter, tahini, avocado) + source of vitamin C (e.g. lemon/lime juice)
*Many commercial 'meat alternative' products are now available, some of which may be suitable for occasional use as main meal foods. Ideally, they should have legumes or soy product as the main ingredient, be fortified with iron and zinc, and be low in sodium.
Supplements: See Table 23.2.

---

## Suggested Amounts of Foods

As infants (under 12 months) obtain a substantial proportion of their nutrition from breastmilk or formula, specific quantities of foods for infants are not always provided in feeding guides. The guidelines in Table 23.1 for children from 12 months of age are designed to meet recommended intakes of essential nutrients as laid down by the European Food Safety Authority (2017), the British Nutrition Foundation (2015), the National Health & Medical Research Council in Australia (2014) and the Institute of Medicine (2006) in the USA.

The amounts are minimums and are expressed in standard metric cups (250 ml) for ease of use. Upper limits are given for iodised salt (due to the need to limit sodium intake), fruit (due to its lower nutrient content and tendency to displace other more nutritious foods) and soy milk (due to its tendency to displace solid food).

**TABLE 23.1** Amounts of foods required to meet recommended intakes of key essential nutrients for one to three-year olds

| Food group | Recommended amount per day* |
| --- | --- |
| Iron-fortified cereals/ other iron-fortified grain-based foods | ½ cup+ |
| Other grain products (eg pasta, rice, bread), potato. (One slice bread equiv. to ½ cup cooked grain) | ½ cup+ |
| Green vegetables | ½ cup+ |
| Red/orange/yellow vegetables | ½ cup+ |
| Tofu, tempeh, legumes | ½ cup+ |
| Nut and seed pastes** | 1 tbsp+ |
| Fresh fruit | ½–1 cup |
| Fortified soy milk | 1.5–2 cups |
| Iodised salt | ¼–1/3 tsp*** |
| Other high fat foods (e.g. avocado, coconut yoghurt/cream, oil) | 0-discretionary/ as required |

*Measured in form eaten (e.g. cooked), 1 cup = 250 ml.
+These are minimum amounts, and more can be offered according to appetite
**Include equivalent of ¼ Brazil nut in areas where soil selenium is low, and 1 tsp ground flaxseeds/chia seeds if DHA is not supplemented regularly
***Amount will depend on local fortification practices

*Source:* European Food Safety Authority (2017), the British Nutrition Foundation (2015), the National Health & Medical Research Council in Australia (2014) and the Institute of Medicine (2006) in the USA.

The lower amounts specified in Table 23.1 provide 35 grams of protein and 3,325 kJ (795 calories). This meets the estimated requirements of a moderately active one-year old. Additional energy can be provided with extra servings of grains, legumes/soy products and high fat foods, as required. The plan provides 18% of energy from protein and 36% of energy from fat and meets the recommended intake for the following nutrients for a one to three-year old: protein, total fat, fibre, vitamins A, B1, B2, B3, B6, B9, B12, C, E, iron, zinc, calcium, phosphorus, magnesium, iodine, selenium, linoleic acid and ALA. The plan does not meet the recommended amount of vitamin D or DHA, and although the fortified soy milk may provide the recommended daily intake (RDI) of vitamin B12, it is recommended that this also be supplemented as a precaution.

## Summary

The diets of infants weaned onto a vegan diet need to be appropriately planned to ensure requirements are met for key nutrients. Vitamins B12 and D should be supplemented, and care taken to ensure an adequate intake of iron, zinc, protein,

**TABLE 23.2** Recommended supplementation for infants and children on a vegan diet to meet recommendations for essential nutrients

| Nutrient | Daily supplementation rate depending on age | | |
|---|---|---|---|
| | 0–6 months | 6–12 months | 1–3 years |
| Vitamin B12 | 5 mcg if maternal pregnancy intake poor | 5 mcg | 5 mcg |
| Vitamin D | 400 IU | 400 IU if breastfed (infant formula usually contains vitamin D in adequate levels, so supplementation is less important in formula-fed infants) | 400 IU – 600 IU |
| Iodine | From breastmilk★ / formula | From breastmilk★ / formula | Approx. 90 mcg from iodised salt / fortified foods / supplement |
| ALA | From breastmilk★ / formula | 0.5 tsp flaxseed oil | 0.5 tsp flaxseed oil or 1 tsp ground flaxseeds or chia seeds |
| DHA+ | | 100 mg | 100–250 mg |
| Calcium | From breastmilk★ / formula | From breastmilk / formula + supplementary foods | From fortified foods (e.g. fortified soy milk, approx. 375 ml/day) |
| Iron | From iron stores / formula | Iron-fortified baby cereal / other iron-fortified foods | Iron-fortified foods/ iron-rich foods at every meal, served with a source of vitamin C; otherwise, supplement may be required |

★It is recommended that lactating women supplement with 150–250 mcg iodine daily.

+ If DHA is not supplemented regularly (e.g. due to cost constraints), increasing the amount of ALA may help compensate.

energy, vitamin A and omega-3 fatty acids. Calcium-fortified soy milk can be given as a drink and iodised salt used from 12 months of age. In some countries, iodine supplements may be required to meet recommended intakes. While flax-seed oil can provide adequate amounts of omega-3 alpha-linolenic acid (ALA), supplementation with docosa-hexanoic acid (DHA) is required to meet WHO recommended intakes. Care should be taken to avoid excessive fibre intake and to provide adequate high fat foods to enhance calorie intake.

## Practice Pointers

- Not all vegan diets are the same and determining the specifics of the parents' eating habits and their intentions for their child is important for making appropriate recommendations.
- Most vegans adhere to their diet due to strongly-held ethical beliefs and suggesting that they compromise their beliefs may result in termination of the relationship with the health professional.
- It cannot be assumed that breastfed infants are protected from nutrient deficiency, as maternal diet and supplementation influence breastmilk composition.
- Nutrient content of foods varies depending on where they were grown and whether fortified, and to what extent.
- It is recommended that specialised advice be sought from nutrition experts well-versed in plant-based nutrition when infants are to be weaned onto a vegan diet.

## References

Alexy, U., Fischer, M., Weder, S., Längler, A., Michalsen, A. et al. (2021) Nutrient intake and status of German children and adolescents consuming vegetarian, vegan or omnivore diets: Results of the VeChi Youth Study. Nutrients, 13(5):1707.

Amit M. (2010) Vegetarian diets in children and adolescents. Paediatrics & Child Health, 15(5):303–314.

Bae, Y. J., Kratzsch, J. (2018) Vitamin D and calcium in the human breast milk. Best Practice and Research: Clinical Endocrinology & Metabolism, 32(1):39–45.

Baroni, L., Goggi, S., Battaglino, R., Berveglieri, M., Fasan, I. et al. (2019) Vegan nutrition for mothers and children: Practical tools for healthcare providers. Nutrients, 11(1):5.

Baroni, L., Goggi, S., Battino, M. (2019a) Planning well-balanced vegetarian diets in infants, children, and adolescents: The VegPlate Junior. Journal of the Academy of Nutrition and Dietetics, 119(7):1067–1073.

BDA (2017) British Dietetic Association confirms well-planned vegan diets can support healthy living in people of all ages. Available at: https://www.bda.uk.com/resource/british-dietetic-association-confirms-well-planned-vegan-diets-can-support-healthy-living-in-people-of-all-ages.html <accessed 14 July, 2020>

British Nutrition Foundation (2015) Nutrient requirements. London: British Nutrition Foundation.

Cardwell, G., Bornman, J.F., James, A.P., Black, L.J. (2018) A review of mushrooms as a potential source of dietary vitamin D. Nutrients, 10(10):1498.

Cherry, P., O'Hara, C., Magee, P.J., McSorley, E.M., Allsopp, P.J. (2019) Risks and benefits of consuming edible seaweeds. Nutrition Reviews, 77(5):307–329.

Dagnelie, P.-C., van Staveren, W.A., van den Berg, H. (1991) Vitamin B-12 from algae appears not to be bioavailable. American Journal of Clinical Nutrition, 53(3):695–697.

Desmond, M. A., Sobiecki, J. G., Jaworski, M., Płudowski, P., Antoniewicz, J., et al. (2021). Growth, body composition, and cardiovascular and nutritional risk of 5-to 10-y-old children consuming vegetarian, vegan, or omnivore diets. The American Journal of Clinical Nutrition, 113(6):1565–1577.

Dror, D.K., Allen, L.H. (2018) Iodine in human milk: A systematic review. Advances in Nutrition, 9(suppl.1): 347S–357S.

European Food Safety Authority (EFSA) (2017) Dietary reference values for nutrients: Summary report. EFSA Supporting Publications, 14:e15121E.

Eveleigh, E.R., Coneyworth, L.J., Avery, A., Welham, S.J.M. (2020) Vegans, vegetarians, and omnivores: How does dietary choice influence iodine intake? A Systematic Review. Nutrients 12(6):1606.

Federal Commission for Nutrition (FCN) (2018) Vegan diets: Review of nutritional benefits and risks. Expert Report of the Federal Commission for Nutrition. Bern, Switzerland.

Fewtrell, M., Bronsky, J., Campoy, C., Domellöf, M., Embleton, N. et al. (2017) Complementary feeding: A position paper by the European Society for Paediatric Gastroenterology, Hepatology, and Nutrition (ESPGHAN) Committee on Nutrition. Journal of Pediatric Gastroenterology and Nutrition, 64(1):119–132.

Honzik, T., Adamovicova, M., Smolka, V., Magner, M., Hruba, E. et al. (2010) Clinical presentation and metabolic consequences in 40 breastfed infants with nutritional vitamin B12 deficiency – What have we learned? European Journal of Paediatric Neurology, 14(6):488–495.

Ierodiakonou, D., Garcia-Larsen, V., Logan, A., Groome, A., Cunha, S. et al. (2016) Timing of allergenic food introduction to the infant diet and risk of allergic or autoimmune disease: A systematic review and meta-analysis. JAMA, 316:1181–1192.

Institute of Medicine (2006) Dietary Reference Intakes: The essential guide to nutrient requirements. Washington, DC: The National Academies Press. Available at: https:// doi.org/10.17226/1153 <accessed 6 September, 2020>

Kondo, H., Binder, M.J., Kolhouse, J.F., Smythe, W.R., Podell, E.R. et al. (1982) Presence and formation of cobalamin analogues in multivitamin-mineral pills. Journal of Clinical Investigation, 70(4):889–898.

Krebs, N.F. (2013) Update on zinc deficiency and excess in clinical pediatric practice. Annals of Nutrition and Metabolism, 62(Suppl. 1):19–29.

Kristensen, N.B., Madsen, M.L., Hansen, T.H., Allin, K.H., Hoppe, C. et al. (2015) Intake of macro- and micronutrients in Danish vegans. Nutrition Journal, 14:article no.:115.

Lazarus, J.H. (2014) Iodine status in Europe in 2014. European Thyroid Journal, 3(1):3–6.

Lemoine, A., Giabicani, E., Lockhart, V., Grimprel, E., Tounian, P. (2020) Case report of nutritional rickets in an infant following a vegan diet. Archives de Pédiatrie, 27(4):219–222.

Leung, A., Pearce, E., Braverman, L., Stagnaro-Green, A. (2014) AAP recommendations on iodine nutrition during pregnancy and lactation. Pediatrics, 134(4):e1282.

Leung, W., Hessel, S., Meplan, C., Flint, J., Oberhauser, V. et al. (2009) Two common single nucleotide polymorphisms in the gene encoding ß-carotene 15, 15'-monoxygenase alter ß-carotene metabolism in female volunteers. The FASEB Journal, 23(4):1041–1053.

Lightowler, H.J., Davies, G.J. (2000) Micronutrient intakes in a group of UK vegans and the contribution of self-selected dietary supplements. Journal of the Royal Society for the Promotion of Health, 120(2):117–124.

Lönnerdal, B. (2000) Dietary factors influencing zinc absorption. Journal of Nutrition, 130(5):1378S–1383S.

Mangels, A.R., Messina, V. (2001) Considerations in planning vegan diets: Infants. Journal of the American Dietetic Association, 101(6):670–677.

Melina, V., Craig, W., Levin, S. (2016) Position of the academy of nutrition and dietetics: Vegetarian diets. Journal of the Academy of Nutrition and Dietetics, 116(12):1970–1980.

Menal-Puey, S., Martínez-Biarge, M., Marques-Lopes, I. (2019) Developing a food exchange system for meal planning in vegan children and adolescents. Nutrients, 11(1):43.

Munns, C., Zacharin, M.R., Rodda, C.P., Batch, J.A., Morley, R. et al. (2006) Paediatric Endocrine Group, Paediatric Bone Australasia. Prevention and treatment of infant and childhood vitamin D deficiency in Australia and New Zealand: A consensus statement. Medical Journal of Australia, 185(5):268–272.

National Health & Medical Research Council (NHMRC) (2010) Public Statement: Iodine supplementation for pregnant and breastfeeding women. Canberra: NHMRC.

National Health & Medical Research Council (NHMRC) (2013) Australian Dietary Guidelines. Canberra: NHMRC.

National Health & Medical Research Council (NHMRC) (2014) Nutrient Reference Values for Australia and New Zealand. Canberra: NHMRC.

Pawlak, R., Vos, P., Shahab-Ferdows, S., Hampel, D., Allen, L.H. et al. (2018) Vitamin B-12 content in breast milk of vegan, vegetarian, and nonvegetarian lactating women in the United States. American Journal of Clinical Nutrition, 108(3):525–531.

Pearce, E.N., Andersson, M., Zimmermann, M.B. (2013) Global iodine nutrition: Where do we stand in 2013? Thyroid, 23(5):523–528.

Redecillas-Ferreiro, S., Moráis-López, A., Moreno-Villares, J.M. (2020) Position paper on vegetarian diets in infants and children. Committee on Nutrition and Breastfeeding of the Spanish Paediatric Association. Anales de Pediatría (English Edition), 92(5):306.e1–306.e6.

Richter, M., Boeing, H., Grünewald-Funk, D., Heseker, H., Kroke, A. et al. (2016) Vegan diet. Position of the German Nutrition Society (DGE). Ernährungs Umschau, 63(04):92–102.

Saraf, R., Morton, S.M.B., Camargo Jr., C.A., Grant, C.C. (2016) Global summary of maternal and newborn vitamin D status – A systematic review. Maternal and Child Nutrition, 12(4):647–668.

Shubham, K., Anukiruthika, T., Dutta, S., Kashyap, A.V., Moses, J.A. et al. (2020) Iron deficiency anemia: A comprehensive review on iron absorption, bioavailability and emerging food fortification approaches. Trends in Food Science & Technology, 99:58–75.

Shulkin, M., Pimpin, L., Bellinger, D., Kranz, S., Fawzi, W. et al. (2018) N–3 fatty acid supplementation in mothers, preterm infants, and term infants and childhood psychomotor and visual development: A systematic review and meta-analysis. Journal of Nutrition, 148(3):409–418.

Springmann, M., Godfray, H.C.J., Rayner, M., Scarborough, P. (2016) Analysis and valuation of the health and climate change cobenefits of dietary change. Proceedings of the National Academy of Sciences, 113 (15):4146–4151.

Sutter, D, Bender, N. (2021) Nutrient status and growth in vegan children. Nutrition Research, 91:13–25.

Untoro, J., Mangasaryan, N., De Benoist, B., Darnton-Hill, I. (2007) Reaching optimal iodine nutrition in pregnant and lactating women and young children: Programmatic recommendations. Public Health Nutrition, 10(12A):1527–1529.

Vandenplas, Y., Castrellon, P.G., Rivas, R., Gutiérrez, C. J., Garcia, L.D. et al. (2014) Safety of soya-based infant formulas in children. British Journal of Nutrition, 111(8):1340–1360.

West, C. (2017) Introduction of complementary foods to infants. Annals of Nutrition and Metabolism, 70(Suppl. 2):47–54.

Wiseman, E.M., Bar-El Dadon, S., Reifen, R. (2017) The vicious cycle of vitamin A deficiency: A review. Critical Reviews in Food Science and Nutrition, 57(17):3703–3714.

Young, V.R., Pellett, P.L. (1994) Plant proteins in relation to human protein and amino acid nutrition. American Journal of Clinical Nutrition, 59(5 Suppl.):1203s–1212s.

# 24

# A RELATIONSHIP-BASED FRAMEWORK FOR EARLY CHILDHOOD MEDIA USE

*Jenny S. Radesky and Katherine Rosenblum*

This chapter reviews the research evidence about media, parent–child interaction, and child social–emotional development and then seeks to translate evidence into action-oriented guidance within a relationship-based intervention framework. This framework aims to complement World Health Organization and other guidelines for family screen use by highlighting the ways media use intersects with parent–child relationships in the context of everyday experiences that we hope will be relevant to early childhood interventionists.

★

From the time of its invention, the radio took 38 years to reach 50 million households. TV took 14 years to achieve the same reach. Although each of these technologies felt disruptive at the time it was introduced (e.g., the radio replacing oral storytelling), society had decades in which to adjust to them. In contrast, the Internet took four years to reach 50 million households; iPads only 80 days, and Pokemon Go only 19 days to reach the same number. Digital disruption of the ways people communicate, consume information, and stay entertained has occurred at such a rapid pace that parents understandably describe feeling that they cannot keep up. Mobile communication scholars call this a stage of 'technologic determinism', when users feel more controlled by technology than they feel control over it (Ling, 2004).

Parents sense this lack of control in regard to their children's media usage as well. In in-depth interviews (Radesky et al., 2016a), low-income parents particularly described feeling little control over how they or their children were using technology; they said that their devices had a 'hook' that kept them coming back again and again, or that their children always found a way around their technology limit-setting. Parents therefore wanted limit-setting to be programmed into

DOI: 10.4324/9781003223771-29

the device (such as a timer or filter), rather than needing to behaviorally manage their child's media usage (Radesky et al., 2016b). Yet, even motivated parents report simply not knowing how to enable parent controls or privacy filters on home devices (Common Sense Media, 2019).

## Practice Pointers

- Many parents, teachers, and clinicians feel an unease with how rapidly technologies are coming into their children's lives. Without up-to-date evidence about the best ways to use or limit technology in early childhood, parents are left to figure it out for themselves, which has contributed to a polarized idea of being a 'low-tech' or 'high-tech' parent (Kamenetz, 2018). It is important to recognize that this can lead to feelings of judgment, which closes off opportunities for open conversation and reflection.
- Early childhood providers may feel a mismatch between their own technology use habits and those of the families they serve; it is therefore important to recognize any implicit reaction to others' media habits and maintain an open, inquisitive stance as to why parents use different technologies (e.g., do they find background TV noise soothing? do they want their child to learn from apps?) which will allow a productive conversation.
- Helping restore parents' internal locus of control about technology may include sympathizing with the universal feeling that technology adoption is moving so quickly, it's hard to keep up with. Also, provide concrete resources that can support decision-making and deliver effective strategies (e.g., Common Sense Media, www. commonsensemedia.org, a free website with well-reasoned and useful tips for parents).

## The Presence of Media in Family Routines

It is important to consider not only the amount of 'screen time' children use per day, but also how media are used through daily activities and family routines. Family routines such as meals, bedtimes, and travel (e.g., car or bus rides) offer times for parent–child conversation, emotional connection, and co-regulation; yet, with the portability and instant accessibility of mobile devices, it has become common for parents or children to use technology during family routines (McDaniel & Radesky, 2018; Raman et al., 2017). Moreover, family downtime – when play, exploration, synchrony, and countless other positive parent–child experiences can occur – may be perceived as 'boring' by parents and a trigger for media use (Radesky et al., 2016a). Parents who describe their children as having social–emotional delays (Raman et al., 2017) or who have lower perceived control about parenting (Radesky et al., 2016c) are more likely to give their toddler a mobile device during family routines or to keep things quiet.

Family meals are an important daily routine that facilitates parent–child conversation and emotional connection (Fiese et al., 2006). Watching TV during family meals has been linked with higher weight status (Vik et al., 2013), possibly due to lower response to satiety cues. Recent research from videotaped family mealtimes suggests that as the number of mealtime media devices increases, the healthfulness of children's meals decreases (Robinson et al., 2021).

Bedtime is another opportunity to teach children self-regulatory skills, but in a recent survey, (Rideout, 2017), about half of young children were reported to use media to watch videos or play games in the hour before bedtime, with 17% doing so 'often' and 32% 'sometimes'. Although use of media before bed is associated with later onset of sleep, more overnight awakenings, and shorter duration of sleep from infancy to adolescence (Hill et al., 2016), many families find this a challenging habit to break.

## Practice Pointers

- By examining how media is interwoven into daily routines and parent–child interactional cascades, clinicians can also identify points of intervention that will be most relevant to parents' everyday experiences and to their personal reasons for use of media. Encourage parents to think about their day. Where does media come in, and did you plan it that way, or did it just happen? What was the feeling right before use – distress from you, or your child? Boredom? What other strategies have helped the parent address these concerns in the moment?
- In addition to antecedents of media use, help parents reflect upon what happened during or after media use. Was it helpful, in that you got the information or social connection you were seeking, or did it stress you out more? Did media use contribute to conflict or displace time that could have been spent doing a routine you enjoy with your child, such as reading or dancing? This type of conversation can provide a launching point for finding alternative strategies for dealing with distress, boredom, or problematic child behaviors during meals or bedtime, for example.
- It might also be helpful to increase parents' awareness and understanding that modern interactive technologies are designed to be habit-forming – meaning that the designers intend for the user to be inseparable from the phone, want to watch another video, or read more. This constant engagement provides more revenue for digital products and allows the collection of digital 'breadcrumbs' about the user's behavior, which can be used to create an advertising profile. Parents may feel more willing to unplug during family routines if they are aware of these design motives.

## Parent Media Use and Parent–Child Interaction

Parents now have devices pinging for their attention, providing tailored news-feeds, informing them when others have given approval through 'likes' or shares, and delivering more information than human brains can likely process effectively

(Levitin, 2014). These aspects of interactive design are effective in drawing parents' attention to devices, which parents say they often use to escape from stressful parenting moments (Torres et al., 2021). Multi-tasking between mobile devices and child social bids is described as highly challenging by many parents (Radesky et al., 2016a) and has been observed to lead to harsher parent responses (Radesky et al., 2014a) or less response altogether (Hiniker et al., 2015; Radesky et al., 2015).

There are several mechanisms by which parent mobile device use might negatively impact parent–child interaction quality:

- When parents use mobile devices, there is less verbal exchange with children (Radesky et al., 2015) which has implications for the quantity and quality of language exposure – both important for early language development and conversational skills.
- When parent–child teaching interactions were interrupted with a brief phone call or text, children showed less effective learning, thought to be due to reduced joint attention and reciprocity (Reed et al., 2017).
- With frequent or long duration of mobile device use, there may be a displacement of opportunities for reading social cues (Uhls et al., 2014) or developing mentalization capacities about children's thoughts and feelings (Radesky et al., 2018). A recent modified 'still face' study involving mothers looking at their mobile device showed that infants of mothers who were frequent mobile device users had more difficulty during the repair phase, with less emotional co-regulation (Myruski et al., 2018).
- Finally, parents report frequent emotional arousal from news or information received via their mobile device, sometimes unexpectedly, which may influence downstream interaction with children (Radesky et al., 2016a).

Although parents describe using media as a stress reliever during challenging moments with their children (Radesky et al., 2016c), evidence suggests that this does not help the child's behavior in the long term: When parents used more technology during parent–child activities due to stress about their child's problem behaviors, their children developed more problem behaviors in subsequent months (McDaniel & Radesky, 2018).

## Practice Pointers

- It may be helpful to encourage parent insight into how their phone use might be perceived by their child – this can be an opportunity for teaching mind-mindedness. It is difficult to read someone else's mind as they are staring at a device – because users often have a flat facial expression. This opacity of the other's mental state can be reflected upon in relation to adult-to-adult phone snubbing (also termed 'phubbing') and then turned around for the parent to understand how others feel.

- Instead of telling parents to stop using their mobile devices altogether, problem-solve some unplugged spaces and times when the devices stay in another room, so that the parent can feel the ease of single-tasking.
- Providers can also ask parents if there have been times when their phone broke or was lost for a few days, and how this felt – both the good and the bad.

## Child Media Use and Social–Emotional Development: The Importance of Design and Parent–Child Interaction Quality

In the age of TV and infant-directed DVDs such as 'Baby Einstein', multiple studies showed correlations between higher duration of daily media use with lower toddler and preschooler language scores, social–emotional competence, and school readiness (see Hill et al., 2016). Few studies on child mobile device use have been conducted, but they generally support previous findings of higher risk of developmental or behavioral concerns with more daily hours of media use (Madigan et al., 2019) or more interactive app use (McNeill et al., 2019).

The relationship is reciprocal, however; infants and toddlers with more regulatory problems, active temperament, or social–emotional delays are more likely to develop heavier media use habits in early childhood (Nabi & Krcmar, 2016; Radesky et al., 2014b). This may be due to greater parental use of devices for calming (Radesky et al., 2016c) and behavioral regulation purposes (Nikken & Schols, 2015) in children with behavioral difficulties.

In addition to duration, it is important to consider the content or design of the media that children view. Prosocial content such as 'Sesame Street' or 'Mister Roger's Neighborhood', or more recently, 'Daniel Tiger's Neighborhood' (Rasmussen et al., 2016), is associated with better social–emotional outcomes in early childhood through adolescence. Changing from violent entertainment content (such as 'Power Rangers') to prosocial or educational content has been associated with significant reductions in externalizing behaviors in preschoolers, particularly low-income boys (Christakis et al., 2013). Unfortunately, violent and highly commercialized content is easily accessible through streaming platforms such as YouTube (Radesky et al., 2020).

Interactive design, defined as programming that responds to the child's input or guides usage behavior, is also important because it steers children's attention or rewards it with gimmicks such as balloons, cheers, and coins, which can make digital experiences less educational (Meyer et al., 2021). The idea of play as generated within the child to explore the world and come up with their own ideas is now frequently replaced by rote or repetitive play, programmed by app developers rather than the child's interests. Moreover, highly gamified or fast-paced media make it harder for parents to scaffold their child in digital activities (Hiniker et al., 2018), which leaves many parents allowing their child to use her mobile device alone (Domoff et al., 2019).

Interactive design also includes data collection and behavioral marketing, in which ads are targeted at users based upon their past behaviors. A review of apps in the Google Play '5 and Under' category showed high levels of advertising, many with deceptive approaches (such as characters in the app encouraging purchases), ads that popped up unexpectedly, and several with inappropriate privacy policies (Meyer et al., 2019). Indeed, a review of the free apps most likely to collect personal data from devices and share them with third-party marketing groups showed that free children's apps were one of the most common (Binns et al., 2018).

## Practice Pointers

- Media fulfills a strong function for families who are stressed, need their child to be occupied, or who feel low self-efficacy for other activities with children. Its use is interwoven with other family stressors and sources of inequitable opportunity. Therefore, overly simplistic solutions, without teaching replacement strategies, will likely not be effective.
- Providers should encourage parents to be savvy about content, advertising, data collection, and what is inappropriate for young children to view. Parents who want to co-use media with their young children can be encouraged to read recommendations on resources such as Common Sense Media. From a relationship standpoint, parents can be supported in using media that creates a space for them and helps them understand their child more, rather than feeling like a barrier.
- When talking to parents about the limits of digital play, it is worth contrasting the constrained design of many children's tech products to the open, imaginative way children see the world. In contrast to some parents' beliefs that digital content may be 'best' for children's learning, simple toys are really the best for helping children learn and discover the way the world works. Even without toys, parents may recognize the connection they feel to their child during singing/dancing games, telling stories, reading, drawing, or other ways of playing – which can be contrasted with the shut-off feeling that can occur with media.

## Summary: Discussion Guide for Reflective Problem-Solving around Media

It is impossible to address each of the above points about digital media at every visit with families; however, using these positive sets of messages over and over at multiple time points will help demonstrate to families that this is an important topic and worth communicating about. Parents should also be warned that media use can be difficult to change all at once, but problem-solving and encouraging a reflective stance in relation to both their child and to media will help them arrive at feasible, meaningful solutions. They are not in this alone. It may be helpful to let parents know that this is a challenge faced by millions of parents, and that by learning and reflecting on their intentions for media use, they are part of a growing number who are trying to identify healthy and practical approaches to media use with children.

1 Encouraging reflection is the most important first step. Much modern technology design is intended to be 'frictionless', that is, used without pausing or need for conscious thought, in a way that inserts itself into everyday habits. Even uses described above – such as to keep an intense child occupied and quiet, or to calm one's inner distress – may not be fully conscious to the parent or intentional. Therefore, conversations should first focus on pausing and considering the parent's motives for and reactions to media (either their own use, or their child's).

2 Use reflective probe questions that pick up on feelings of ambiguity the parent might have about media and allow the parent to think out loud about their hopes and frustrations with media.

3 It can be tempting to respond to initial parent equivocation about media with a dogmatic set of 'rules' about screen time. Instead, allow the conversation to continue so that the clinician and parent can arrive at a definition of the problem together.

4 To aid in this conversation, use the positive. Ask the parent to reflect upon which activities facilitate the 'serve and return' or back-and-forth exchange between parent and child, and how the presence of technology changes this?

5 Once a problem is defined, engage parents in thinking about substitute activities (as many as possible so that they can land on a truly feasible choice). The solution may not be a reduction in screen time or any behavior change at all. It may just be the parent being more aware of his/her relationship with technology for a week or two, to return with more observations and ideas about the advantages and disadvantages of different solutions.

6 As this awareness increases, it may be helpful to support parents' self-efficacy in being tech-savvy. In the current 'tech-lash' era of increased scrutiny of how technology companies conduct business, as well as users' rights in terms of data protection, many parents may be open to messages about savviness. These may include knowing how to change privacy or notification settings on devices, knowing which online resources and articles provide up-to-date information, or feeling confident in identifying low-quality media (full of ads, too simplistic) that is not worth a parent's or child's attention.

7 We suspect that experiential learning will further help increase self-awareness and self-efficacy. At each visit, determine a small change about media the parent would like to continue or implement before the next visit. Make this a realistic choice so that the parent does not feel guilty if they cannot complete it. Remind parents that the digital world is vying for their attention, so progress can be slow.

# References

Binns, R., Lyngs, U., Van Kleek, M., Zhao, J., Libert, T. et al. (2018) Third party tracking in the mobile ecosystem. Proceedings of the 10th Association for Computing Machinery Conference on Web Science: 23–31.

Christakis, D.A., Garrison, M.M., Herrenkohl, T., Haggerty, K., Rivara, F.P. et al. (2013) Modifying media content for preschool children: A randomized controlled trial. Pediatrics, 131(3):431–438.

Common Sense Media (2019) What's that you say? Smart speakers and voice assistants toplines. Available at: https://www.commonsensemedia.org/sites/ default/files/ uploads/pdfs/2019_cs-sm_smartspeakerstoplines_final-release.pdf <accessed 19 November, 2021>

Domoff, S.E., Radesky, J.S., Harrison, K., Riley, H., Lumeng, J.C. et al. (2019) A naturalistic study of child and family screen media and mobile device use. Journal of Child and Family Studies, 28(2):401–410.

Fiese, B.H., Foley, K.P., Spagnola, M. (2006) Routine and ritual elements in family mealtimes: Contexts for child well-being and family identity. New Directions for Child and Adolescent Development, 111(Special Issue):67–89.

Hill, D., Ameenuddin, N., Reid Chassiakos, Y., Cross, C., Hutchinson, J. et al. (2016) Media and young minds. Pediatrics, 138(5):e20162591.

Hiniker, A., Lee, B., Kientz, J.A., Radesky, J.S. (2018) Let's Play! Digital and analog play between preschoolers and parents. Paper presented at: Proceedings of the 2018 CHI Conference on Human Factors in Computing Systems, Montreal, Canada.

Hiniker, A., Sobel, K., Suh, H., Sung, Y-C., Lee, C.P. et al. (2015) Texting while parenting: How adults use mobile phones while caring for children at the playground. Paper presented at: Proceedings of the 33rd Annual ACM Conference on Human Factors in Computing Systems.

Kamenetz, A. (2018) The Art of Screen Time: How your family can balance digital media and real life. London: Hachette.

Levitin, D.J. (2014) The Organized Mind: Thinking straight in the age of information overload. London: Penguin.

Ling, R. (2004) The Mobile Connection: The cell phone's impact on society. Burlington, Massachusetts: Morgan Kaufmann.

Madigan, S., Browne, D., Racine, N., Mori, C., Tough, S. (2019) Association between screen time and children's performance on a developmental screening test. JAMA Pediatrics, 173(3):244–250.

McDaniel, B.T., Radesky, J.S. (2018) Technoference: Longitudinal associations between parent technology use, parenting stress, and child behavior problems. Pediatric Research, 84:210–218.

McDaniel, B.T., Radesky, J.S. (2018) Technoference: Parent distraction with technology and associations with child behavior problems. Child Development, 89(1):100–109.

McNeill, J., Howard, S.J., Vella, S.A., Cliff, D.P. (2019) Longitudinal associations of electronic application use and media program viewing with cognitive and psychosocial development in preschoolers. Academic Pediatrics, 19(5):520–528.

Meyer, M., Adkins, V., Yuan, N., Weeks, H.M., Chang, Y-J. et al. (2019) Advertising in young children's apps: A content analysis. Journal of Developmental & Behavioral Pediatrics, 40(1):32–39.

Meyer, M., Zosh, J. M., McLaren, C., Robb, M., McCaffery, H. et al. (2021) How educational are 'educational' apps for young children? App store content analysis using the Four Pillars of Learning framework. Journal of Children and Media: 1–23. doi:10 .1080/17482798.2021.1882516

Myruski, S., Gulyayeva, O., Birk, S., Pérez-Edgar, K., Buss, K.A. et al. (2018) Digital disruption? Maternal mobile device use is related to infant social-emotional functioning. Developmental Science, 21(4):e12610.

Nabi, R.L., Krcmar, M. (2016) It takes two: The effect of child characteristics on US parents' motivations for allowing electronic media use. Journal of Children and Media, 10(3):285–303.

Nikken, P., Schols, M. (2015) How and why parents guide the media use of young children. Journal of Child and Family Studies, 24(11):3423–3435.

Radesky, J.S., Eisenberg, S., Kistin, C.J., Gross, J., Block, G. et al. (2016b) Overstimulated consumers or next-generation learners? Parent tensions about child mobile technology use. The Annals of Family Medicine, 14(6):503–508.

Radesky, J.S., Kistin, C., Eisenberg, S., Gross, J., Block, G. et al. (2016a) Parent perspectives on their mobile technology use: The excitement and exhaustion of parenting while connected. Journal of Developmental & Behavioral Pediatrics, 37(9):694–701.

Radesky, J.S., Kistin, C.J., Zuckerman, B., Nitzberg, K., Gross, J. et al. (2014a) Patterns of mobile device use by caregivers and children during meals in fast food restaurants. Pediatrics, 133(4):e843–849.

Radesky, J.S., Leung, C., Appugliese, D., Miller, A.L., Lumeng, J.C. et al. (2018) Maternal mental representations of the child and mobile phone use during parent-child mealtimes. Journal of Developmental & Behavioral Pediatrics, 39(4):310–317.

Radesky, J.S., Miller, A.L., Rosenblum, K.L., Appugliese, D., Kaciroti, N. (2015) Maternal mobile device use during a structured parent-child interaction task. Academic Pediatrics, 15(2):238–244.

Radesky, J.S., Peacock-Chambers, E., Zuckerman, B., Silverstein, M. (2016c) Use of mobile technology to calm upset children: Associations with social-emotional development. JAMA Pediatrics, 170(4):397–399.

Radesky, J., Schaller, A., Yeo, S., Weeks, H.M., Robb, M.B. (2020) Young kids and YouTube: How ads, toys, and games dominate viewing, 2020. Available at: https://d2e111jq13me73.cloudfront.net/sites/default/files/uploads/research/2020_ youngkidsyoutube-report_final-release_forweb.pdf < accessed 19 November, 2021>

Radesky, J.S., Silverstein, M., Zuckerman, B., Christakis, D.A. (2014b) Infant self-regulation and early childhood media exposure. Pediatrics, 133(5):e1172–1178.

Raman, S., Guerrero-Duby, S., McCullough, J.L., Brown, M., Ostrowski-Delahanty, S. et al. (2017) Screen exposure during daily routines and a young child's risk for having social-emotional delay. Clinical Pediatrics, 56(13):1244–1253.

Rasmussen, E.E., Shafer, A., Colwell, M.J., White, S., Punyanunt-Carter, N. et al. (2016) Relation between active mediation, exposure to Daniel Tiger's Neighborhood, and US preschoolers' social and emotional development. Journal of Children and Media, 10(4):443–461.

Reed, J., Hirsh-Pasek, K., Golinkoff, R.M. (2017) Learning on hold: Cell phones sidetrack parent-child interactions. Developmental Psychology, 53(8):1428.

Rideout, V. (2017) The common sense census: Media use by kids age zero to eight. San Francisco, CA: Common Sense Media: 263–283.

Robinson, C.A., Domoff, S.E., Kasper, N., Peterson, K.E., Miller, A.L. (2021) The healthfulness of children's meals when multiple media and devices are present. Appetite, 105800.

Torres, C., Radesky, J., Levitt, K.J., McDaniel, B.T. (2021) Is it fair to simply tell parents to use their phones less? A qualitative analysis of parent phone use. Acta Paediatrica, 110(9):2594–2596.

Uhls, Y.T., Michikyan, M., Morris, J., Garcia, D., Small, G.W. et al. (2014) Five days at outdoor education camp without screens improves preteen skills with nonverbal emotion cues. Computers in Human Behavior, 39:387–392.

Vik, F.N., Bjørnarå, H.B., Øverby, N.C., Lien, N., Androutsos, O. et al. (2013) Associations between eating meals, watching TV while eating meals and weight status among children ages 10–12 years, in eight European countries: The ENERGY cross-sectional study. International Journal of Behavioral Nutrition and Physical Activity, 10(1):58.

# PART VI

# The 'How' of Educating and Supporting Parents

## Introduction

This final section of the book comprises chapters that were originally published primarily as articles about the 'how' of perinatal education rather than the 'what'. The first chapter warns educators of the harm caused by inconsistent advice and of the dangers presented by parenting gurus advocating specific parenting *techniques*. Instead, educators need to be strong and confident to transmit a persistent and consistent message that warmth, responsiveness and setting boundaries are the qualities that both research and the parenting community itself have found to be the bedrock of parenting from babyhood to adolescence.

Educational theorists have much to offer. Tapping into the springs, ancient and modern, that have fed and continue to feed educational practice down the years refreshes practice by stimulating reflection on the way in which we respect the adulthood of learners, care for them and introduce them into a community of parenting practice which parents can both draw on and contribute to.

Women with abnormal fear of childbirth seem to be increasing in number. Helping them understand, express and share their emotions with their peers in a safe group environment minimizes stress that is harmful to their unborn babies, contributes to a less traumatic labor and makes it more likely that they will enjoy a positive, responsive relationship with their newborn babies.

The majority of research into perinatal education has focused on the 'usual suspects', that is parents who are WEIRD: White, Educated, living in post-Industrial countries, 'Rich' (by contrast with most of the world's parents) and living in Democratic societies. As issues of diversity and inclusion shout out for a hearing in the twenty-first century, it is overdue that we should start to include, work with and learn from marginalized groups. Currently, parenting programs are often not relevant to – and therefore not attended by – many groups who find

DOI: 10.4324/9781003223771-30

them oblivious to their particular interests, way of life and needs. Muslim parents often seek an antenatal education program that is founded on their faith values. LGBTQ+ parents may avoid programs which are unthinkingly hetero- and cis-normative. Pregnant adolescents may be deterred from coming to a group composed of much older parents-to-be who are at a different stage of life from themselves. Even fathers (who do now appear in the literature) continue to feel ignored or relegated to the role of 'mother's little helper' by antenatal educators and professionals, while their unique experience of pregnancy, labor, birth and early parenthood is not acknowledged.

Chapters in this section examine how perinatal education can respect and cater for the interests and needs of these poorly served groups. Authors repeatedly stress the importance of *asking* parents what they want from their birth and parenting education; of seeing every topic from their point of view; and of seeking their feedback, or better still, inviting them to co-design and deliver programs of education that truly support their particular journeys into parenthood.

To end the book, we acknowledge the rise of online antenatal and early parenting education and look at best practice guidelines. Much research remains to be done on whether online groups are effective in increasing knowledge and building confidence in parents-to-be, and how best they can prepare parents for the physical, emotional and spiritual experience of having and caring for a baby. At this point, we are learning from each other. In all honesty, for childbirth and parenting educators, this has always been the case.

We wish you the very best in your work.

# 25

# COMMENTARY

## Tug of War – Could Polarized Parenting Advice Cause Harm?

*Kathleen Hodkinson, Tara Acevedo and Katrin Kristjansdottir*

Should you use controlled crying techniques or will this damage your child's emotional development? When your child misbehaves, should you 'connect and reflect' or send them to their room? Parents today are inundated with an overwhelming mass of conflicting emotive information about how to parent (Eisenberg et al., 2015; Sanders & Calam, 2016; Strahan et al., 2009). This comes from the internet (Germic et al., 2021; Porter & Ispa, 2013), parenting books (e.g. Green, 2014; Siegel & Bryson, 2014a) and even from healthcare professionals. Some of this advice is lacking in empirical support, and some is actually contrary to scientific evidence (McInnes et al., 2015). Much of it is presented in a polarized and moralistic way, reflecting a culture of 'combative mothering' (Abetz & Moore, 2018). So, how do parents know what to believe? Knowing which advice is sound and which is little more than opinion can be a challenge, even for professionals.

The reality is that there has never been, nor is there currently, a consensus on exactly 'how to parent', even within the scientific community. At present, two very different theoretical approaches are prominent both within scientific discourse and the wider media: Behaviorism and attachment parenting (Troutman, 2015). These approaches can seem to generate opposite recommendations about how best to parent. Simply put, behaviorism focuses mainly on strengthening certain behaviors through reinforcements (rewards) and reducing others through extinction (ignoring) (e.g. Skinner, 1953, 1974). Over the last 50 years, behaviorism has led the field of parenting research and currently forms the basis of the majority of evidence-based parenting intervention programs (e.g. Sanders, 1999; Webster-Stratton, 2005). By contrast, attachment parenting (Sears, 1982; Sears & Sears, 2001) is a somewhat more recent parenting philosophy that has become increasingly popular. The focus of attachment parenting approaches is usually on the development of a secure parent–child relationship

DOI: 10.4324/9781003223771-31

and emotion-regulation skills in children. This is achieved through the presence of sensitive responsiveness on the part of the parent and respecting children's choices (Miller & Commons, 2010).

So, which approach should parents follow? Perhaps surprisingly, there is very little research evaluating the relative benefits of specific parenting *techniques* on parent and child outcomes. Most scientific research examines the efficacy of overall parenting programs in families who need support, and not the specific components within each program or the mechanisms leading to improvement (Troutman, 2015). Nevertheless, discourse about the 'right way to parent' has become increasingly dogmatic and polarized in popular media (Moore & Abetz, 2016). To make matters even more confusing, parenting advice given by experts can be misleading. Scientists who present parenting advice in the form of popular literature may publish work that reflects a greater amount of opinion than scientific evidence (Strahan et al., 2009) or in which nuances are lost within oversimplified headlines (e.g. Siegel & Bryson, 2014b; 2014c).

What effect does this conflicting information have on parents? If parents are frequently exposed to inconsistent information about how to parent, this may (i) reduce parenting confidence (self-efficacy) and (ii) lead to more inconsistent parenting. Parenting self-efficacy is a predictor of both parental competence and child adjustment (Jones & Prinz, 2005), and research has repeatedly shown that inconsistent parenting practices are associated with negative behavioral outcomes in children (e.g. Stormshak et al., 2000). There is, as yet, no concrete experimental evidence that exposure to inconsistent parenting information leads parents to feel less confident or to parent more inconsistently. However, studies from other fields support such a conjecture (Carpenter et al., 2014; Kai, 1996; Marshall, 2013). Recent evidence has also shown that receiving parenting advice from internet sources is associated with lower parenting self-efficacy (DeGroot & Vik, 2019), and qualitative research reveals that the conflicting and confusing nature of such information can lead to parents feeling inadequate and anxious (Strange et al., 2018). Finally, there are indications that parenting self-efficacy is significantly lower in recent years than it was at the end of the 1990s and conflicting information is a potential key contributor to this decline (Glatz & Buchanan, 2021).

## Toward a Solution

Behavioral and attachment approaches are often presented in the media as polar opposites, with the message that parents must choose one or the other (Troutman, 2015). Of course, factors such as parent and child temperament mean that a one parenting style fits all approach is far from optimal (O'Connor & Scott, 2007). Polarized advice ignores heterogeneity and fails to consider key variables such as parents' capacity for emotional regulation, their own developmental experiences, the cultural and social context or neurodiversity of parent and/or child. How can we transition to a more evidence-based, nuanced and inclusive discourse?

Despite their differences, behavioral and attachment parenting approaches actually share a number of similar principles, many of which fall within the construct of *authoritative parenting*. This term, coined by Diane Baumrind in 1966, refers to an emphasis on warmth and responsiveness, in the context of clear limits and helping children to understand the reasons behind rules and the consequences of behavior (Baumrind, 1966). There is overwhelming evidence that the authoritative parenting style is a consistent predictor of both parental wellbeing and child outcomes (Hoskins, 2014). When analyzed more closely, parenting advice from ostensibly very different theoretical perspectives actually places a primary emphasis on authoritative parenting. This is encouraging, given that the main ingredients of authoritative parenting – warmth and responsiveness combined with consistent limit setting – appear to be the most evidence-based approach toward parenting today. When these factors are present in a consistent way, the precise parenting tools used are not so important. In an age of increasingly polarized debate and judgment about 'correct' parenting practices, much of which is based on opinion rather than science, this is a key message to convey to parents.

## References

Abetz, J., Moore, J. (2018) 'Welcome to the Mommy Wars, Ladies': Making sense of the ideology of combative mothering in mommy blogs. Communication Culture & Critique, 11. doi:10.1093/ccc/tcy008

Baumrind, D. (1966) Effects of authoritative parental control on child behavior. Child Development, 37(4):887–907.

Carpenter, D.M., Elstad, E.A., Blalock, S.J., DeVellis, R.F. (2014) Conflicting medication information: Prevalence, sources, and relationship to medication adherence. Journal of Health Communication, 19(1):67–81.

DeGroot, J., Vik, T. (2019) 'Fake smile. Everything is under control': The flawless performance of motherhood. Western Journal of Communication, 85:1–19.

Eisenberg, S.R., Bair Merritt, M.H., Colson, E.R., Heeren, T.C., Geller, N.L., et al. (2015) Maternal report of advice received for infant care. Pediatrics, 136(2):e315–22.

Germic, E., Eckert, S., Vultee, F. (2021) The impact of instagram mommy blogger content on the perceived self-efficacy of mothers. Social Media + Society, 7(3). doi:10.1177/20563051211041649.

Glatz, T., Buchanan, C.M. (2021) Trends in parental self-efficacy between 1999 and 2014. Journal of Family Studies. doi:10.1080/13229400.2021.1906929.

Green, C. (2014) Toddler Taming. Australia: Random House.

Hoskins, D. (2014) Consequences of parenting on adolescent outcomes. Societies, 4(3):506–531.

Jones, T., Prinz, R. (2005) Potential roles of parental self-efficacy in parent and child adjustment: A review. Clinical Psychology Review, 25:341–363.

Kai, J. (1996) Parents' difficulties and information needs in coping with acute illness in preschool children: A qualitative study. British Medical Journal, 313(7063):987–990.

Marshall, L.H. (2013) What should I do now? Impact on self-efficacy of seeing conflicting medical information online. Chapel Hill: University of North Carolina.

McInnes, R.J., Arbuckle, A., Hoddinott, P. (2015) How UK internet websites portray breast milk expression and breast pumps: A qualitative study of content. BMC Pregnancy and Childbirth, 15:article no. 81.

Miller, P.M., Commons, M.L. (2010) The benefits of attachment parenting for infants and children: A behavioral developmental view. Behavioral Development Bulletin, 16(1):1–14.

Moore, J., Abetz, J. (2016) 'Uh oh Cue the [new] mommy wars': The ideology of combative mothering in popular US newspaper articles about attachment parenting. Southern Communication Journal, 81(1):49–62.

O'Connor, T.G., Scott, S. (2007) Parenting and Outcomes for Children. York: Joseph Rowntree Foundation.

Porter, N., Ispa, J.M. (2013) Mothers' online message board questions about parenting infants and toddlers. Journal of Advanced Nursing, 69(3):559–568.

Sanders, M.R. (1999) Triple P-Positive Parenting Program: Towards an empirically validated multilevel parenting and family support strategy for the prevention of behavior and emotional problems in children. Clinical Child and Family Psychology Review, 2(2):71–90.

Sanders, M.R., Calam, R. (2016) Parenting information and advice and the mass media. In: Durkin, K., Schaffer, H.R. (Eds.) The Wiley Handbook of Developmental Psychology in Practice. Chichester: John Wiley & Sons, Ltd: 100–120.

Sears, W. (1982) Creative Parenting: A continuum of child care from birth through adolescence. Manchester: Dove.

Sears, W., Sears, M. (2001) The Attachment Parenting Book: A common-sense guide to understanding and nurturing your baby. Boston, MA: Little Brown & Co.

Siegel, D.J., Bryson, T.P. (2014a) No Drama Discipline: The whole brain way to calm the chaos and nurture your child's developing mind. Victoria: Scribe Publications.

Siegel, D., Bryson, T.P. (2014b) 'Time-outs' are hurting your child. Time: September 23.

Siegel, D., Bryson, T.P. (2014c) You said WHAT about time-outs?! Huffington Post: October 21.

Skinner, B.F. (1953) Science and Human Behavior. Cambridge: The Free Press.

Skinner, B.F. (1974) About Behaviorism. New York: Alfred A. Knopf.

Stormshak, E.A., Bierman, K.L., McMahon, R.J., Lengua, L.J. (2000) Parenting practices and child disruptive behavior problems in early elementary school. Journal of Clinical Child Psychology, 29(1): 17–29.

Strahan, E.Y., Dixon, W.E., Banks, J.B. (2009) Parenting with Reason: Evidence-based approaches to parenting dilemmas. Abingdon: Taylor & Francis.

Strange, C., Fisher, C., Howat, P., Wood, L. (2018) 'Easier to isolate yourself… there's no need to leave the house' – A qualitative study on the paradoxes of online communication for parents with young children. Computers in Human Behavior, 83:168–175.

Troutman, B. (2015) Comparison of attachment and behavioral parenting perspectives. In: Troutman, B. (Ed.) Integrating Behaviorism and Attachment Theory in Parent Coaching. New York: Springer International Publishing: 43–51.

Webster-Stratton, C. (2005) The Incredible Years: A training series for the prevention and treatment of conduct problems in young children. In: Hibbs, E.D., Jensen, P.S. (Eds.) Psychosocial Treatments for Child and Adolescent Disorders: Empirically based strategies for clinical practice. American Psychological Association: 507–555.

# 26

# EXPLORING THE APPLICATION (OR USE) OF EDUCATIONAL THEORY IN PERINATAL TEACHING THROUGH FOUR THEORISTS

*Shona Gore and Kay Cram*

Lifelong learning is composed of many experiences that involve incorporating new knowledge or concepts into one's understanding of the world. Becoming a parent is a transformative experience and a period of potential disjuncture, presenting 'disorientating dilemmas' (Jarvis, 2009; Mezirow, 1981). Exploring theories of adult education can help the practitioner to support new parents through this extraordinary time of change and meet the aims of perinatal education as outlined below:

- To build self-efficacy for normal birth
- To strengthen the relationship between the parents and their unborn baby
- To reduce stress in parents and improve mental health
- To strengthen the couple relationship
- To create social support
- To build strong, healthy communities based on strong healthy families
- To ameliorate social inequalities (Nolan, 2020).

This chapter will demonstrate how the ideas of four key figures in educational theory can inform the practice of childbirth and early parenting educators and help them create an effective learning environment.

## Socrates (Died 399 BC) Greek Philosopher and Teacher

Much of what we know about Socrates comes indirectly from writings by his pupil, Plato, from Xenophon and the plays of Aristophanes. Socrates believed that learning came through 'discourse', through listening and talking, and that both teacher and student could learn from each other. In Plato's *Theaetetus*, Socrates likens his way of philosophising to the occupation of his mother who was a

DOI: 10.4324/9781003223771-32

midwife: Not pregnant with ideas himself, he assists others with the delivery of their ideas:

> I ask questions of others and have not the wit to answer them myself....the reason is that the gods compel me to be a midwife, but do not allow me to bring forth. And therefore, I am not myself at all wise, nor have I anything to show which is the invention or birth of my own soul, but those who converse with me profit. The many fine discoveries to which they cling are of their own making.

> *Plato's Theaetetus (translation by Jowett, 2009: 97)*

Socrates' way of asking and answering questions to stimulate critical thinking has become known as the 'Socratic Method'. Questioning allows learners to examine critically their prior knowledge and ideas and to gain new understanding through discussion.

As outlined by Socrates, a variety of questions might be posed:

- Questions of clarification
- Questions that probe assumptions
- Questions that probe reasons
- Questions about viewpoints or perspectives
- Questions that probe implications and consequences
- Questions about the question.

According to Paul and Elder (1997), a Socratic questioner/facilitator should keep the discussion focused and ensure that it is intellectually responsible (i.e. that the discussion is logical and reasonable). The questioner/facilitator should stimulate discussion with probing questions and periodically summarise what has been said and which issues remain unresolved. It is important to draw as many students as possible into the discussion.

★★★

TEACHING ACTIVITY based on Socratic inquiry, questioning, small group discussion to enable parents to learn from each other, and teacher as facilitator not 'expert'.

## The Quest for Perfect Pain Management during Labour and Birth

### Aims

- To enable parents to explore their ideas and concerns around the management of pain during labour and birth and to discover their preferences in the light of information gained.

## Learning Outcomes

As a result of participating in this activity, parents will be better able to:

- State the advantages and disadvantages of the various pain management options available to them (information gained through Socratic inquiry)
- Identify their preferences for pain management in labour (through the use of Socratic questioning and discussion)
- Recognise some circumstances that may affect their choices during labour (Socratic uncertainty – 'no knowledge is certain').

## Activity

Brainstorm: Facilitator asks parents what they think are 'The Attributes of Perfect Pain Management for Labour & Birth'. Parents write their ideas on post-its and place on flipchart. Facilitator reads out all the contributions and then opens up a discussion:

- Why is it important to you that the pain management strategy you choose in labour should be … (insert whatever the parents have said is important for them).

Parents are then given a blank table with the five main pain management options available to them written at the head of each column. Down the left-hand side, they are invited to fill in the attributes of pain management that are most important to them. In small groups, they then visit tables/displays of information about the main options for pain management. After exploring the information, they mark their sheets according to whether each option fulfils their criteria. The facilitator moves around the room asking open questions and offering guidance if required.

**TABLE 26.1** Our pain management preferences Tick the boxes according to whether each form of pain relief meets your requirements

| Our priorities (examples) | Self-help methods | Tens | Water | Epidural | Pethidine |
|---|---|---|---|---|---|
| To have no pain | | | | | |
| No negative effect on baby | | | | | |
| Non invasive | | | | | |
| Natural | | | | | |
| No negative effect on breastfeeding | | | | | |
| No needles | | | | | |

The parents come together for a plenary session during which the facilitator opens up a discussion to enable them to explore concerns arising from the information they have gathered and to share and reflect on their feelings and thoughts.

## Resources

Flipchart, post-its, pens, pro-forma tables (on clip boards), displays of evidence-based and up-to-date information on pain management options, including visual aids – for example a Tens machine, epidural pictures, an epidural catheter, birth pool photographs, aids to self-help such as birth balls, massage tools, videos of epidural, and water birth.

## Malcolm Knowles (1913–1997) American Adult Educator

Malcolm Knowles is often described as the 'father of andragogy'. He was influenced by the work of Eduard Lindeman, a German-American author and educator who published *The Meaning of Adult Education* in 1926. Knowles' conclusions about how adults learn were first published in his 1973 book, 'The Adult Learner – A Neglected Species', in which he described andragogy as the art and science of helping adults learn and proposed four characteristics of adult learners. He later added two further characteristics: Motivation to learn and the need to know.

Knowles' Characteristics of Adult Learners (1973, 1984, 1990)

1  The need to know: Adults need to know why they need to learn something before undertaking to learn it.
2  Self-concept: As a person matures, his/her self-concept moves from one of dependence to one of being self-directed.
3  Experience: As people mature, they accumulate a reservoir of experience that becomes an increasing resource for learning.
4  Readiness to learn: Readiness to learn is increasingly linked to the developmental tasks of social roles.
5  Orientation to learning: The orientation towards learning shifts from being subject-centred to problem-centred and from postponed application of knowledge to immediacy of application.
6  Motivation to learn: As a person matures, the motivation to learn is internal rather than external.

Knowles' theory of andragogy has been challenged (Merriam et al., 2007), although its underlying principles of self-direction, experience, relevance, and motivation have been helpful in describing learning at different ages and stages across the life span and can certainly be usefully applied to parent education (Merriam, 2001).

Knowles advised educators that adults need to be involved in planning their own learning, and in evaluating it, and that the basis for learning activities is drawn from adult learners' experiences, including the mistakes they have made during their lives. Adults are most interested in information and skills that have immediate relevance to their circumstances and can help them address current or anticipated problems and challenges in their lives.

Parents-to-be have strong motivation to learn how best to approach birth and early parenting. Educators meet these adults at a uniquely 'teachable' moment when they feel an urgent need to become more independent and responsible and are seeking relevant information and skills to apply in the near future.

★★★

TEACHING ACTIVITY based on the characteristics of adult learners as described by Knowles.

## Pass the Pelvis

### Aim

To develop parents' understanding of the benefits of movement in labour and use of different positions for comfort and to support the process of labour and birth.

### Learning Outcomes

As a result of participating in this activity, parents will be able to:

- Describe how the shape of the pelvis, the flexibility of the pelvic joints, and the pelvic floor muscles influence the descent of the baby during labour and birth
- Demonstrate the movements of the baby as (s)he moves through the pelvis during labour
- Describe the effect that movement and gravity have on the passage of the baby during labour and thus on the progress of labour and the comfort of the mother
- Use upright, forward, and open positions during labour.

### Activity

#### Fathers'/Partners' Group

Invite the fathers/birth partners to examine a model pelvis, note interesting features, and take measurements of the internal dimensions. Ask them to pass a ball through the pelvis with the pelvis in a horizontal position as if the woman were lying on her back and note the ease of movement of the ball and its direction. Ask them to try again with the pelvis in an upright position, again noting the direction of movement and ease of passage of the ball.

## Mothers'/Birthing Persons' Group

Invite the women/birthing persons to discuss the role of the pelvic floor muscles during labour and birth and practise pelvic floor exercises with them.

## Whole Group Plenary

Ask the fathers/birth partners to share the findings of their exploration of the pelvis with the whole group. Ask questions (if needed) to draw out key information:

- What did they notice about the pelvis, for example, its flexibility and movement of the coccyx?
- What did they notice about the way in which the ball passed through the pelvis?
- From their research and experimentation, what do they think the mother/birthing person can do to aid the process of labour and birth?
- What can they do to help and support her?

## Couples Work

Applying the knowledge they now have, ask couples to practise positions for labour and birth. Suggest a contraction by timing a 45/60-second period and talking through how the contraction may feel, or by increasing and then decreasing the intensity of 'white noise', or by rattling a maraca. Encourage couples to try a variety of positions and decide which they feel will help the progress of their labour and which they feel comfortable using.

## Resources

Model pelvis, small soft-bodied doll to fit through the pelvis, drawing of a female pelvis, ball of similar diameter to the head of a newborn, tape measure, diagrams of positions for labour and birth.

## ABRAHAM MASLOW (1908–1970) American Psychologist

Maslow explored human motivation and proposed a Hierarchy of Needs (Maslow, 1943). This is most often presented as the familiar 'pyramid'.

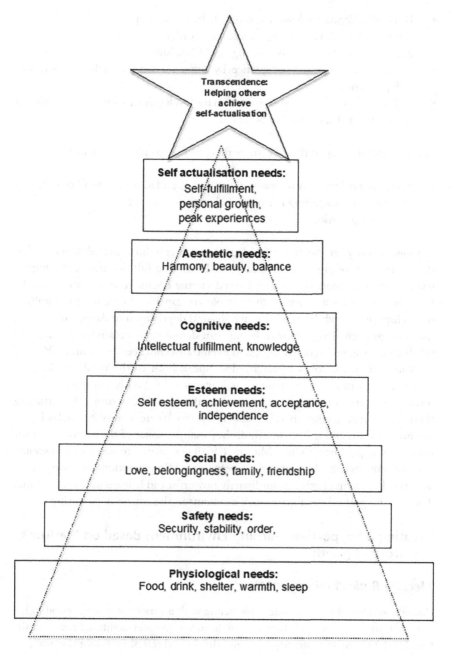

**FIGURE 26.1** Maslow's Hierarchy of Needs.
*Source*: Derived from Maslow (1943).

- Basic *physiological needs* such as food, shelter, and sleep
- *Safety needs* such as security, stability, and order
- *Social needs* such as love, belonging, and friendship
- *Esteem needs* including acceptance by others, a sense of achievement, and independence
- *Self-actualisation needs*, the goal of human development which occurs when a person meets his or her full potential.

Maslow later developed this five-stage model of motivation to include:

- *Cognitive needs* such as intellectual fulfilment and acquisition of knowledge
- *Aesthetic needs* including harmony, balance, and beauty
- *Transcendence needs*.

Maslow's theory has been criticised in that a hierarchical model suggests that the lower levels of physical and safety needs must be fulfilled before the higher level of self-actualisation can be achieved via the cognitive and aesthetic levels. However, it has been observed that people are capable of creative and intellectual achievements whilst experiencing physical deprivation or danger and that at times of great challenge, human beings can demonstrate creativity and achieve fulfilment, love, self-actualisation, and even transcendence (Tennant, 2006).

Nonetheless, Maslow's hierarchy does speak both to the needs of the new infant, and to those of the parents as learners – for bodily comfort, security, interaction and communication, acceptance, affection, and learning. By nurturing their adult learners, educators also model how to nurture infants' needs. By keeping both parents and infants in mind, they may lay some of the groundwork for later 'peak experiences' which Maslow (1970) considered to be those transcendent moments in life when humans experience sublime emotions of ecstasy, awe, and wonder, feeling both extraordinarily powerful and helpless at the same time. There is the possibility of many such moments in the course of parenting.

## Creating a Supportive Learning Environment Based on Maslow's Hierarchy of Needs

### Meeting Basic Physiological Needs

Provide an accessible and comfortable venue with a variety of seating, good lighting, fresh air, appropriate heating, accessible and clean toilet facilities. Provide cushions for the pregnant women/people and drinks and refreshments for the group.

### Meeting Safety Needs

Create a welcoming and accepting environment where parents feel comfortable to share their thoughts and concerns, to ask questions that they might be reluctant to ask elsewhere, to make mistakes and not feel belittled or silly. Show respect, trust, and empathy and value the experiences that parents bring to the group. Agree 'ground-rules' to secure a safe environment, for example about the use of mobile phones and social media.

## Meeting Social Needs

Entrust ownership of the group to the group members, offering parents time and opportunity for socialising and discussion, encouraging the development of a support network and opening up communication channels.

## Meeting Esteem Needs

Build self-esteem by demonstrating a non-judgemental attitude, inviting parents' contributions and valuing them, acknowledging individual experiences and achievements. Give parents the freedom to express feelings and thoughts. Draw out the knowledge parents already have, thereby enhancing their self-esteem. Provide multiple opportunities to acquire practical baby care skills and self-help skills for labour and birth so that parents feel they have competency to meet the practical challenges ahead.

## Meeting Cognitive Needs

Provide evidence-based information and opportunities for parents to demonstrate their knowledge and share information. Ask parents to research information on specific issues. Signpost them to sources of information and support.

## Meeting Aesthetic Needs

Create a pleasant learning environment with pictures on the walls and by using a variety of colourful and engaging visual and teaching aids. Use music for relaxation sessions.

## Meeting Self-Actualisation Needs and Transcendence Needs

By providing an optimal learning environment and demonstrating respect for parents' experiences, by adding to their knowledge and skills, and supporting the emergence of a peer-support group for after the babies are born, educators may help the parents in their groups to achieve self-actualisation and transcendence needs. These needs may be met long after the antenatal sessions are finished by developing parents' awareness of their babies as individuals with minds of their own through exploration of attachment and bonding, baby communication and baby development, and babies' learning. Educators can build parents' confidence to achieve sensitive and joyful parenting.

★★★

## Etienne Wenger (1952–) Swiss Educational Theorist

Etienne Wenger worked with Jean Lave, a social anthropologist, looking at apprenticeship as a way of learning. Their book, 'Situated Learning' (1991), introduced the concept of 'communities of practice'. Wenger went on to write 'Communities of Practice: Learning, Meaning, and Identity' (1998) in which he developed the idea that people in communities or groups learn with and from each other. He suggested that communities of practice occur naturally through a shared interest or may be formed intentionally for the purpose of gaining and sharing knowledge and expertise in a particular area (Lave & Wenger 1991). Whilst many take place in face-to-face environments, online communities of practice also exist where members can communicate and share experiences and gain new knowledge and skills through virtual learning environments, discussion boards, and social media groups.

In order to be a 'community of practice', there needs to be a common purpose or task (the domain), a particular set of skills or knowledge (the practice), and a group of practitioners who share their practice and knowledge (the community). Parents can be seen as one such 'community of practice' as can the antenatal educators who offer them the opportunity to explore their entry into the new community of parents and parenting. Antenatal education brings together a group of strangers, the parents-to-be, who have a common goal, namely to gain knowledge and practise the skills of parenting and to become familiar with the language, culture, and roles of parents today supported by a group of peers. As they make the transition to parenthood, they assimilate aspects of their new identity and begin to 'belong' to their new community. Antenatal education can play a major part in developing that identity and growing that community of practice.

For example, parents attending antenatal education sessions often state that they want to learn about changing a baby's nappy. This learning may be facilitated in small groups with the parents-to-be investigating the advantages and disadvantages of different makes and kinds of nappies, gaining new knowledge of babies' patterns of elimination, sharing previous knowledge and cultural and social differences around baby care. During this activity, they will not only have acquired skills of nappy changing, but will also have had the opportunity to discuss baby care choices and learn some new vocabulary relevant to the early postnatal period, for example 'meconium'. The surprise of changing a nappy worn by a doll that contains mock 'poo' is often much more memorable than photographs. Thus, this simulated activity enables parents-to-be to move towards full membership of the new community they are about to join. Resources you may need for this activity – nappies disposable and cloth (with nappy covers), cotton wool, wipes, nappy disposal bags, laundering suggestions, dolls (plastic bodied) wearing nappies containing mock poo made from mustard, chocolate sauce, damp nappies, photographs showing how baby excretion changes.

## Teaching Activity

Parents-to-be can gain confidence and skills to become part of the new 'community of practice' they are joining by practising the skills of the community and becoming aware of its special 'lingo'. Antenatal sessions can also increase awareness of sources of support accessible to them as members of this new community. There is an old saying that 'It takes a village to raise a child' and knowing how and where to access support is reassuring.

## 'It Takes a Village to Raise a Child'

### Aim

To develop awareness of the resources and community of support available to parents.

### Learning Outcomes

By participating in this learning activity, parents will be better able to:

- Identify appropriate resources and sources of support available to the community of parents
- Name the people and resources in their own 'village' community
- Integrate more confidently into the community of parents.

### Activity

Introduce the concept of 'It Takes a Village to Raise a Child'. Explain that this activity will help parents identify who is there for them after their babies are born and enable them to feel part of their new community.

Place 'village' cards on the floor, each one labelled with common sources of support for new parents, for example midwife, GP, health visitor, breastfeeding counsellor, family, friends, antenatal group. Have a few blank cards so that parents can label these themselves. A card labelled 'Instincts' can be included as these can be a valuable resource for new mothers and fathers!

Organise parents into small groups. Give each group a few postnatal scenario cards (different for each group) and ask them to discuss from whom or from where support can be found in each situation.

### Examples of Postnatal Scenarios

Our baby is 6 weeks old and has started crying inconsolably for hours in the evening. Nothing seems to make him feel better – we have tried

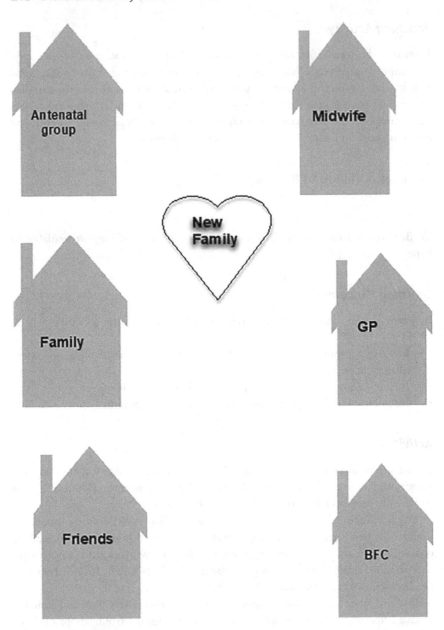

**FIGURE 26.2** It Takes a Village to Raise a Child: Activity.
*Source*: Authors.

rocking and walking, bathing and soothing. We are really worried – what can we do to help him and who can help us?

My baby is breastfed and is now 3 weeks old. She seems to be constantly hungry and wants to feed all the time – now my nipples are sore as well.

Does she need more milk – how can I know she is getting enough? Who can I turn to for some help?

Come back into the whole group and give each couple (or parent) their own village handout so that they can start to populate it with sources of support during the next part of the activity. Ask the small groups to feedback to the whole group by reading out their scenarios and identifying where they thought parents might access support in these situations. Ask them to place the relevant 'village building' cards around the postnatal scenario card to illustrate the community of support for parents. After several scenarios have been discussed, parents will be able to recognise the range of support available to them.

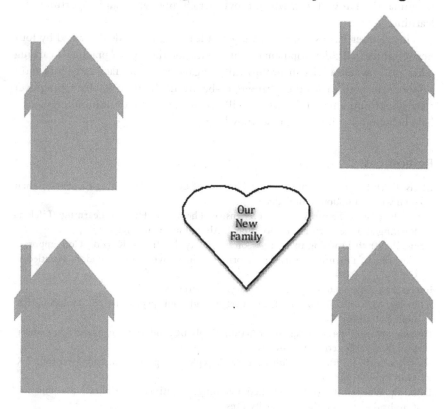

FIGURE 26.3 Our Support Contacts.

At the end of the activity, provide a handout with relevant contact details of local and national support organisations and websites.

## Resources

'Village' cards and postnatal scenario cards, Local support resources handout.

★★★

## In Conclusion

True learning has been identified as involving the whole person (Jarvis, 2006) leading to permanent and ongoing change (Illeris, 2009), transforming the individual and his or her life (Jarvis, 2009). Becoming a parent has been described as a major life transition and a life crisis (McCourt, 2006). It is a 'disorienting dilemma' (Mezirow, 1981), which provides rich motivation and opportunity for learning.

This chapter has explored teaching and learning methods described by four major figures in the development of adult education theory and practice. Learning takes place when adults in groups fully engage with the facilitator and most importantly with each other. Parents-to-be are in the process of stepping over a threshold into a new role, which will involve critically examining previously held beliefs and assimilating new knowledge.

## References

Illeris, K. (Ed.) (2009) Contemporary Theories of Learning. Learning theorists in their own words. London: Routledge.

Jarvis, P. (2006) Towards a Comprehensive Theory of Human Learning: Lifelong learning and the learning society. Vol. 1. Abingdon: Routledge.

Jarvis, P. (2009) Learning to be a person in society. In: Illeris, K. (Ed.) Contemporary Theories of Learning: Learning theorists in their own words. London: Routledge: Ch. 2.

Jowett, B. (2009) Plato's Theaetetus. Maryland: Serenity Publishers.

Knowles, M.S. (1973) The Adult Learner: A neglected species (1st ed). Houston, TX: Gulf Publishing Co.

Knowles, M.S. (1984) Andragogy in Action. Applying modern principles of adult education. San Francisco, CA: Jossey Bass.

Knowles, M.S. (1990) The Adult Learner: A neglected species (4th ed.). Houston, TX: Gulf Publishing Co.

Lave, J., Wenger, E. (1991) Situated Learning: Legitimate peripheral participation. Cambridge: Cambridge University Press

Lindeman, E.C. (1926) The Meaning of Adult Education (1989 ed.) Norman: University of Oklahoma.

Maslow, A.H. (1943) A theory of human motivation. Psychological Review, 50(4):370–396.

Maslow, A. (1970) Motivation and Personality (2nd ed.). New York: Harper and Row.

McCourt, C. (2006) Becoming a parent. In: Page L. (Ed.) The New Midwifery: Science and sensitivity in practice. Edinburgh: Churchill Livingstone: 49–71.

Merriam, S. (Ed.) (2001) The New Update on Adult Learning Theory: New directions for adult and continuing education. San Francisco, CA: Jossey Bass.

Merriam, S., Caffarella, R., Baumgartner, L. (2007) Learning in Adulthood. A comprehensive guide. San Francisco, CA: Jossey Bass.

Mezirow, J. (1981) A critical theory of adult learning and education. Adult Education, 32:3–24.

Nolan, M. (2020) Parent Education for the Critical 1000 Days. London: Routledge.

Paul, R., Elder, L. (1997) Foundation for Critical Thinking. Available at: www.criticalthinking.org

Wenger, E. (1998) Communities of Practice: Learning, meaning, and identity. Cambridge: Cambridge University Press.

# 27

# GROUP INTERVENTION TO TREAT FEAR OF CHILDBIRTH WITH PSYCHO-EDUCATION AND RELAXATION EXERCISES

*Riikka Airo, Terhi Saisto, and Hanna Rouhe*

Severe fear of childbirth (FOC) causes emotional suffering during pregnancy and interferes with the normal psychological growth towards childbirth and motherhood (Sydsjö et al., 2014; Veringa et al., 2016). In addition, FOC also increases the complication rate in labour, if untreated (Rouhe et al., 2013), and the risk of post-traumatic stress reactions and depression after childbirth (Räisänen et al., 2013; Söderquist et al., 2009). Pregnant women with FOC often have very negative images of and emotions about childbirth (Serçekus & Okumus, 2009). To enable more positive experiences of childbirth and the transition to parenthood, there is a need for effective ways to treat women with FOC. This chapter discusses a group intervention consisting of psycho-education with relaxation exercises, which has been shown to be an effective way to treat nulliparous women with FOC.

★

Being afraid of childbirth is natural, as childbirth per se involves most likely severe pain, loss of control, dependence on caregivers, and worry regarding the well-being of the baby. Up to 10% of women suffer from severe fear of childbirth (FOC) which manifests as anxiety, nightmares, physical complaints, difficulties in concentrating on work or on family activities during pregnancy, and a wish to have a caesarean section (Saisto & Halmesmäki, 2003; Storksen et al., 2012). Women with FOC are usually motivated to get help, because their due-date is approaching and childbirth has to be faced. Receiving treatment for FOC offers benefits to general well-being during pregnancy, increases the likelihood of a more positive childbirth experience (Rouhe et al., 2015a; Saisto et al., 2006), and facilitates better early interactions with the infant (Rouhe et al., 2015a). It is important to learn how to regulate negative emotions such as anxiety and

DOI: 10.4324/9781003223771-33

fear, as anxiety has been found to predict pain during childbirth (Carvalho et al., 2014).

There is no consensus on how, where, and by whom FOC and request for caesarean section should be treated. However, a number of studies that have explored FOC and request for caesarean have shown that with treatment, 50–85% of women can prepare themselves for vaginal delivery and caesarean by maternal request can be avoided (Rouhe, 2011). Most treatments have been based on psychological support, short-term therapy, and relaxation training. A recent study has shown promising results from internet-based treatment (Nieminen et al., 2016). Most of these studies were not randomized trials, thereby compromising their reliability.

## Group Intervention: Theory

The idea of providing treatment in a therapeutic group situation and using specific exercises to help women meet the challenges of childbirth is underpinned by various studies.

- The core factors of psychological change are therapeutic alliance, empathy, goal consensus and collaboration, positive regard and affirmation, congruence/genuineness, mentalization and emotional experience and can be achieved in short-term group treatment (Nahum et al., 2019).
- Using a psycho-educative orientation can provide information while simultaneously meeting the psychological needs of patients (Petch & Halford, 2008).
- Promoting mentalizing skills through mentalization-based discussions can increase the ability to reflect on one's own emotional states and those of others (Allen et al., 2008).
- Teaching relaxation techniques and mindfulness-based exercises can strengthen the body–mind connection and increase self-regulatory skills (Duncan, 2010).

A therapeutic group can provide a safe setting for emotional change. The decrease in FOC is possible through gaining a better capacity to regulate emotions, especially negative ones (Airo et al., 2018). Being able to share difficult emotions concerning childbirth with women who are in the same situation may decrease feelings of isolation, guilt, and shame, which are typical of women with FOC. Dealing with current emotions and thoughts in a 'here-and-now'-situation is an essential component of group therapy (Yalom & Leszcz, 2005).

Psycho-education integrates and synergizes psychotherapeutic and educational interventions. In a psycho-educational intervention, participants are supported to self-observe and create a new, more flexible relationship with their original difficulty (Lukens & McFarlane, 2004). With an improved understanding of the causes and effects of their problems, psycho-education can broaden clients' perceptions and interpretations of their problem. Women with FOC benefit from psycho-educative information on the mind–body bridge; how emotions affect the body and how the experience of pain is affected by the interpretation of sensations. Visual material showing the muscle cells during contractions, how dilatation occurs and what causes the pain of contractions, is helpful. Understanding how vaginal birth enables positive adaptation of the infant to extra-uterine life may promote empathy with the infant's situation, helping to relieve the fear of pain and making it possible to see labour pain as meaningful instead of dangerous.

## Group Intervention to Promote Mentalization

A group intervention consisting of psycho-education and relaxation exercises to treat nulliparous women with FOC was developed in Finland in 1998 (Saisto et al., 2006). The goal was to combine different approaches that had been shown to be effective in treating FOC. The intervention aims to promote participants' capacity to mentalize. Mentalizing can be defined as the ability to understand the mental states of oneself or others that underlie overt behaviour (Allen et al., 2008).

The three domains of mentalizing emotions are:

1   Identifying emotions – finding the words and labels
2   Modulating emotions – achieving the capacity to regulate emotions
3   Expressing emotions, which is predicated on the earlier steps of identifying and modulating, outwardly to others and also inwardly to oneself.

These three steps confer inner strength and flexibility, and achieving them increases the likelihood of being understood by others. Women with FOC appear to have difficulties in all of these three domains.

- Firstly, identifying their fear in detail requires moving beyond stating that they have 'an awful feeling', or 'horror of losing control' or 'don't want to give birth'.
- Secondly, modulating emotions is especially hard if fear is overwhelming. Finding meaning is key as when emotions become more meaningful, they are easier to regulate (Allen et al., 2008). Women with FOC may see childbirth as painful to no purpose. With treatment, their understanding of childbirth can be modified so that they see it as something natural, meaningful, and manageable, thereby helping them to trust their capacity to handle and regulate the sensations and pain.
- Thirdly, sharing emotions, fears, and hopes in a group situation helps women to express their feelings about and needs in relation to childbirth.

The body–mind connection is supported with relaxation and mindfulness-based exercises to increase self-regulatory skills which, in turn, increase the experience of safety during childbirth (Melender, 2002). Mindfulness may be defined as 'awareness that arises from paying attention to the present moment, non-judgmentally' (Kabat-Zinn, 2003). Through mindfulness exercises, it is possible to learn to observe sensations, pain, and emotions during childbirth. One can learn to respond (subject-position) to the pain instead of to react (object-position) to it. Mindfulness-practice provides the opportunity to relate to fear and pain in such a way that the sensory component is uncoupled from the emotional component.

Mindfulness interventions have been shown to be effective for a variety of psychological and physical conditions, including depression, anxiety, stress (Khoury et al., 2013), and chronic pain (Reiner et al., 2013). They have been shown to reduce parental stress, parental psychopathology, child psychopathology and to improve parenting and co-parenting (Bögels et al., 2014). Mindfulness interventions can reduce perinatal anxiety, depression, and the severity of labour pain (Dunn et al., 2012). Guided imagery exercises have been shown to be effective in reducing pain and stress in childbirth (Duncan, 2010).

To be effective, the group intervention needs to be delivered by professionals with psychotherapeutic and group-dynamic expertise and knowledge of pregnancy issues. The atmosphere at the group sessions has to be confidential, safe, and attentive, so that sharing difficult emotions is possible. It is as important to help participants to share emotions arising from past traumatic experiences that may be linked to the impending childbirth (such as experiences of painful procedures), as to bring them back to the actual moment and introduce new, alternative ways of reacting, in preparation for labour.

## Finnish FOC Group Intervention with Psycho-Education and Relaxation Exercises

The group intervention with psycho-education and relaxation exercises (Airo et al., 2018; Rouhe et al., 2015a; Saisto et al., 2006) consists of six group sessions during pregnancy (starting at around the 28th week) and one session with the infants 6–8 weeks after delivery. Each group consists of between six and eight nulliparous women. Sessions are led by a psychologist who specializes in group therapy and pregnancy issues. Each session lasts about two hours. The sessions are semi-structured, starting with sharing current emotions, connecting and empathizing with the infant, and sharing thoughts that came up after previous sessions. Each session has a focused topic (Table 27.1) related to childbirth and parenthood. The sessions end with a 30-minute guided relaxation/mindfulness-based exercise.

At the start of the sessions, most of the participants hope to have a caesarean birth. They are supported to leave the decision about mode of birth until after the intervention but are reassured that they will be able to have a caesarean, if they still request it following the intervention. The primary goal of the intervention

---

**GOALS FOR EACH SESSION**

(1) To create an environment of trust and security where women are able to discuss and deal with difficult emotions and fear around childbirth and parenthood
(2) To give psycho-educational information about childbirth, the stages of labour, and parenthood
(3) To normalize emotions related to childbirth and FOC
(4) To develop self-regulation skills through breathing, relaxation, and mindfulness exercises, building a bridge between emotions and bodily sensations and making it easier to recognize and to express needs during childbirth.

---

is not to support women to choose vaginal birth, but to provide a safe space in which to deal with emotions and information about childbirth and parenthood. Empathizing with the infant is encouraged throughout the group process with questions and exercises aiming to arouse curiosity about the infant's experiences. The goal of the relaxation and mindfulness exercises is to learn new ways to calm and regulate emotions and to strengthen the body–mind connection.

## Session Topics and the Mindfulness/Relaxation Exercises

Session 1. When a group of fearful pregnant women meet, the first requirement of therapeutic work is to ensure a safe and secure atmosphere and help the participants to trust each other. The leader creates this atmosphere with her calm and warm presence, while normalizing the experience of FOC. To promote feelings of safety, sharing experiences and emotions concerning pregnancy and childbirth takes place in couples or small groups. The mechanism of contraction pain in labour, and the link between emotions and experience of pain intensity, are taught using visual material and with exercises that help participants learn the difference between tension and relaxation and how to connect breathing to releasing tension.

Session 2. This session covers the stages of childbirth, which are discussed from the viewpoint of the parturient: How the different stages feel, what happens and why, and how to help and calm herself. Special attention is also paid to the infant's point of view: What is known about the physical and psychological impact of childbirth on the infant. A special audio tape developed for this group is used to guide participants through an imaginary labour, with calming and restorative suggestions and releasing tension with the out-breath.

Session 3. This session is held on the delivery ward with a midwife attending. The whole process of labour is explained in detail, and participants can ask any questions they like. Pain-relief methods and the equipment used for labour are

**TABLE 27.1** Manual for psycho-educative group therapy intervention Every session includes discussion around a focused topic (90-minutes) and 30-minute guided relaxation.

| Group session | Weeks of pregnancy | Topic | Agenda | In attendance |
|---|---|---|---|---|
| 1 | 28 | Introductions<br>Pregnancy and feelings about childbirth<br>Normalization of fear<br>Connection between fear and pain<br>Effects of relaxation | Getting to know each other<br>Building a safe environment<br>Sharing feelings about childbirth<br>Psycho-education on links between pain and emotions | Therapist |
| 2 | 29 | Stages of labour, especially psychological link between emotions and pain | Psycho-education about fear<br>Education about stages of labour<br>How to regulate emotions with breathing techniques | Therapist |
| 3 | 30 | Hospital routines<br>The birth process<br>Pain relief | Introduction by midwife who goes through the process of the birth, what happens in hospital, stages of labour, and methods of pain relief | Therapist, Midwife |
| 4 | 31 | Partner communication<br>Building a family | Strengthening the connection between parents<br>Empathizing with the emotional needs of the baby | Therapist, Partner |
|  |  |  |  | *(Continued)* |

| Group session | Weeks of pregnancy | Topic | Agenda | In attendance |
|---|---|---|---|---|
| 5 | 32 | Transition to motherhood<br>Attachment and bonding with the infant<br>Signs of postnatal depression and its treatment | Psycho-education about the time after birth<br>Sharing emotions about motherhood<br>Emotional bonding with the infant | Therapist |
| 6 | 33 | Final preparations for labour<br>Childbirth wishes addressed to the midwife | Getting prepared for delivery<br>Obtaining support<br>Encountering setbacks | Therapist |
| 7 | 6–8 weeks after delivery | Delivery experiences<br>Mother–infant relationship and positive parenthood | Information about motherhood<br>Introduction of infants<br>Sharing the birth stories<br>Summarizing the group experience<br>Discussion of the joys and difficulties of being a mother<br>Building feelings of being good enough mothers<br>Information on how to get help if needed<br>What messages would this group send to the next group? | Therapist, Babies |

explained in detail. The delivery ward environment arouses a lot of tension; thus, a short body-scan mindfulness exercise is essential.

Session 4. The topic for this session is becoming a family and the women are accompanied by their partners. Couples discuss with each other and in the larger group their hopes and fears about labour and birth and also about impending parenthood and their relationship as parents. The viewpoint of the infant is explored with an exercise highlighting her/his psychological and emotional needs from the parents. The session ends with an exercise in which couples synchronize their breathing to strengthen the bond between them so that partners have a strategy for helping the labouring woman to calm her emotions.

Session 5. The topic is the psychological process of transition to motherhood and life after childbirth. Participants are asked to bring something they have acquired for their infant and talk about it. Psycho-educative information about the importance of early interaction and attachment is presented and discussed. Ways to promote secure attachment and bonding with the infant are highlighted. Prevention, signs, and treatment of postnatal depression are introduced.

Session 6. The last antenatal session is about expressing emotions and needs during labour and birth. Participants fill in a form, a 'letter' to the midwife about their thoughts and wishes for childbirth. The letters are shared with the group and discussed to practise expressing emotions, wishes, and needs. Participants are guided through an imaginary trip to the future in which they hold their newborn in their arms. They send a message from this imaginary-future with their infant to their pregnant selves. As they invoke all their senses as they imagine holding their infant, typical messages are: 'You will do fine'; 'Everything will work out'; and 'Your baby is worth everything you have been through'.

Session 7. The group meets again with their infants aged 6–8 weeks. Their childbirth stories, varying from the very positive to the traumatic, are shared in detail. Participants give and receive support from each other. The infants are introduced and their physical and emotional features discussed. If a need for further psychological assistance is obvious, follow-up is available. (For summary of sessions, see Table 27.1.)

## Benefits of Group Intervention for FOC

To demonstrate the benefits of group intervention to treat FOC, our randomized study and an earlier study are discussed here. The extra costs due to group psycho-education during the antenatal period were more than compensated for by reduced delivery costs (Rouhe et al., 2015b).

In the study by Saisto et al. (2006), nulliparous women (n = 102) referred because of FOC (most of them requesting caesarean section) were invited to participate in a group intervention with psycho-education and relaxation exercises between 1998 and 2002. Women who attended the group intervention were compared to women (n = 85) who had been referred for FOC just before the group psycho-education intervention was developed. These women had met a midwife or obstetrician for guidance on one to three occasions. Participants in the group intervention chose vaginal birth more often than women who had conventional treatment for FOC (82% vs. 67%; p = 0.02). Women participating in the group psycho-education intervention were more satisfied with their childbirth experience; their labours were shorter, and they also had fewer interventions and fewer emergency caesareans than the average primiparous woman birthing at the hospital.

In the study by Rouhe et al. (2013), 4,575 women were screened for FOC using the Wijma Delivery Expectancy Questionnaire (W-DEQ). Women with W-DEQ sum score ≥ 100 (n = 371, 8% of the screened nulliparous women) were randomized in proportion 1:2 into the intervention group (n = 131) and the control group (n = 240). Of those in the control group, 76 women were later referred to special maternity care because of FOC and 30 attended focused childbirth preparation classes. Women who participated in the group intervention chose trial of vaginal birth more often than the women who were treated in the special maternity care unit because of their FOC (88% vs. 65%; p = 0.002). They also achieved a vaginal delivery more often, with the rate of emergency caesarean and vacuum extraction being higher in the control group. The incidence of haemorrhage was significantly higher in the control group than in the intervention group.

Experience of childbirth was measured in two ways, using the Wijma Delivery Experience Questionnaire B which is a postnatal version of W-DEQ and the Delivery Satisfaction Scale (DSS). The intervention group women had a less fearful childbirth experience compared to the women in the control group (W-DEQ B sum score 63 vs. 74; p = 0.016), and this difference was seen across all delivery modes. More women in the intervention group had a very positive experience of delivery, measured by the DSS, compared with control women (36% vs. 23%; p = 0.04) (Rouhe et al., 2013).

## Psychological Benefits

In our study (Rouhe et al., 2015a), maternal adjustment was measured using the Maternal Attitudes and Attachment (MAMA) scale. Women in the intervention group showed better adjustment three months after childbirth compared to women in the control group (MAMA sum score 38.1 vs. 35.7; p = 0.001). Depressive symptoms were measured using the Edinburgh Postnatal Depression Scale (EPDS). There were fewer postnatal depressive symptoms in the intervention group compared to the control group (EPDS mean sum score 6.4 vs. 8.0; p = 0.02).

## Conclusion

Group intervention with psycho-education and relaxation exercises has proven to be an effective treatment for nulliparous women with FOC, offering a safe setting to explore the difficult and often contradictory emotions concerning the impending labour and birth.

Group intervention for FOC does not only affect delivery mode, it also improves the experience of childbirth and maternal adjustment, promotes the transition to parenthood, and diminishes the risk of postnatal depression. Based on our results, the group intervention protocol has been used in clinical practice in Helsinki and the Southern District of Finland, which together are responsible for a third of births in Finland. All nulliparous women referred with FOC to special maternity care are recommended to participate in the group intervention. Our research and clinical experience in treating nulliparous women with FOC using the psycho-educative group intervention with mindfulness and relaxation exercises lead us to believe that the intervention would be useful in other Western countries.

## Practice Pointers

- Group intervention improves the experience of childbirth and maternal adjustment, promotes the transition to parenthood, and diminishes the risk of postnatal depression.
- A therapeutic group can provide a safe setting for emotional change.
- The leader of the group has to have knowledge in group dynamics, psychotherapy, and basics of physiology of pregnancy and childbirth.
- The decrease in FOC is possible through gaining a better capacity to regulate emotions, especially negative emotions.

## References

Airo, R., Korja, R., Saisto, T., Rouhe, H., Muotka, J. et al. (2018) Changes in emotions and personal goals in primiparous pregnant women during group intervention for fear of childbirth. Journal of Reproductive and Infant Psychology, 36(4):363–380.

Allen J.G., Fonagy P., Bateman A.W. (2008) Mentalizing in Clinical Practice. Washington, DC: American Psychiatric Publishing Inc.

Bögels, S.M., Hellemans, J., van Deursen, S., Römer, M., van der Meulen, R. (2014) Mindful parenting in mental health care: Effects on parental and child psychopathology, parental stress, parenting, coparenting, and marital functioning. Mindfulness, 5(5):536–551.

Carvalho, B., Zheng, M., Aiono-Le Tagaloa, L. (2014) Evaluation of experimental pain tests to predict labour pain and epidural analgesic consumption. Survey of Anesthesiology, 58(2):75–76.

Duncan, L.G., Bardacke N. (2010) Mindfulness-based childbirth and parenting education: Promoting family mindfulness during the perinatal period. Journal of Child and Family Studies, 19(2):190–202.

Dunn, C., Hanieh, E., Roberts, R., Powrie, R. (2012) Mindful pregnancy and childbirth: Effects of a mindfulness-based intervention on women's psychological distress and well-being in the perinatal period. Archives of Women's Mental Health, 15(2):139–143.

Kabat-Zinn, J. (2003) Mindfulness-based interventions in context: Past, present, and future. Clinical Psychology: Science and Practice, 10(2):144–156.

Khoury, B., Lecomte, T., Fortin, G., Masse, M., Therien, P. et al. (2013) Mindfulness-based therapy: A comprehensive meta-analysis. Clinical Psychology Review, 33(6):763–771.

Lukens, E.P., McFarlane, W.R. (2004) Psycho-education as evidence-based practice: Considerations for practice, research, and policy. Brief Treatment and Crisis Intervention, 4(3):205.

Melender, H. (2002) Fears and coping strategies associated with pregnancy and childbirth in Finland. Journal of Midwifery & Women's Health, 47(4):256–263.

Nahum, D., Alfonso, C. A., Sönmez, E. (2019) Common factors in psychotherapy. In: Javed, A., Fountoulakis, K.N. (Eds.) Advances in Psychiatry. New York: Springer: 471–481.

Nieminen, K., Andersson, G., Wijma, B., Ryding, E., Wijma K. (2016) Treatment of nulliparous women with severe fear of childbirth via the internet: A feasibility study. Journal of Psychosomatic Obstetrics & Gynecology, 37(2):37–43.

Petch, J., Halford, W.K. (2008) Psycho-education to enhance couples' transition to parenthood. Clinical Psychology Review, 28(7):1125–1137.

Räisänen, S., Lehto, S.M., Nielsen, H.S., Gissler, M., Kramer M.R. et al. (2013) Fear of childbirth predicts postpartum depression: A population-based analysis of 511 422 singleton births in Finland. British Medical Journal Open, 3(11):e004047-2013-004047.

Reiner, K., Tibi, L., Lipsitz J.D. (2013) Do mindfulness-based interventions reduce pain intensity? A critical review of the literature. Pain Medicine, 14(2):230–242.

Rouhe H. (2011) Should women be able to request a caesarean section? No. British Medical Journal, 343:d7565.

Rouhe, H., Salmela-Aro, K., Toivanen, R., Tokola, M., Halmesmäki, E. et al. (2013) Obstetric outcome after intervention for severe fear of childbirth in nulliparous women – Randomised trial. British Journal of Obstetrics & Gynaecology, 120(1):75–84.

Rouhe, H., Salmela-Aro, K., Toivanen, R., Tokola, M., Halmesmäki, E. et al. (2015a) Group psycho-education with relaxation for severe fear of childbirth improves maternal adjustment and childbirth experience – A randomised controlled trial. Journal of Psychosomatic Obstetrics & Gynecology, 36(1):1–9.

Rouhe, H., Salmela-Aro, K., Toivanen, R., Tokola, M., Halmesmäki, E. et al. (2015b) Life satisfaction, general well-being and costs of treatment for severe fear of childbirth in nulliparous women by psychoeducative group or conventional care attendance. Acta Obstetricia et Gynecologica Scandinavica, 94(5):527–533.

Saisto, T., Halmesmäki, E. (2003) Fear of childbirth: A neglected dilemma. Acta Obstetricia et Gynecologica Scandinavica, 82(3):201–208.

Saisto, T., Toivanen, R., Salmela-Aro, K., Halmesmäki, E. (2006) Therapeutic group psycho-education and relaxation in treating fear of childbirth. Acta Obstetricia et Gynecologica Scandinavica, 85(11):1315–1319.

Serçekus, P., Okumus, H. (2009) Fears associated with childbirth among nulliparous women in Turkey. Midwifery, 25(2):155–162.

Söderquist, J., Wijma, B., Thorbert, G., Wijma, K. (2009) Risk factors in pregnancy for post-traumatic stress and depression after childbirth. British Journal of Obstetrics & Gynaecology, 116(5):672–680.

Storksen, H.T., Eberhard-Gran, M., Garthus-Niegel, S., Eskild, A. (2012) Fear of childbirth: The relation to anxiety and depression. Acta Obstetricia et Gynecologica Scandinavica, 91(2):237–242.

Sydsjö, G., Bladh, M., Lilliecreutz, C., Persson, A.M., Vyöni, H. et al. (2014) Obstetric outcomes for nulliparous women who received routine individualized treatment for severe fear of childbirth - A retrospective case control study. BMC Pregnancy and Childbirth, 14:article no.:126.

Veringa, I.K., de Bruin, E.I., Bardacke, N., Duncan, L.G., van Steensel, F.J. et al. (2016) 'I've changed my mind.' Mindfulness-based childbirth and parenting (MBCP) for pregnant women with a high level of fear of childbirth and their partners: Study protocol of the quasi-experimental controlled trial. BMC Psychiatry, 16(1):377.

Yalom, I.D., Leszcz, M. (2005) Theory and Practice of Group Psychotherapy. New York: Basic Books.

# 28

# COMMENTARY

## Parenting Programmes Are Not Culturally Relevant to Many Communities

*Hanan Hussein, Kathryn Thomson and Kathleen Roche-Nagi*

Participating in group parenting programmes can result in a range of benefits, including helping relieve parental stress and anxiety (Barlow et al., 2002), targeting early child conduct problems (Borden et al., 2010) and improving family relations (Sanders, 2008).

### The Importance of Culturally Appropriate Interventions

Bornstein (2013) describes culture as 'a set of distinctive patterns of beliefs and behaviour that are shared by a group of people and that serve to regulate their daily living' and argues that culture therefore shapes parenting practices, with noted differences, for example, in the parenting of traditionally collectivist vs. individualistic societies.

As most universal family prevention programmes have been researched within Western countries, their applicability to all cultural groups has been questioned (Kumpfer et al., 2002). Prior research has concluded that people from minority backgrounds are under-served due to parenting programmes being inaccessible and not culturally relevant, with poorer outcomes than for families from other socio-cultural groups (Dumas et al., 2011; Short & Johnston, 1994). Parenting programmes lacking cultural adaptation risk high attrition and poor engagement of parents from ethnic minority groups (Barlow, 1999; Davis et al., 2012). Short and Johnston (1994) identify the main participation barriers as language issues, fear of stigmatisation, and lack of culturally compatible content owing to differences in child-rearing practices and values.

### Adapting Parenting Programmes

Efforts have been made to adapt parenting programmes for different cultural backgrounds. For example, the 'Strengthening Families' programme is a US

DOI: 10.4324/9781003223771-34

family skills training programme designed for preventing drug use that has been culturally adapted for African American, Hispanic, Asian, Pacific Islander and Indian American families, with successful outcomes (Kumpfer et al., 2008). However, research into relevant evidence-based programmes has not kept pace with the greater diversity within society (Castro et al., 2010).

Interventions adapted for specific cultural groups may have fidelity issues and cost implications (Castro et al., 2010). Webster-Stratton (2009) argues that using core programmes, with facilitators trained in culturally sensitive practices to improve outcomes for ethnic minorities, off-sets costs and manages fidelity. Morawska et al. (2011) found that the core principles of the Triple P programme (Sanders et al., 2003) were acceptable to a group of culturally diverse parents, although practical considerations hindered attendance. As for fidelity, poorer outcomes are found if key skills within a programme are omitted when making cultural adaptations; therefore, identifying and retaining these components appears important (Kumpfer et al., 2008).

The adapted programmes' efficacy depends on the degree of adaptation carried out. Surface-level adaptations relate to feasibility, such as changing the language of the programme or location. Deep structural adaptations determine the impact of an intervention by ensuring it fits a specific culture through incorporating important cultural values (Resnicow et al., 2000). In a meta-analysis, van Mourik et al. (2017) found that deep structural adaptations were most effective in improving parenting in programmes for ethnic minority parents. However, Schilling et al. (2021) recently critiqued the literature around culturally adapted parenting programmes and noted that only half of studies had a control group. They concluded that more studies need to specify the adaptations made before the most effective level of adaptation can be ascertained.

## Co-Producing a New Programme

Creating a new programme for a specific population is an alternative to adapting an existing evidence-based programme; this potentially overcomes the fidelity and fit problem that culturally adapted programmes may experience. Becher and Hussain (2003) state that the needs of parents from ethnic minorities should be built into an original programme, rather than added on once developed. This is supported by the British Psychological Society which encourages co-production by involving ethnic minority families in the creation of parenting programmes (Davis et al., 2012). Co-production gives ownership of the programme to the community and enhances its meaning, thereby yielding stronger results (Wainberg et al., 2007; Wingood & DiClemente, 2008). It may also be hypothesised that such programmes will draw on the 'deeper' values described by Resnicow et al. (2000) forming a mechanism for change.

Muslim parents have traditionally been hard to reach and retain in universal parenting programmes. This led Approachable Parenting, a social enterprise providing parenting courses and parent-coaching to Muslim families, to develop the '5 Pillars of Parenting' programme. Initial data from the programme for parents of 4- to 11-year olds shows improvements in child behaviour, parenting style and parental mental health (Thomson et al., 2018). The importance of valuing religious beliefs alongside cultural considerations in parenting programmes has also been noted by the Family Links parenting course (Scourfield & Nasiruddin, 2015).

## Conclusion

As Lau (2006) states, benefits of cultural adaptation of parent education programmes include greater effectiveness and providing insights into adaptations that may also benefit other minority groups. It is hugely important to consider the underlying values of a community, alongside proven psychological parenting principles, when creating or adapting parent education programmes to ensure their acceptability and good outcomes.

## References

Barlow, J. (1999) Systematic Review of the Effectiveness of Parent-Training Programmes in Improving Behaviour Problems. Oxford: Health Services Research Unit.

Barlow, J., Coren, E., Stewart-Brown, S. (2002) Meta-analysis of the effectiveness of parenting programmes in improving maternal psychosocial health. British Journal of General Practice, 52(476):223–233.

Becher, H., Hussain, F. (2003) Supporting Minority Ethnic Families - South Asian Hindus and Muslims in Britain: Developments in family support. London: National Family and Parenting Institute.

Borden, L.A., Schultz, T.R., Herman, K.C., Brooks, C.M. (2010) The Incredible Years parent training program: Promoting resilience through evidence-based groups. Group Dynamics: Theory, Research and Practice, 14(3):230–241.

Bornstein, M. (2013) Cultural approaches to parenting. Parenting Science and Practice, 12(2–3):212–221.

Castro, F., Barrera, M., Steiker, L. (2010) Issues and challenges in the design of culturally adapted evidence based interventions. Annual Review of Clinical Psychology, 6:213–239.

Davis, F.A., McDonald, L., Axford, N. (2012). Technique Is Not Enough: A framework for ensuring that evidence-based parenting programmes are socially inclusive. Leicester: The British Psychological Society.

Dumas, J.E., Arriaga, X.B., Begle, A.M., Longoria, Z.N. (2011) Child and parental outcomes of a group parenting intervention for Latino families: A pilot study of the CANNE program. Cultural Diversity and Ethnic Minority Psychology, 17(1):107–115.

Kumpfer, K.L., Alvarado, R., Smith, P., Bellamy, N. (2002) Cultural sensitivity and adaptations in family-based prevention interventions. Prevention Science, 3(3):241–246.

Kumpfer, K., Pinyuchon, M., Whiteside, H.O., de Melo, A.T. (2008) Cultural adaptation process for international dissemination of the Strengthening Families program. Evaluation and the Health Professions, 31(2):226–239.

Lau, A. (2006) Making the case for selective and directed cultural adaptations of evidence based treatments: Examples from parent training. Clinical Psychology Science and Practice, 13(4):295–310.

Morawska, A., Sanders, M., Goadby, E., Headley, C., Hodge et al. (2011) Is the Triple P-Positive Parenting Programme acceptable to parents from culturally diverse backgrounds? Journal of Child and Family Studies, 20:614–622.

Resnicow, K., Soler, R., Braithwaite, R.L. (2000) Cultural sensitivity in substance use prevention. Journal of Community Psychology, 28(3):271–290.

Sanders, M.R. (2008) Triple P-Positive Parenting Program as a public health approach to strengthening parenting. Journal of Family Psychology, 22(4), 506–517.

Sanders, M.R., Cann, W., Markie-Dadds, C. (2003) The Triple P – Positive Parenting Programme: A universal population-level approach to the prevention of child abuse. Child Abuse Review, 12(3):155–171.

Schilling, S., Mebane, A., Perreira, K.M. (2021) Cultural adaptation of group parenting programs: Review of the literature and recommendations for best practice. Family Process. doi:10.1111/famp.12658

Scourfield, J., Nasiruddin, Q. (2015) Religious adaptation of a parenting programme: Process evaluation of the Family Links Islamic Values course for Muslim fathers. Child: Care, Health and Development, 41(5):697–703.

Short, K., Johnston, C. (1994) Ethnocultural parent education in Canada: Current status and directions. Canadian Journal of Community Mental Health, 13:43–54.

Thomson, K., Hussein, H., Roche-Nagi, K., Butterworth, R. (2018) Evaluating the impact of the 5 Pillars of Parenting programme: A novel parenting intervention for Muslim families. Community Practitioner, 91(2):45–47.

van Mourik, K., Crone, M.R., de Wolff, M.S., Reis, R. (2017) Parent training programs for ethnic minorities: A meta-analysis of adaptations and effect. Prevention Science, 18(1):95–105.

Wainberg, M. L., Alfredo González, M., McKinnon, K., Elkington, K. S., Pinto, D. et al. (2007) Targeted ethnography as a critical step to inform cultural adaptations of HIV preventions for adults with severe mental illness. Social Science and Medicine, 65:296–308.

Webster-Stratton, C. (2009) Affirming diversity: Multi-cultural collaboration to deliver the Incredible Years parent programme. International Journal of Child Health and Human Development, 2(1):17–32.

Wingood, G.M., DiClemente, R.J. (2008) The ADAPT-ITT model: A novel method of adapting evidence-based HIV interventions. Journal of Acquired Immune Deficiency Syndrome, 47(1):S40–S46.

# 29

# APPROACHABLE PARENTING

## The Five Pillars of Parenting Pregnancy and Beyond Programme for Muslim Families

*Kathleen Roche-Nagi and Yasmin Shikara*

Approachable Parenting is a UK-registered not-for-profit Community Interest Company that provides parent education courses and coaching mainly to Muslim families. Its inspiration came from Muslim families who wanted help with parenting issues from an organisation that understood them and their faith, beliefs and culture. However, Approachable Parenting works with parents from all backgrounds, offering support to people from many different cultures and faiths and to those of no faith. It has been delivering parenting programmes since 2007, with a range of programmes from pregnancy to the teenage years. This chapter looks specifically at its Pregnancy and Beyond programme.

*

The Five Pillars of Parenting suite of programmes was written by Muslim clinical psychologists and parenting experts. They integrate psychological models based on attachment, bonding and attunement within an Islamic framework that respects the attitudes of Muslim families and understands their motivation as Muslim parents. The Five Pillars which scaffold all Approachable Parenting's programmes are:

- Character: Identifying the importance of good character, morals, personality and behaviour
- Knowledge: Learning new skills
- Action: Putting learning into practice to achieve results
- Steadfastness: Commitment to overcoming difficulties in parenting
- Relationships: Strengthening family bonds and creating lasting positive relationships through improved parenting.

DOI: 10.4324/9781003223771-35

## The Pregnancy and Beyond Programme

The Five Pillars of Parenting Pregnancy and Beyond programme is delivered in two-hour sessions, over four weeks in an antenatal clinic or community setting and is always facilitated by two trainers. Parents are invited from 16 weeks' gestation onwards. Groups comprise of between 8 and 16 parents. Although the programme was developed with Muslim parents in mind, it has attracted many parents from other 'seldom heard communities'.

The Pregnancy and Beyond programme aims to help parents raise their children in a loving and supportive environment. It enables parents to understand the importance of developing a good relationship with their child from pregnancy onwards and introduces the concepts of bonding, attachment and attunement. The programme also explores changes in family relationships when a baby arrives, parental mental health and the importance of looking after oneself.

Engaging fathers in parenting programmes is an ongoing challenge. Approachable Parenting has been proactive in promoting the importance of a father's role, in keeping with the Islamic faith, and there is increasing demand from fathers for the 4 to 11 years parenting programme and the teenage programme. In the Pregnancy and Beyond programme, we make explicit reference to the ways in which fathers can bond and foster a secure attachment with their child.

## The Faith Base of the Birth and Beyond Programme

Religious references support psychological concepts which enables parents to understand theories that underpin the Birth and Beyond programme. Reference is made to verses from the holy book of Islam, the Quran, and to Hadith which is a record of the traditions or sayings of the Prophet Muhammad.

In the course of the programme, various Islamic concepts are discussed, including 'Adab' – having good manners and conducting oneself in the correct way – and 'Akhlaq' – being of good character and interacting appropriately with others:

'And verily, you (O Mohammed) are of an exalted standard of character' (Quran 68:4).

Group discussions tend to be varied according to the attendees. Muslim parents are often keen to discuss the spiritual development of the foetus, rights and responsibilities and the importance of intentions alongside actions. Every good intention is rewarded: 'Verily deeds are by their intentions' (40 Hadeeth).

Parents reflect on their intention, their responsibilities and what they want to gain from the programme. They develop techniques and skills to enable them to be better parents. Raising children is considered a trust and a form of worship, which places responsibilities upon them. These responsibilities are balanced by the status and rewards given to parents when they raise righteous children: 'And know that your possessions and your children are but a trial and that surely with Allah is a mighty reward' (Quran 8:28).

## Approachable Parenting Trainers

It is important that trainers delivering Approachable Parenting programmes are from the Muslim faith so that they are able to establish trusting relationships with parents and facilitate more open discussions about parenting concepts. Our partners from Children's Centres and other services also feel this shared faith experience is important to the fidelity of the programme.

To become an Approachable Parenting trainer, individuals need to have suitable knowledge and skills from a psychological or family support background. Trainers undergo a four-day in-house training followed by assignments and compiling a portfolio to gain the Award in Education and Training. They then deliver Approachable Parenting programmes alongside a senior trainer before gaining their licence to practise.

Community languages such as Urdu, Bengali and Arabic are spoken by trainers enabling them to explain concepts to parents in their own languages.

---

### BOX 29.1 – EVALUATION

Approachable Parenting gathers and publishes qualitative and quantitative evaluations (see Thomson et al., 2018). Parents complete a series of questionnaires pre and post the programme. These have shown an improvement in spousal relationships, in the security of attachment between parents and their babies and improved mental health and wellbeing.

#### PARENTS' FEEDBACK: PREGNANCY AND BEYOND PROGRAMME

- Helped me to understand what is expected of me as a parent and how to communicate with my baby
- Will communicate with husband to discuss family values, how to implement them, have more fun and play with my baby
- Learning about ways to bond with baby, learning the importance of play
- Every aspect of the course was most beneficial and I learnt so many new techniques and key skills to make the journey to motherhood easier.

---

### Respecting Different Models of Parenting

Research informs us that pregnancy and the early years of life have a huge impact on babies' development. Pregnancy is a critical 'window of opportunity' when many parents are receptive to advice and support. Sanders et al. (2003) observe that parenting interventions should be tailored in such a way as to respect and not undermine the cultural values, aspirations, traditions and needs of different ethnic groups. Approachable Parenting's Five Pillars of Parenting programmes demonstrate respect for models of parenting within different cultures, while at the same time recognising the commonalities shared by parents within the Islamic faith.

## Practice Pointers

* Create connections to help parents feel respected, valued and understood by using community settings and workers from community backgrounds.
* Make course materials relevant to parents, through the inclusion of cultural and religious themes in parenting that parents are able to relate to.

## References

Sanders, M.R., Cann. W., Markie-Dadds, C. (2003) The Triple P-Positive Parenting Programme: A universal population-level approach to the prevention of child abuse. Child Abuse Review, 12(3):155–171.

Thomson, K., Hussein, H., Roche-Nagi, K., Butterworth, R. (2018) Evaluating the impact of the 5 Pillars of Parenting programme: A novel parenting intervention for Muslim families. Community Practitioner, 91(2):45–47.

# 30

# HETERONORMATIVE OBSTACLES IN REGULAR ANTENATAL EDUCATION, AND THE BENEFITS OF LGBTQ-CERTIFIED OPTIONS

## Experiences among Prospective LGBTQ Parents in Sweden

*Anna Malmquist and Sofia Klittmark*

Prospective parents in Sweden are offered antenatal education led by midwives. The composition of some classes is based on the family situation, and some LGBTQ prospective parents are offered separate classes. People who attend such separate classes are generally highly satisfied with the programme. They emphasize that they feel comfortable and find the discussed topics relevant to them. On the contrary, LGBTQ people who attend regular antenatal education reflect on hetero- and cis-normativity in the education, where midwives focus on stereotypic gender roles. In particular, non-pregnant mothers and pregnant transmasculine people feel excluded.

*

Prospective parents in Sweden are offered antenatal education free of charge in public or private healthcare, and the classes are led by midwives (Pålsson et al., 2019). The education generally focuses on giving birth, pain relief and lactation. Other topics concern how life changes once the child is born and what the participants expect of their upcoming roles as parents. Antenatal education is typically attended during the last trimester of the first pregnancy. Some classes are oriented to participants in specific family situations, e.g. to young parents or single mothers. Some classes have been offered specifically to lesbian, gay, bisexual, transgender and queer (LGBTQ) prospective parents. A private antenatal clinic (Mama Mia) in Stockholm has for the past two decades offered separate antenatal education classes for this group, and during the past two years, RFSL (The Swedish Federation for Lesbian, Gay, Bisexual, Transgender, Queer and Intersex Rights) has held antenatal parental preparation groups, both online and as physical meetings (RFSL, 2021).

DOI: 10.4324/9781003223771-36

Childbearing opportunities for LGBTQ people in Sweden have increased in the past decades. Female same-sex couples have had access to fertility treatment in public healthcare since 2005, and both parents are registered as the child's legal parents (Malmquist, 2015). Fertility treatment has been accessible for transgender men since 2013 and for singles with a childbearing capacity since 2016. With an increasing number of expecting LGBTQ people, their experiences of antenatal care in Sweden have been discussed in several previous studies (for an overview, see Wells & Lang, 2016). These studies describe how staff and routines at antenatal clinics are experienced as respectful and competent by some people, yet as prejudicial and condescending by others. Pregnant transmasculine people are, in particular, exposed to ignorance and prejudice (Falck et al., 2021). LGBTQ people who suffer from fear of childbirth are also particularly vulnerable (Malmquist et al., 2019).

Experiences of antenatal education are highlighted in some previous studies. Lesbian parents often experience antenatal class leaders as non-inclusive, and classes as being generally oriented towards heterosexual participants (Klittmark et al., 2019; Larsson & Dykes, 2009). Non-birth mothers are put in awkward situations when the groups are divided into gendered subgroups, in that they neither belong to the group of pregnant mothers nor the fathers' group (Dahl & Malterud, 2015). In addition, pregnant transmasculine people generally feel excluded when pregnant persons are referred to as 'mothers' (Malmquist et al., 2019).

The present chapter draws on two different data sets. The first is a study of Swedish female same-sex couples' parenting experiences, with their reflections on antenatal education being the focus in this chapter. The interviews were conducted in 2009–2010 with 96 mothers in 51 families, each couple raising children conceived in a same-sex relationship (for more details about the study, see Malmquist, 2015). All participants resided in southern and central Sweden, and a large minority (23 families) lived in the Stockholm region. At the time of the interviews, an LGBTQ-certified antenatal clinic was accessible in Stockholm, but no such options existed in other parts of Sweden. Accordingly, most of the Stockholm-based parents had attended the LGBTQ-certified clinic, while parents from other parts of Sweden had attended their local regular antenatal clinics.

The second data set summarizes participants' experiences from RFSL's midwifery-led parental preparation groups. Objectives for these groups were to create a community for continued contact between LGBTQ parents and offer a non-heteronormative space where the prospective parents could exchange experiences. Further, the groups aimed to strengthen and support the prospective parents and offer LGBTQ-competent and norm-conscious information. In total, 188 self-identified LGBTQ people from 97 families participated in the groups in 2019–2021 (for more details on the programme, see RFSL, 2021). Each group consisted of about five families who met on four occasions. Parents from all over Sweden participated, but a majority resided in larger cities.

Nine families had at least one parent with trans experience. Most families were two-parent constellations: 79 same-sex mothers, four same-sex fathers and six parent couples were of different sex and/or trans. Eight families consisted of single parents or three-parent families, half of them with trans experience. In total, 20 groups were arranged. Most meeting were held on digital platforms due to the COVID-19 pandemic. The participants were offered this participation in addition to the antenatal education offered at their regular antenatal unit.

In the following, participant experiences of regular antenatal care will be described, followed by experiences of LGBTQ-certified options.

## Hetero- and Cis-Normativity in Regular Antenatal Education

When describing their encounters with antenatal clinics during pregnancy, most participants stated that they had been met with care and positive attitudes. They emphasized the warmth in midwives' treatment and claimed that they had not been discriminated against. Despite the overall positive descriptions, several also discussed deficiencies in their treatment, where professionals' lack of knowledge about LGBTQ families and the primacy of hetero- and cis-normative routines affected them negatively. Hetero- and cis-normative deficiencies were particularly present in the participants' descriptions of antenatal education. Three themes summarize the participants' reflections on regular antenatal education: 'Irrelevant gender stereotypes', 'Non-pregnant mothers and pregnant fathers are overlooked' and 'Adjustments for the LGBTQ couple'.

## Irrelevant Gender Stereotypes

Participants who attended regular antenatal education were generally the only LGBTQ couple in the class. They claimed that the topics brought up for discussion lacked relevance to their social situation. Ida described how heteronormative gender stereotypes were the midwives' point of departure in the group discussions:

> They start from the idea that having a child is a fundamentally different experience for women compared to men. You see, it's this basic idea that makes the healthcare system bad at this – because the woman is acknowledged in one way and the man in another. [...] And when another woman is involved – then all that collapses.

Ida described a heteronormative framing that did not suit her and her partner as two women. The course leader expected men and women to share household tasks in accordance with traditional gender roles, but such stereotypes did not apply to Ida and her partner. When topics are not adjusted to the LGBTQ participants, there is a risk that the discussion becomes irrelevant and excluding. Ida and her partner decided to stay in the class despite these deficiencies, but another lesbian couple, Vanja and Stine, skipped antenatal education because they assumed the discussions would not be relevant to them.

TANJA: We sensed that it was, that it didn't suit us, there was lots of hetero talk and...

STINE: Anyway, we felt that that's what it would be all about.

According to Tanja and Stine, their assumption that antenatal education would focus on 'hetero talk' was enough for them to decide not to attend. The birth mother, Stine, was a physician and felt well prepared for the delivery, based on her previous knowledge. Tanja, on the other hand, described the delivery as a shocking experience for her and stated that she would have benefitted from being more prepared.

## Non-Pregnant Mothers and Pregnant Fathers Are Overlooked

While the excerpts above highlight a risk that antenatal education will exclude both mothers in a lesbian couple, several participants pointed out that it is mainly the non-birth mothers who are overlooked. They described how midwives labelled the non-pregnant partners as 'fathers', despite the lesbian couple's presence in the group. The non-birth mothers were also excluded when the class was divided into gendered subgroups. Non-birth mother, Elsa, described her experience:

'But wait: where should I be, am I Mum or Dad?'... I just joked about it sort of [...] I thought it was a bit, the second time when she still divided us into 'mums' and 'dads', then I think, really she hadn't advanced very much.

As a non-birth mother, Elsa had to explicitly highlight her presence to become visible, in this case by using humour, when she asked whether she counted as a mum or a dad. Despite pointing out the problem, Elsa described how the midwife continued to divide the parents into gender-based subgroups.

Similarly, for pregnant transmasculine people, the labelling of pregnant people as 'mothers' is excluding. Ture, a pregnant father, reflected on his experiences:

The antenatal class leader was, in my opinion, trans-excluding. [...] I tried to explain, like, 'Well, you know everyone who has a child is not a woman' and explained like, 'We do not force sterilizations on transgender people any longer – you can be pregnant'. She didn't get it at all.

Because of the class leader's ignorance, Ture had felt urged to educate her about transmasculine people's reproductive opportunities.

## Adjustments for LGBTQ Participants

Some participants described how midwives had adjusted the education in an effort to be inclusive to the LGBTQ couple in the class. Ida explained how the midwife had addressed the non-pregnant parents as 'Dads, and then you', referring to her as the non-birth mother. She said that this explicit focus on her had felt uncomfortable. Another couple, Ellen and Jessica, were happier about the adjustment made in their class:

ELLEN: In the [antenatal] parent group, they changed and stopped saying, 'Dad, dad' all the time.
JESSICA: Right, they started the first time we were there – they started with saying 'Dad', but then...
ELLEN: Then they changed to 'Parent'... for our sake.

Ellen and Jessica appreciated the change from 'dad' to 'parent', as this had included both partners.

## Separate Antenatal Education for LGBTQ People

As mentioned previously, several participants had attended separate antenatal classes for prospective LGBTQ parents, either at an LGBTQ-certified antenatal clinic in Stockholm or in RFSL's antenatal groups. Three themes summarize the participants' reflections on attending such classes: 'Feeling comfortable', 'Discussing relevant topics' and 'Any class would be fine'.

## Feeling Comfortable

Several participants emphasized how attending an LGBTQ-certified maternity clinic, antenatal education, or delivery ward had made them comfortable. Birth mother, Inger, depicted the programme she attended as a 'luxury' and reflected on its benefits:

It was so natural then that, you know, they treated us like a couple, no problems and no questioning.

One major benefit of LGBTQ-oriented antenatal units is that they signal to parents that they will meet well-informed and competent caregivers. Knowing in advance that they will not be discriminated against enables the parents to feel safe. Inger pointed out that other clinics may also treat LGBTQ people well, but attending a certified clinic had felt like an insurance that they would not have to fear deficient treatment.

## Discussing Relevant Topics

Another benefit of the separate LGBTQ antenatal education classes is the opportunity to discuss topics of specific relevance to prospective LGBTQ parents. One participant, Ellinor, had appreciated the discussion about minority stress in her antenatal class:

> Minority stress is an interesting and important concept. I have probably felt this, in general, about being a lesbian and having a girlfriend. I think there will be a risk of more minority stress when the child is born.

For Ellinor, expectancies of future minority stress as same-sex parents had been an important topic to reflect on with the other participants. Further, many participants appreciated the opportunity to discuss their expectations of becoming a non-normative family, including specific experiences as the non-genetic and/or non-pregnant parent. To discuss their relationship with their families of origin and their attitudes to the LGBTQ family formation had also been important for some participants. Other topics of relevance were about having a donor-conceived child and concerns about future meetings with authorities, child healthcare and preschool.

Many LGBTQ people have a long journey towards pregnancy. Therefore, many appreciated talking about this journey with others who understood the unique obstacles they had faced when opting for parenthood.

Some participants explained how they had stayed in contact with other parents from the class when their children were born and reflected on the benefits of continued contact with LGBTQ families.

## Any Class Would Be Fine

For most of the participants, access to an LGBTQ antenatal class had been important. Others, however, claimed that they would probably have been fine in any antenatal class. Desireé appreciated the discussions she had with other LGBTQ parents but assumed that similar topics would probably have been discussed in an antenatal class with heterosexual parents:

> I don't know if I think it would have been different compared to a mixed group, you know, with hetero and lesbian couples. I think the questions are just about the same; everyone wonders about the delivery and what it will be like to be parents. I don't think the differences are all that great.

The participants varied in their opinions about the desirability of having separate LGBTQ classes. One participant, Frida, said that she was very happy with the LGBTQ-certified antenatal care and delivery ward, but the antenatal education group had not suited her. A few participants also claimed that they did not have much in common with other LGBTQ people. Nonetheless, the majority of the parents who had access to the LGBTQ antenatal classes expressed satisfaction.

## Discussion

Based on the participants' experiences, it is clear that prospective parents who attended the LGBTQ-certified antenatal education felt more comfortable, while those who attended regular classes often felt excluded: In particular, the non-pregnant mothers and the transmasculine pregnant persons. Topics raised during the group discussions in regular antenatal education focused on the social situation of normative families and had felt irrelevant to LGBTQ participants. In contrast, those who attended the LGBTQ antenatal education classes were happy about the opportunity to discuss topics of relevance to their situation.

Participants in separate LGBTQ classes had felt strengthened by the contact with other LGBTQ persons. They expressed gratitude for being able to reflect together with people who had had similar experiences.

Separate antenatal education classes for prospective LGBTQ parents can strengthen and prepare participants to encounter a hetero- and cis-normative environment. Ultimately, the classes can reduce minority stress and enable prospective parents to feel more secure before childbirth and in making the transition to parenthood. Separate antenatal classes for LGBTQ people can be offered as physical or digital meetings, depending on the number of prospective parents in the region. They can be offered as a substitute or complement to a regular antenatal class. Regardless of the offers of any separate class for LGBTQ participants, it is still of major importance that regular antenatal classes are made inclusive and relevant for parents in various family situations.

## Practice Pointers

- Clinicians in regular antenatal clinics must consider a variety of family forms when planning their antenatal education programmes. In a mixed group, with different family constellations, it is crucial to adjust the content to suit all present. Class leaders need to consider the topics they select for group discussion and how they could be adjusted to include all families attending their class. It may be wise to avoid gendered subgroups. Language must be inclusive of all participants; therefore, gender-neutral language should be used when referring to pregnant as well as non-pregnant prospective parents.
- It is valuable to offer LGBTQ people separate antenatal classes. If possible, separate classes can also be directed to subgroups of LGBTQ parents, such as transgender people or single LGBTQ parents. Participation can be

offered online to address distance issues. Collaboration with nearby clinics can be used to identify LGBTQ people who are expecting children at the same time. However, sometimes, the estimated date of birth can be of less importance than the opportunity of sharing experiences with those in similar family situations.

• When it is not possible to organize a separate group for prospective LGBTQ parents, make sure that there is more than one LGBTQ family attending the regular antenatal class or offer an extra individual meeting. Make sure to cover topics relevant for prospective LGBTQ parents, such as minority stress, norms in society and non-genetic parenthood.

## References

Dahl, B., Malterud, K. (2015) Neither father nor biological mother: A qualitative study about lesbian co-mothers' maternity care experiences. Sexual & Reproductive Health Care, 6(3):169–173.

Falck, F., Frisén, L., Dhejne, C., Armuand, G. (2021) Undergoing pregnancy and childbirth as transmasculine in Sweden: Experiencing and dealing with structural discrimination, gender norms and microaggressions in antenatal care, delivery and gender clinics. International Journal of Transgender Health, 22(1–2):42–53.

Klittmark, S., Garzón, M., Andersson, E., Wells, M. (2019) LGBTQ competence wanted: LGBTQ parents' experiences of reproductive health care in Sweden. Scandinavian Journal of Caring Sciences, 33(2):417–426.

Larsson, A-K., Dykes, A-K. (2009) Care during pregnancy and childbirth in Sweden: Perspectives of lesbian women. Midwifery, 25(6):682–690.

Malmquist, A. (2015) Pride and prejudice: Lesbian families in contemporary Sweden. Doctoral thesis. Linköping: Linköping University.

Malmquist, A., Jonsson, L., Wikström, J., Nieminen, K. (2019) Minority stress adds an additional layer to fear of childbirth in lesbian and bisexual women, and transgender people. Midwifery, 79:102551.

Pålsson, P., Kvist, L. J., Persson, E. K., Kristensson Hallström, I., Ekelin, M. (2019) A survey of contemporary antenatal parental education in Sweden: What is offered to expectant parents and midwives' experiences. Sexual and Reproductive Healthcare, 20:13–19.

RFSL (2021) *Hbtq-kompetens - för dig som arbetar med blivande och nyblivna föräldrar.* [LGBTQ Competence - For you who work with expectant and new parents] Stockholm: RFSL.

Wells, M., Lang, S. (2016) Supporting same-sex mothers in the Nordic child health field: A systematic literature review and meta-synthesis of the most gender-equal countries. Journal of Clinical Nursing, 25(23–24):3469–3483.

# 31

# A PSYCHODYNAMIC APPROACH TO WORKING WITH PREGNANT TEENAGERS AND YOUNG PARENTS

*Hen Otley*

Many healthcare providers may have an intuitive understanding of how to help teenage parents. However, few get specific training and may take on a Young Parents' Clinic with no specialist education. Professor Joan Raphael-Leff's handbook (2012) introduces an approach to this work which may be helpful in influencing thinking and practice in such clinics.

★

When I started specialising as a Young Parents' Midwife, I felt I had only my colleagues' advice, my personal memories of adolescence and my experience of my own teenage children to draw on when working out how to engage with the particular needs of this client group. Wanting to develop my skills, I found Psychoanalyst and Social Psychologist Joan Raphael-Leff's psychodynamic insights very helpful.

Her book, 'Working with teenage parents: Handbook of theory and practice' (2012), presents a psychodynamic approach to working with teenage parents, recommending that the practitioner should be mindful of what she is bringing to encounters with her clients and what the young person's emotional experience might be. Based on psychoanalysis, psychodynamic thinking recognises how people's responses and mental states are affected by forces beyond our awareness and often developed in early childhood.

Midwives and health visitors are not offering psychotherapy, but an awareness of the frame of mind in which we meet our clients can be an essential first step to providing them with perhaps their first experience of a safe and separate place to explore their feelings. Raphael-Leff points out that healthcare providers have a significant impact on young clients, even when it may appear that everything we say is being disregarded. Advice may be followed unquestioningly

DOI: 10.4324/9781003223771-37

or a small comment may be felt to be a brutal accusation. Helpful suggestions inappropriately voiced may be received as domineering or patronising. It is, therefore, crucial to consider how best to approach interactions with young clients. If we can help them to express themselves, to notice their own emotions and to recognise the importance of holding others' feelings in mind, we are facilitating skills which adolescents are still developing and which are fundamentally important in good parenting.

Psychoanalytic thinking recognises the sometimes conflicting existence of conscious and unconscious motivations for feelings and behaviour. We cannot hope to get to the bottom of a teenager's unconscious reasons for having a child, but it is worth considering that these will diverge significantly from one person to another and are invariably more complex than mere ignorance, accident and a chaotic lifestyle, as people can often assume. I have been interested in the desire or need to become a mother that many young women have told me about, while also being aware of the emotional, practical, financial and social struggles likely to lie before them. With sex education and access to contraception and terminations widely available, the fact that young women continue to have babies in adolescence suggests that needs are fulfilled by becoming a mother at this point in their lives. It has been my understanding in my clinic that having a baby serves emotional and practical functions and is likely to represent a choice in some form, conscious or otherwise. It may be that the young mother has experienced attachment and relationship issues within her own family and she is enacting a 'doll's house' fantasy of being able to create a 'real' or 'perfect' family (Waddell, 2009). She might be seeking a purpose and an identity, looking for somebody to love or who will love her. Perhaps she is attempting to preserve a failing relationship or wanting to prove her fertility. There may be subtle unconscious impulses at play, such as a desire to become fully adult, to recapture lost elements of her baby self or even an attempt to continue the mother–daughter relationship by 'becoming

## BOX 31.1: CASE STUDY

Seventeen-year-old 'Natalie' told me that she was happy to be pregnant. Although she was taking the contraceptive pill, she had missed a few days, aware of the possible consequences. Neither she nor her boyfriend, 'Joe', was working or in college. She was hurt by her uncle's suggestion that they were hoping to get housed by the council. Natalie went on to tell me her sadness about her difficult relationship with her mum and the loss she felt now that her mother, who had recently given birth herself, was planning to move away with her new husband. Natalie did not feel ready to move into a flat with Joe and instead was trying to find a way to persuade her mum not to move and to let her stay at home when the baby came so they could be a family again.

the mother in order not to lose her' (Raphael-Leff, 2012). Considering each situation individually and starting to grasp the tangled reasons that might lead a particular young woman to become pregnant can offer a way to give clients more meaningful support.

## Pregnancy in Adolescence

In psychoanalytic thinking, adolescence is considered a time for replaying the unresolved struggles of early childhood, perhaps exploring passionate feelings for one parent and hostility towards the other (Raphael-Leff, 2012). Anxiety, loneliness, confusion and frustration from earlier childhood experiences may re-emerge. The psychoanalyst, Anna Freud (1895–1982), Sigmund Freud's daughter, called adolescence 'a second chance', an opportunity to find new solutions to old problems, to question assumptions and explore boundaries, with the tempestuous emotions of adolescence representing a creative search for change (Freud, 1958). It is generally recognised that the teenage years are a time for inquiry when full adult responsibility does not need to be taken. The successful outcome, after all the turmoil, is a well-adjusted, realistic, empathetic young adult with good self-esteem. It is easy to see, therefore, how pregnancy, childbirth and parenthood in adolescence might be construed as a double conflict which both derails and escalates this important developmental process (Raphael-Leff, 2012).

A crucial task of adolescence is to try to find a way to separate and differentiate ourselves from our parents (Pines, 2010), so becoming a parent when a young person is so close to their own childhood is a complex situation. At a time when independence and exploration are such strong drives, it is particularly hard to find yourself unable to spend time having fun with your peers and instead to be beholden to your parents for help and support. Child psychotherapist Margot Waddell (2009) highlights the tension between a young mother's act of getting pregnant as both a rejection of her own mother and a fierce expression of needing her mother. As with Natalie (see Case Study), becoming a parent may ignite intense feelings of yearning, disappointment, resentment and rage. This offers some insight into why young parents are at particular risk of mental distress and why self-harm (Raphael-Leff [2012] suggests this can be a disguised attack on the body of the mother-to-be's mother) is so prevalent among pregnant adolescents.

## What Teenagers Need from Health Professionals and Educators

The challenges some young parents face combined with an often high level of risky behaviour can make it difficult for a practitioner to remain non-judgemental and emotionally accessible in their clinical work. A reflective approach, where ingrained prejudices or assumptions are recognised and set aside, can make encounters with a young parent more helpfully open-minded.

Raphael-Leff (2012) gives a useful list of what a teenage client needs from healthcare practitioners and educators:

- Reliability and trustworthiness
- Non-judgemental listening
- Empathy without intrusion (being neither under-involved nor over-identified)
- Presentation of realistic options
- Engagement of fathers-to-be and other family members (as appropriate)
- Help to increase self-confidence, aspirations and a sense of agency.

She advises that we should support young parents by:

- Acknowledging the difficulties of pregnancy and parenthood
- Being honest and setting boundaries
- Asking our clients what they would want in their ideal world
- Helping them to build reasonable expectations
- Offering a role model in our own engagement with them
- Not giving solutions to family problems but encouraging clients to talk about their worries and find their own way forward.

Using these basic psychodynamic skills, we can help prepare young parents and parents-to-be to offer responsive and loving care to their children. For practitioners as well as clients, nurturing another person is something that needs thought in order to avoid blindly repeating the care we received ourselves as babies (Raphael-Leff, 2012). As professionals, we also need to be able to contain our own feelings since over-identification with clients will hamper our ability to support them.

There are a number of ways we can validate a client's experience and make her feel heard and considered. We can check to see if we've understood correctly by using tentative wording such as, 'I get the impression that…' or, 'Is it possible that…?' A phrase such as 'I wonder if you might be feeling…' gives an opportunity both to demonstrate empathy and to invite people to think about their reactions. We also need to examine and challenge misconceptions if these seem detrimental, such as believing that a craving for energy drinks or crisps is the baby 'demanding' these, or a father-to-be discounting postnatal contraceptive advice as his girlfriend 'owes' him another baby. Other ideas, for example being told by a pregnant young woman that her baby kicks a lot in bed at night because he doesn't like her partner, clearly merit further exploration.

## Conclusion

Adolescents are very much in the throes of their own developmental processes and require significant support to build the internal resources they will need to care for a child. We can help to prepare a young person for the challenges ahead by improving their self-esteem, by encouraging the development of a sense of agency by setting realistic goals, and by guiding them to be curious about their own feelings. As Raphael-Leff (2012) describes, pregnant teenagers and young mums and dads are having to deal with the collision of the challenging demands of both adolescence and parenthood. If through the connections we are able to make in providing maternity care, we can offer an opportunity for reflection and an experience of being understood, we can nurture invaluable emotional skills needed for parenting.

## Practice Pointers

Raphael-Leff (2012) suggests healthcare professionals can help young parents and parents-to-be by:

- Identifying and reinforcing clients' strengths
- Offering a model for thinking about feelings
- Attempting to name and summarise the problems and worries that clients bring up
- Helping clients to think about concerns and to find their own solutions
- Increasing clients' confidence and enabling them to cope with uncertainty and frustration
- Emphasising that their child will also experience these feelings.

## References

Freud, A. (1958) The Psychoanalytical Study of the Child: Adolescence. New York: International Universities Press: 255–278.

Pines, D. (2010) A Woman's Unconscious Use of Her Body (2nd edition). New York: Routledge.

Raphael-Leff, J. (2012) Working with Teenage Parents: Handbook of theory and practice. London: Anna Freud Centre.

Waddell, M. (2009) Why teenagers have babies. Journal of Infant Observation, 12(3):271–281.

# 32

# FATHERS' PRENATAL RELATIONSHIP WITH 'THEIR' BABY AND 'HER' PREGNANCY – IMPLICATIONS FOR ANTENATAL EDUCATION

*Richard Fletcher, Chris May, and Jennifer St George*

In parallel with technological and psychological changes surrounding pregnancy, there has been an expansion of research examining fathers' views of labour and birth as well as increased consideration of co-parenting and father–infant relationships. We now have a body of evidence to draw on when considering how services aiming to improve family health and wellbeing might approach fathers. In this chapter, our current understanding of how fathers relate to their unborn babies and fathers' experience of pregnancy will be described to suggest how fathers may be effectively included in antenatal programmes.

★

According to a national survey of 4,616 women in England (Redshaw & Henderson, 2013), more than 50% of the fathers were present for the pregnancy test. Most of the fathers also attended at least one antenatal check and were present for ultrasound examinations and for the birth. Similar figures were reported in a study of 600 Danish fathers (Madsen et al., 2002, cited in Plantin et al., 2011) and in a longitudinal study of 205 Australian mothers and their partners (Svensson et al., 2006). In non-western settings, evidence of fathers' antenatal involvement is difficult to gauge. Salvadorian expectant fathers report similar rates to those quoted above (Carter & Speizer, 2005); however, among Kenyan fathers, cultural prohibitions strongly discourage fathers' involvement in birth-related activities (Kwambai et al., 2013).

Men's attendance at key processes surrounding pregnancy, at least in western industrialised countries, is an indication of fathers' interest in being involved with their baby's development. To understand a father's relationship to the foetus, however, requires exploring his interior world, his mental picture of the

DOI: 10.4324/9781003223771-38

developing baby and his idea of being a father to this particular infant. We would also wish to track his feeling states over the course of the pregnancy,

A first indicator is fathers' acceptance of pregnancy. In the survey by Redshaw and Henderson (2013) for example, mothers reported that over 80% of the men were 'pleased' or 'overjoyed' when the pregnancy was confirmed. Another indication of the strength of a father's connection to his unborn infant is his reaction to a calamitous outcome such as stillbirth or neonatal death. From a systematic review of quantitative and qualitative studies on the psychological effects of stillbirth and neonatal death, Aydin and Kabukcuoğlu (2020) found that fathers were shocked by the loss and felt useless, sad, guilty and empty. While fathers' grief reactions are found in most cases to be less than mothers', the strongest factor in fathers' grief is their connection to their infant – a connection gained without having the direct experience of pregnancy (Obst et al., 2020).

What are the ways that men connect to the foetus without the direct physical reality of the pregnancy? Interview studies have asked men to describe their experience of getting to know the growing foetus. Their ideas about their infant in the womb may be vague and unformed prior to the 'visual proof' provided by the ultrasound images of the infant. As a father interviewed by Walsh et al. (2014:25) explained:

> Obviously she's pregnant, but then when you actually get to see it you're like - holy cow, you know I'm going to be holding that thing in my arms in like you know six months or less ...

Another avenue for investigating men's relation to the foetus is to examine their responses to statements such as, 'I imagine myself taking care of the baby', and 'I try to picture what the baby will look like'. Men's and women's answers to such questions (using gender-appropriate wording) were obtained from expectant couples in Sweden (Seimyr et al., 2009). Analysis suggested that concern for the foetus was equally strong for both mothers and fathers, although men's thoughts about the developing infant were focused on the baby's life post-birth, whereas women's responses to similar questions indicated a focus on the foetus's current health.

The strength of a father's love for his unborn child can be measured by the Paternal Antenatal Attachment Scale (PAAS) (Condon, 1993) which assesses the expectant father's sense of closeness or distance from the foetus and his feelings of tenderness or irritation. The scale also attempts to capture the father's mental picture of the growing foetus with questions on how often the father thinks about, dreams about or talks to the foetus. In one study, fathers' attachment from pregnancy to live birth was consistent, suggesting a stable bond between father and child over time. As would be expected though, attachment scores were lower for depressed expectant fathers (Condon et al., 2013). This finding implies that those fathers who will struggle to form an attachment with their infant may be readily identified before the birth.

In summary, we have evidence that, at least in western industrialised societies where social norms strongly favour father-involvement with children, fathers are motivated to form a relationship with their unborn child. The expectant father's curiosity about the foetus, his mental engagement and preoccupation with the wellbeing, activities and personality of the foetus are markers of the strength of this relationship.

## Fathers' Experience of Pregnancy

Related to a father's commitment to the unborn child is his own personal experience of the pregnancy. These experiences include his role as support to the mother, his changing relationship to others and to self and hormonal changes that influence his attitudes and behaviour.

Fathers can influence the course of pregnancy through the effect that their behaviours have on the health and wellbeing of their partner. Women whose partners remain involved and reside with them during their pregnancy are more likely to attend antenatal care, take better care of their health and deliver healthier babies (Martin et al., 2007; Padilla & Reichman, 2001; Perriera & Cortes, 2006). Paternal behaviours in relation to the consumption of tobacco and alcohol also are important. Partners can assist women's efforts to cease smoking (Campbell et al., 2018). One study found that both mothers and fathers reduce their alcohol consumption during pregnancy (Mellingen et al., 2013). Links between paternal and maternal behaviour during the pregnancy in relation to such substances provide powerful examples of the responsibility that fathers share in the health of a pregnancy.

However, the father can also expect to have a personal experience of the pregnancy which is characterised by turmoil. Indeed, the pregnancy period can be more stressful than either the labour-birth or postnatal periods (Genesoni & Tallandini, 2009). Some fathers describe confusion during the pregnancy due to changing relationships (Barclay et al., 1996). Changes in relationships can be triggered by interactions with an array of health professionals, changes in mothers' behaviours and sexuality (Bogren, 1991) and the involvement of extended family, most usually from the maternal lineage (Pollet et al., 2006). These changes occur while the father's relationship with his partner is transforming from one primarily founded on companionship, to a relationship in which he has an unfamiliar and poorly defined supporting role (Cowan & Cowan, 2019). Many fathers feel that there are not enough resources to support their education or spaces to support their involvement, and that there is a lack of recognition of their experiences and feelings about pregnancy, labour, birth and fathering (StGeorge & Fletcher, 2011). It is no wonder then that fathers' growing connection to the pregnancy may be accompanied by emotional responses such as fear, anxiety and curiosity (Hildingsson et al., 2013).

In fact, a father's maladjustment to the pregnancy can lead to a range of dysfunctional behaviours, including the misuse of alcohol, which in turn increases the risk of intimate partner violence (Helmith et al., 2013). In a study by Gartland et al. (2011), for example, a significant minority of mothers reported fear of an intimate partner and experienced physical and/or emotional abuse in the perinatal period. However, a father's developing relationship with the pregnancy may also be a powerful incentive to give up violence in relationships (Maxwell et al., 2012).

Some of the most profound findings concerning a father's experience of pregnancy come from hormonal studies. Hormonal changes during pregnancy indicate that fathers also experience physiological responses to pregnancy. Fathers living with their pregnant partners during the pregnancy have been found to experience lower levels of testosterone and cortisol and higher levels of oestradiol than matched controls whose partners were not pregnant (Berg & Wynne-Edwards, 2001). The oestradiol hormones appear to enhance fathers' sensitivity and responsiveness to their infant's cry; also, fathers with lower levels of testosterone are found to have higher sympathy for their crying infant and are more likely to attend to the infant than fathers with higher levels of testosterone (Fleming et al., 2002). This biochemical adaptation may account for the interest that fathers develop in learning about relationships, baby care and parenting during this time (Deave & Johnson, 2008). These neurologic and physiologic changes indicate that men may be biologically primed by their partner's pregnancy for roles as both a parent and a support to their partner in the transition to parenthood.

## Including Fathers in Antenatal Programmes

Antenatal class content tends to centre on maternal concerns, which is understandable as mothers are often clear about what they want from classes while fathers are carefully vague about their expectations (Jones et al., 2019). However, expectant mothers usually want their partners to attend, and partners also want to attend as a way to signal their support and investment in the pregnancy (Redshaw & Henderson, 2013). This presents a rare opportunity to provide men, an otherwise hard to reach population, with important information and positive experiences of health service delivery (Fletcher et al., 2014).

Addressing fathers' expectations of antenatal programmes is important. Several studies show that fathers find antenatal programmes deficient, particularly as preparation for relationship changes (Deave & Johnson, 2008; Fletcher et al., 2004; Goodman, 2005). However, their expectations and needs have been explored. A small survey of Scottish fathers found that the father's role, care of the baby after delivery and 'what could go wrong' were the most popular topics; least popular were bottle feeding technique and the discomforts of pregnancy (McElligott, 2001). Similarly, when 105 Australian fathers selected topics for an online antenatal education programme, information on father–infant interaction was the most commonly selected topic followed by work–family balance and postnatal depression. As in the Scottish sample, breastfeeding knowledge was accorded a low priority (Fletcher et al., 2008). Six domains of appropriate content for paternal antenatal programmes were synthesised by May and Fletcher (2013) from this and other research:

1 Fathers' role and relationship changes
2 Father as a support person
3 Parenting alliance
4 Paternal depression
5 Infant crying
6 Infant communication.

These domains provide an evidence-supported rationale for paternal content that addresses the key issues of constructing a new identity, supporting his partner and preparing to father a newborn.

Addressing fathers' role as support person is also critical. Emotional and functional support are central to the characterisation of the father's role: This support builds strong foundations in emerging parenting partnerships and enhances child and maternal outcomes (May & Fletcher, 2019; May & Perrin, 1985). May and Fletcher (2019) conclude that educators could feel confident in refining their discussion to four types of supportive behaviour – building the mother's self-esteem (e.g. by telling her, 'You are doing a great job'; 'I am so lucky to have you as a partner in parenting'), and through companionship, functional support and getting help. However, it is also important that educators include discussion on factors that trigger conflict in emerging parenting partnerships, because conflict is likely to erode trust (Cutrona et al., 2005) which has been described as the foundation stone of successful relationships (Hall & Wittkowski, 2006).

As a signal of support and investment in the pregnancy, fathers' presence at ultrasound examinations and participation at the birth are now accepted practice in western nations. However, their involvement in father-focused antenatal education remains less commonplace (Redshaw & Henderson, 2013). Father-focused SMS programmes, compared to online programmes, appear to achieve engagement and participation while providing fathers with relevant and timely information (Fletcher et al., 2017; May et al., 2021). Considering how men use technology may be particularly important in reaching rural and remote fathers in developed and developing nations where the importance of paternal engagement is receiving greater recognition (Chikalipo et al., 2018; Head et al., 2013).

## Conclusion

Fathers have both psychological and physiological responses to pregnancy as they develop complex relationships with their unborn child and negotiate a new relationship with their parenting partner. These responses indicate a need to support fathers through their transition to parenthood. Fathers' antenatal preparation can have a positive influence on maternal, paternal and child outcomes. Antenatal programmes should therefore avoid framing the father's role simply in terms of a helper at the birth. Programmes aiming to enhance fathers' bond to their unborn child, build their support of the mother and lay the groundwork for effective co-parenting of the new baby are likely to be more appealing to expectant fathers and more effective in promoting family wellbeing. Programme content will also need to take into account the man's changing relationships with his partner and society, his own physiological and psychological responses to pregnancy and his emerging awareness of the unborn child. While delivery of antenatal education may be enhanced by use of interactive e-technologies or male educators, we have limited information on how these approaches might work. Effective engagement of fathers in antenatal education is unlikely to require a completely new workforce using a novel skill set. Current educators, using their clinical competencies, aided by information on fathers' needs and a flexible service delivery model, should be able to develop father-inclusive practices to benefit both parents and their newborns.

## Practice Pointers

- Fathers want to form a relationship with their unborn child.
- Fathers experience physiological and psychological changes during pregnancy.
- Clinicians can help fathers build a mental picture of the growing foetus.
- During pregnancy, a father's central role is support of his partner.
- It will be important to help fathers find ways to support their partners postnatally, build trust and manage conflict.

## References

Aydin, R., Kabukcuoğlu, K. (2020) Fathers' experiences of perinatal loss: A sample meta-synthesis study. Journal of Family Issues, 42(9):2083–2110.

Barclay, L., Donovan, J., Genovese, A. (1996) Men's experiences during their partner's first pregnancy: A grounded theory analysis. Australian Journal of Advanced Nursing, 13(3):12–24.

Berg, S.L., Wynne-Edwards, K.E. (2001) Changes in testosterone, cortisol and estradiol in men becoming fathers. Mayo Clinic Proceedings, 76(6):582–592.

Bogren, L.Y. (1991) Changes in sexuality in women and men during pregnancy. Archives of Sexual Behaviour, 20(1):35–45.

Campbell, K.A., Fergie, L., Coleman-Haynes, T., Cooper, S., Lorencatto, F. et al. (2018) Improving behavioral support for smoking cessation in pregnancy: What are the barriers to stopping and which behavior change techniques can influence them? Application of theoretical domains framework. International Journal of Environmental Research and Public Health, 15(2):359.

Carter, M.W., Speizer, I. (2005) Salvadoran fathers' attendance at prenatal care, delivery, and postpartum care. Revista Panamericana de Salud Pública, 18:149–156.

Chikalipo, M.C., Chirwa, E.M., Muula, A.S. (2018) Exploring antenatal education content for couples in Blantyre, Malawi. BMC Pregnancy and Childbirth, 18:article no. 497.

Condon, J.T., (1993) The assessment of antenatal emotional attachment: Development of a questionnaire instrument. British Journal of Medical Psychology, 66:167–183.

Condon, J., Corkindale, C., Boyce, P., Gamble, E. (2013) A longitudinal study of father-to-infant attachment: Antecedents and correlates. Journal of Reproductive and Infant Psychology, 31:15–30.

Cowan, C.P., Cowan, P.A. (2019) Enhancing parenting effectiveness, fathers' involvement, couple relationship quality, and children's development: Breaking down silos in family policy making and service delivery. Journal of Family Theory & Review, 11(1): 92–111.

Cutrona, C.E., Russell, D.W., Gardner, K.A. (2005) The Relationship Enhancement Model of social support. In: Revenson, T.A., Kayser, K., Bodenmann, G. (Eds.) Couples Coping with Stress: Emerging perspectives on dyadic coping. American Psychological Association: 73–95.

Deave, T., Johnson, D. (2008) The transition to parenthood: What does in mean for fathers? Journal of Advanced Nursing, 63(6):626–633.

Fleming, A.S., Corter, C., Stallings, J., Meir, S. (2002) Testosterone and prolactin are associated with emotional responses to infant cries in new fathers. Hormones and Behavior, 42(4):399–413.

Fletcher, R., May, C., Lambkin, F.K., Gemmill, A.W., Cann, W. et al. (2017) SMS4dads: Providing information and support to new fathers through mobile phones - A pilot study. Advances in Mental Health, 15(2):121–131.

Fletcher, R., May, C., StGeorge, J. M. (2014) Fathers' prenatal relationship with 'their' baby and 'her' pregnancy – Implications for antenatal education. International Journal of Birth and Parent Education, 1(3):23–27.

Fletcher, R., Silberberg, S., Galloway, D. (2004) New fathers' post-birth views of antenatal classes: Satisfaction, benefits, and knowledge of family services, The Journal of Perinatal Education, 13(3):18–26.

Fletcher, R., Vimpani, G., Russell, G., Keatinge, D. (2008) The evaluation of tailored email and web-based information for new fathers. Child Care Health & Development, 4(4):439–446.

Gartland, D., Hemphill, S.A., Hegarty, K., Brown, S.J. (2011) Intimate partner violence during pregnancy and the first year postpartum in an Australian pregnancy cohort study. Maternal and Child Health Journal, 15:570–578.

Genesoni, L., Tallandini, M.A. (2009) Men's psychological transition to fatherhood: An analysis of the literature, 1989–2008. Birth, 36:305–318.

Goodman, J.H. (2005) Becoming an involved father of an infant. Journal of Obstetric, Gynecologic, & Neonatal Nursing, 34(2):190–200.

Hall, P.L., Wittkowski, A. (2006) An exploration of negative thoughts as a normal phenomenon after childbirth. Journal of Midwifery & Women's Health, 51(5):321–330.

Head, K.J., Noar, S.M., Iannarino, N.T., Grant Harrington, N. (2013) Efficacy of text messaging-based interventions for health promotion: A meta-analysis. Social Science & Medicine, 97:41–48.

Helmith, J.C., Gordon, K.C. Stuart, G.L., Moore, T.M. (2013) Risk factors for intimate partner violence during pregnancy and postpartum. Archives of Women's Mental Health, 16:19–27.

Hildingsson, I., Johansson, M., Fenwick, J., Haines, H., Rubertsson, C. (2013) Childbirth fear in expectant fathers: Findings from a regional Swedish cohort study. Midwifery, 30(2):242–247.

Jones, C., Wadephul, F., Professor, J. J. (2019). Maternal and paternal expectations of antenatal education across the transition to parenthood. British Journal of Midwifery. 27(4):235–241.

Kwambai, T.K., Dellicour, S., Desai, M., Ameh, C.A., Person, B. et al., (2013) Perspectives of men on antenatal and delivery care service utilisation in rural western Kenya: A qualitative study. BMC Pregnancy and Childbirth, 13:134.

Martin, T.L., McNamara, M.J., Milot, A.S., Halle, T., Hair, E.C. (2007) The effects of father involvement during pregnancy on receipt of prenatal care and maternal smoking. Maternal Child Health Journal, 11:595–602.

Maxwell, N., Scourfield, J., Holland, S., Featherstone, B., Lee J. (2012) The benefits and challenges of training child protection social workers in father engagement. Child Abuse Review, 21:299–310.

May, C., Fletcher, R. (2013) Preparing fathers for the transition to parenthood: Recommendations for the content of antenatal education. Midwifery, 29:474–478.

May, C., Fletcher, R. (2019) Helping him to support her: Building trust and minimising distress through the facilitation of partner support across the transition to parenthood. International Journal of Birth & Parent Education, 7(1):5.

May, C., StGeorge, J., Lane, S. (2021) From presence to participation: Engagement with an SMS program for fathers of children on the autism spectrum. Journal of Child & Family Studies, 30:29–37.

May, K.A., Perrin, S.P. (1985) Prelude: Pregnancy and birth. In: Hanson, S.M.H., Bozett, F.W. (Eds.) Dimensions of Fatherhood. Beverly Hills, CA: Sage Publications:64–91.

McElligott, M. (2001) Antenatal information wanted by first-time fathers. British Journal of Midwifery, 9:556–558.

Mellingen, S., Torsheim, T., Thuen, F. (2013) Changes in alcohol use and relationship satisfaction in Norwegian couples during pregnancy. Substance Abuse Treatment, Prevention and Policy, 8(1):1–11.

Obst, K.L., Due, C., Oxlad, M., Middleton, P. (2020) Men's grief following pregnancy loss and neonatal loss: A systematic review and emerging theoretical model. BMC Pregnancy and Childbirth, 20(1):1–17.

Padilla, Y.C., Reichman, N.E. (2001) Low birthweight: Do unwed fathers help? Children and Youth Services Review, 23(4/5):427–452.

Perriera, K.M., Cortes, K.E. (2006) Alcohol and tobacco use in pregnancy. American Journal of Public Health, 96(9):1629–1636.

Plantin, L., Olukoya, A.A., Ny, P. (2011) Positive health outcomes of fathers' involvement in pregnancy and childbirth paternal support: A scope study literature review. Fathering: A Journal of Theory, Research, and Practice about Men as Fathers, 9:87–102.

Pollet, T.V., Nettle, D., Nelissen, M. (2006) Contact frequencies between grandparents and grandchildren in a modern society: Estimates of the impact of paternity uncertainty. Journal of Cultural and Evolutionary Psychology, 4:203–213.

Redshaw, M., Henderson, J. (2013) Fathers' engagement in pregnancy and childbirth: Evidence from a national survey. BMC Pregnancy and Childbirth, 13:70.

Seimyr, L., Sjögren, B., Welles-Nyström, B., Nissen, E. (2009) Antenatal maternal depressive mood and parental-fetal attachment at the end of pregnancy. Archives of Women's Mental Health, 12:269–279.

StGeorge, J.M., Fletcher, R.J. (2011) Fathers online: Learning about fatherhood through the internet. The Journal of Perinatal Education, 20:154.

Svensson, J., Barclay, L., Cooke, M. (2006) The concerns and interests of expectant and new parents: Assessing learning needs. Journal of Perinatal Education, 15(4):1827.

Walsh, T.B., Tolman, R.M., Davis, R.N., Palladino, C.L., Romero, V.C. et al. (2014) Moving up the 'magic moment': Fathers' experience of prenatal ultrasound. Fathering, 12(1):18–37.

# 33

# TIPS FOR FACILITATING ANTENATAL EDUCATION ONLINE

*Helen Knight and Isabelle Karimov*

During the COVID pandemic, many services moved their antenatal classes online. This required educators to develop a level of technological competence that they may not have had previously, and to adapt their inter-personal and facilitation skills to a virtual environment. In this article, the authors offer brief guidelines on how to ensure a competent and effective online educational experience for parents.

★

## Prior to Delivering Sessions

- Make sure you are on top of the IT. If you're new to facilitating Zoom sessions, practise with colleagues or your family.
- Become confident with breakout rooms.
- Ask the parents who have signed up for your session/course whether they are familiar with Zoom. If not, send them links to YouTube videos such as: https://www.youtube.com/watch?v=QOUwumKCW7M <4 October 2021>
- Rethink your visual aids: Will they work in the online environment? You can photograph your resources and embed them in your PowerPoint presentation.
- It's important to have great visual aids and great internet connection but if clients can't see you, they will soon get frustrated. Invest in a ring light. (They are not expensive and you may be able to offset against your income for tax purposes.)
- Try to find out prior to your session/course what the parents who will be attending are especially interested in.
- Send parents some pre-session course reading and/or video clips to watch. Explain that you will be referring to these during the session.

DOI: 10.4324/9781003223771-39

## The First Session

- Make sure you open any additional documents you want to share before you start the Zoom call.
- Agree ground rules/Zoom etiquette:
  - Participants may have to mute if there is too much background noise
  - Be patient when trying to speak
  - Take turns.

Acknowledge that learning on Zoom comes with challenges for participants and for you as a teacher. Say that it is easy for participants to go into 'watching TV' mode but that this is not the best way to learn! Promise to have regular breaks.

## During the Session

- Deliver topics in bite size chunks.
- Don't try to do too much – it's easy to be unrealistic about how much can be covered in an online session.
- Keep the session interactive.
- Use different teaching approaches and remember that people will become weary if you simply repeat what is on your PowerPoint presentation. Share slides for no more than five minutes and then remember to turn them off and enjoy some free-flowing discussion about what the parents have learned. Maybe divide them into breakout rooms and set a question for discussion (via the 'Broadcast All' message function).
- Encourage couples to discuss their feelings privately, too – remind them to mute whilst they check in with their partner about what they have just learned. Maybe follow up after your Zoom sessions with some 'homework', for example, to watch a video about mental health, research the different methods for induction, talk together about how a caesarean birth might be made as baby-friendly as possible. Ensure that you encourage the free sharing of participants' findings at the beginning of the next session.
- Don't be afraid to use the whiteboard – it's pretty easy to use and fun if the parents can annotate. BUT learn how to delete their annotations; otherwise, all of their drawings, etc. will overlay your next slide!
- Be more directive with questions than perhaps you would face–to–face, for example, 'Dave, you're nodding – what are your thoughts?'
- Give the group the chance just to chat.
- Mix up the breakout rooms so parents get a chance to know everyone in the group. Invite video off-time for relaxation and massage practice.
- Introduce your pets/children who may wander into view (draw parallels with parenting being a series of interruptions for the next 18 years!)

## What to Do about the Participant Who Stays off Video?

This is a unique challenge for you as the teacher and for others on the call. It is the equivalent of someone in a face-to-face group sitting in the circle with a blanket over their head. How would that feel?

Consider why some people might not want to use their video. Maybe they have poor WiFi and turning the video off can be very handy in maintaining their connection? Maybe they are shy? Maybe they live in surroundings that they do not want to share (crowded accommodation/poor accommodation)? Maybe they have disabilities, either physical or mental, that they are not ready to share with the group? Maybe they are famous and wish to maintain their privacy?

Consider how this impacts on the group. Having an unseen member may feel intimidating to other participants and they may start to speculate as to why the person is not revealing themselves. Some teachers have felt extremely uncomfortable with the 'black rectangle' and have taken the view that it has affected the class to such an extent that they have been unable to continue teaching.

One option for addressing this problem is to have something in the ground rules (sent out prior to the course). You could say that people will be expected to have their videos on to facilitate group learning and understanding. If this is going to cause a problem for any participant, invite them to contact you for a one-to-one discussion prior to the start of the session or course.

## Feedback

It's important to check in with participants regularly – is the session working for them? What do they need from the next session? Be clear that you welcome honest feedback. Have a channel for private feedback, too. A WhatsApp group running alongside Zoom is helpful for this. However, it also needs ground rules which include being clear about when you are available to answer questions and at what point you will leave the group.

# INDEX

Printed in the United States
by Baker & Taylor Publisher Services

Printed in the United States
by Baker & Taylor Publisher Services